D1492594

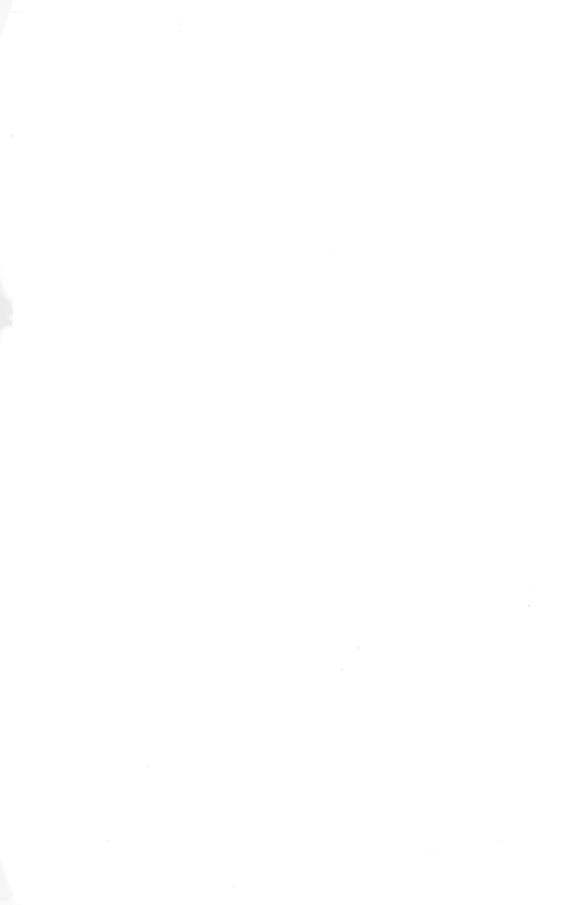

Drug Treatment of Migraine and Other Headaches

Monographs in Clinical Neuroscience

Vol. 17

Series Editor   *M. Fisher*, Worcester, Mass.

Advisory Board   *W.G. Bradley*, Miami, Fla.
                   H.P. Hartung, Würzburg
                   M.A. Moskowitz, Charlestown, Mass.

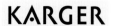
KARGER   Basel · Freiburg · Paris · London · New York ·
               New Delhi · Bangkok · Singapore · Tokyo · Sydney

Drug Treatment of Migraine and Other Headaches

Volume Editor *Hans Christoph Diener*, Essen

36 figures, and 58 tables, 2000

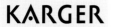

Basel · Freiburg · Paris · London · New York ·
New Delhi · Bangkok · Singapore · Tokyo · Sydney

....
Hans Christoph Diener, MD
Department of Neurology
University Essen
Germany

Library of Congress Cataloging-in-Publication Data

Drug treatment of migraine and other headaches / volume editor, Hans Christoph Diener.
      p.   cm. – (Monographs in clinical neuroscience; vol. 17)
      ISBN 3–8055–6971–8 (hard cover)
      1. Migraine – Chemotherapy. 2. Headache – Chemotherapy. I. Diener, H. C.
      (Hans Christoph), 1951. II. Series.
      [DNLM: 1. Migraine – drug therapy. 2. Headache – drug therapy. WL 344 D794 2000]
    RD392.D78 2000
    616.8′57061–dc21

                                  00–023381

© Copyright 2000 by S. Karger AG, P.O. Box, CH–4009 Basel (Switzerland)
www.karger.com
Printed in Switzerland on acid-free paper by Reinhardt Druck, Basel
ISSN 1420–2441
ISBN 3–8055–6971–8

....

Contents

Preface

There are plenty of books on headache. Why do we need another one? As editor I had been missing a book that concentrated on the drug treatment of migraine and other headaches based on pharmacological knowledge and evidence-based medicine. I was happy to be able to recruit the top experts on headache to contribute to this book. Some of the invited authors were unable to meet the deadline thereby forcing the editor to write more chapters than he had planned. The chapters on the pharmacology of the triptans are in most cases written by the pharmacologist who either developed the substance or was involved in the program in a major way. In contrast, the chapters on treatment are written by clinicians who participated in clinical trials and have extensive experience with the use of these substances in clinical practice. Authors were asked to review the literature and provide practical advice at the end of the chapter. The reader will immediately recognize that many studies in the migraine prophylaxis dating before 1992 are difficult to evaluate due to constraints in trial methodology. In both the parts on acute therapy and prophylaxis of migraine, the reader is confronted with the important issues of trial design. The last part concentrates on drug treatment of other headaches. The editor is aware that there is no proven drug treatment for cervicogenic headache, but nevertheless felt that this important headache variant should not be neglected. The book opens with 2 contributions on the epidemiology of migraine and classification of headache. I consider nonmedical treatment very important. Including this topic, however, would have been too much to cover in one volume which could still be carried around and read while traveling or sitting on the terrace.

The reader is invited to have another look at one of the older books on headache therapy. This will show the incredible advances in headache research and pharmacology within the last 15 years.

I thank all the authors for their cooperation and the time they invested in this project. I hope that the data provided in this book will serve to enable our headache patients to get a better treatment.

H.C. Diener

Treating the Acute Migraine Attack

Diener HC (ed): Drug Treatment of Migraine and Other Headaches.
Monogr Clin Neurosci. Basel, Karger, 2000, vol 17, pp 2–15

······················
Epidemiology of Migraine

Richard B. Lipton [a], *Walter F. Stewart* [b], *Ann I. Scher* [c]

[a] Departments of Neurology, Epidemiology and Social Medicine, Albert Einstein
College of Medicine and Headache Unit, Montefiore Medical Center, Bronx N.Y.
and Innovative Medical Research, Stamford, Conn.;
[b] Department of Epidemiology, The Johns Hopkins University, Baltimore, Md. and
Innovative Medical Research, Towson, Md., and
[c] Department of Epidemiology, The Johns Hopkins University, Baltimore, Md. and
Neuroepidemiology Branch, National Institute for Neurological Disorders and
Stroke, National Institutes of Health, Bethesda, Md., USA

Migraine headache is an extremely common condition affecting about
11% of adult populations in Western countries. Because migraine sufferers
usually do not consult physicians for headache [1–3], clinic-based studies are
prone to significant selection bias.

This chapter reviews recent epidemiologic studies of migraine. We begin
by discussing some methodologic issues in epidemiologic research, including
case definition and selection bias [4–6]. We then summarize studies of migraine
incidence and prevalence and close with discussions of health care and the
natural history of migraine.

Migraine Epidemiology: Methodological Considerations

Classification of migraine is complicated by the episodic and heterogeneous nature of the illness. In the absence of reliable biological markers and
diagnostic tests for migraine, diagnosis is based on self-reported symptoms
and on the exclusion of other disorders. Migraine attacks vary between individuals in frequency, severity, and associated headache features. Even within
individuals, attacks may vary considerably. Most migraineurs experience more
than one type of headache and may have difficulty recalling which features
occur with each headache type. The imperfect demarcation among the primary
headache disorders further complicates the classification of individual head-

ache attacks. In fact, there is some controversy as to whether migraine and tension-type headache are distinct disorders [7, 8] or opposite ends of a continuum of severity [9–11].

The International Headache Society (IHS) classification system has made major contributions to epidemiologic research. The IHS criteria provide categories and explicit criteria which specify features required for diagnosis as well as features which exclude particular headache disorders [4]. Although some argue these criteria are limited, particularly in the classification of daily headaches, the IHS criteria represent an enormous advance in headache classification [12].

Epidemiologic studies should be conducted in representative samples of defined populations. This is particularly important for migraine, as the modest rates of consulting create substantial opportunities for selection bias. It is also important to use well-established, uniform methods for ascertaining the clinical features used for diagnosis.

Migraine Incidence

Incidence refers to the rate of onset of a particular disease in a defined population. It is preferable to estimate incidence prospectively by following individuals free of migraine over time. In one prospective study which was designed to assess the relationship of major depression or anxiety disorders and migraine [13], a group of 848 21–30-year-olds recruited from a large managed care organization were followed for incident migraine. Seventy-one developed migraine over the 5-year follow-up period, corresponding to an incidence rate of 17 per 1,000/person years (24 female, 6 male). This excellent study is limited primarily by the narrow age range of the samples; incidence below the age of 21 could only be estimated.

Longitudinal studies are expensive and time-consuming. An alternative is to use cross-sectional studies. Without adjustment, incidence may be overestimated as individuals tend to recall events in the past as occurring more recently than they actually occurred (telescoping) [14]. In a Danish population-based study, Rasmussen [15] estimated the incidence of migraine at 3.7 per 1,000 person years (5.8 female, 1.6 male). This study did not have adequate power to assess age-specific incidence and did not adjust for telescoping. Reported rates represent the average of young adults with high rates and older adults with very low rates. In a telephone interview survey of 10,000, Stewart et al. [16] found that after adjusting for telescoping, the peak age of onset was at ages 5–10 for males and 12–13 for females for migraine with aura and 10–11 for males and 14–17 for females for migraine without aura. Peak incidence rates for migraine with aura were 6.6/1,000 person years for males and 14.1/1,000 person years for females and 10.1/1,000 person years for males and

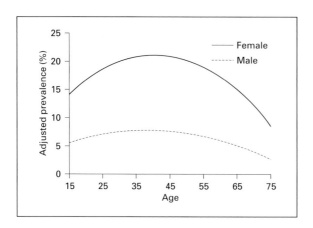

Fig. 1. Gender- and age-specific prevalence estimates of migraine based on 21 population-based studies that used International Headache Society (IHS) diagnostic criteria. Estimates are model-based and shown for North America [20].

18.9/1,000 person years for migraine without aura. Thus, males had an earlier
onset than females and, for both males and females, migraine with aura had
an earlier onset than migraine without aura. For both males and females,
onset was usually before age 20.

Migraine Prevalence

Prevalence refers to the proportion of a given population that has a disease
over a defined period of time. A large number of migraine prevalence surveys
have been published and summarized elsewhere [15, 17–19]. Table 1 presents
the results from recent population-based studies that: (1) used IHS criteria
and (2) were based on representative populations. Most of these studies measured one-year period prevalence, that is, respondents reporting a migraine
attack within 1 year of the interview are counted as a prevalent case.

There is considerable variation among these studies. Recent meta-analyses
suggest that much of this variability is due to differences in the sociodemographic profiles of the study subjects, including gender, age, race, and geographic region [6, 20]. These demographic factors are discussed below.

Age. Most studies on migraine prevalence have reported variation by
age, with prevalence following an inverted U-shaped distribution. Figure 1
illustrates this pattern, with peak prevalence occurring in the late 30s and
early 40s.

Gender. The prevalence of migraine is the same or greater in boys than
in girls prior to puberty. Three studies (table 1) [21–23] based on pediatric or

Table 1. Gender-specific prevalence estimates of migraine from 25 population-based studies using IHS diagnostic criteria

Author (Year of publication)	Country	Source	Method	Sample size	Time frame	Age range	Migraine prevalence (%) Female	Male	Total	Comments
Abu-Arefeh (1994) [21]	Scotland	School	Clin interview	1,754	1 yr	5–15	11.5	9.7	10.6	Prevalence is higher in boys prior to age 12 (1.14:1). After age 12, more common in girls (2.0:1)
al Rajeh (1997) [83]	Saudi Arabia	Community	Face-to face/ Clin interview	22,630		All	6.8	3.2	5.0	
Alders (1996) [84]	Malaysia	Community	Face-to face	595	1 yr	5+	11.3	6.7	9.0	
Arregui (1991) [85]	Peru	Community	Clin interview	2,257		All	12.2	4.5	8.4	
Barea (1996) [22]	Brazil	School	Clin interview	538	1 yr	10–18	10.3	9.6	9.9	2–48-h duration allowed
Breslau (1991) [34]	US	Community	Face-to-face/ Telephone	1,007	1 yr	21–30	12.9	3.4	9.2	
Cruz (1995) [86]	Ecuador	Community	Clin interview	2,723	Lifetime	All	7.9	5.6	6.9	Community endemic for cysticercosis
Cull (1992) [87]	UK	Community	Face-to-face	16,002	1 yr	16+	11.0	4.3	7.8	Without aura only
Göbel (1994) [32]	Germany	Community	Mail SAQ	4,061	Lifetime	18+	15.0	7.0	11.0	
Haimanot (1995) [88]	Ethiopia	Community	Face-to-face/ Clin interview	15,000	1 yr	20+	4.2	1.7	3.0	
Henry (1992) [89]	France	Community	Face-to-face	4,204	1 yr	15+	11.9	4.0	8.1	
Jabbar (1997) [90]	Saudi Arabia	Community	Face-to-face	5,891	Lifetime	15+			8.0	
Jaillard (1997) [91]	Peru	Community	Clin interview	3,246	1 yr	15+	7.8	2.3	5.3	
Merikangas (1993) [92]	Switzerland	Community	Clin interview	379	1 yr	28–29	32.6	16.1	24.5	Weighted prevalence
Michel (1995) [50]	France	Community	Mail SAQ	9,411	3 month	18+	18.0	8.0	13.0	
O'Brien (1994) [33]	Canada	Community	Telephone	2,922	1 yr	18+	21.9	7.4	15.2	
Raieli (1994) [23]	Italy	School	Clin interview	1,445	1 yr	11–14	3.3	2.7	3.0	
Rasmussen (1992) [93]	Denmark	Community	Clin interview	740	1 yr	25–64	15.0	6.0	10.0	
Russell (1995) [94]	Denmark	Community	Clin interview	3,471	Lifetime	40	23.7	11.7	17.7	
Sakai (1996) [72]	Japan	Community	Mail SAQ	4,029	1 yr	15+	12.9	3.6	8.4	Female:Male prevalence ratio = 3.6. Regional differences
Stewart (1992) [28]	US	Community	Mail SAQ	20,468	1 yr	12–80	17.6	5.7	12.0	
Stewart (1996) [27]	US	Community	Telephone	12,328	1 yr	18–65	19.0	8.2	14.7	Racial differences
van Roijen (1995) [51]	Netherlands	Community	Face-to-face	10,480	1 yr	12+	12.0	5.0	9.0	
Wang (1997) [95]	China	Community	Clin interview	1,533	1 yr	65+	4.7	0.7	3.0	
Wong (1995) [96]	Hong Kong	Community	Telephone	7,356	1 yr	15+	1.5	0.6	1.0	

adolescent populations show almost equal prevalence rates in boys and girls. After adolescence, the gender prevalence ratios (female to male) range between 2.0 and 3.6 (table 1). The gender prevalence ratio varies with age, increases from 12 to 42 and declining thereafter. However, prevalence remains elevated in females relative to males even at age 80.

Socioeconomic Status (SES). Migraine was once considered to be a disease of the affluent. Bille found no support for this idea in a study of school children [24, 25]. Studies using intelligence testing and occupation as SES measures also failed to find an association between migraine prevalence and social class or intelligence [26]. As noted earlier, migraine prevalence in inversely related to household income and education in US population-based studies [27, 28]. However, those with higher income are more likely to receive a migraine diagnosis from a physician, presumably due to higher rates of consultation [28–30].

Studies outside of the US have not supported the association of low SES (as measured by education, occupation, or income) with headache prevalence [21, 31–33]. This lack of association outside the US may be influenced by differences in access to health care or cultural differences in medical consultation.

Geography and Race. The American Migraine Study showed that migraine prevalence was lower in African Americans than Caucasians, although differences were statistically significant for males only [28]. An independent US study found that prevalence was higher in Caucasians than Africans, with the lowest prevalence in Asians [27]. Consistent geographic differences in migraine prevalence were found in a recent meta-analysis of 21 population-based surveys using IHS criteria [20]. Although these studies reported wide variation in their prevalence estimates, most of this variability was accounted for by the age distributions of the study populations and, most strongly, by the geographic area in which the surveys were conducted. In particular, age-adjusted migraine prevalence was lower in Africa and Asia and higher in Europe, Middle East, and the Americas (fig. 2). As there were relatively few African and Asian surveys which used the IHS criteria in this analysis, these results must be interpreted with caution. Further, there may be geographic variation within the Americas, Europe, Africa, and Asia based on either biological or environmental risk factors. Whether these apparent geographic differences in headache prevalence are real remains an area of future research.

Comorbidity of Migraine

A number of conditions are more likely to occur in individuals with migraine than in the general population. Population-based studies demonstrate that migraine is comorbid with depression, anxiety disorders, and manic de-

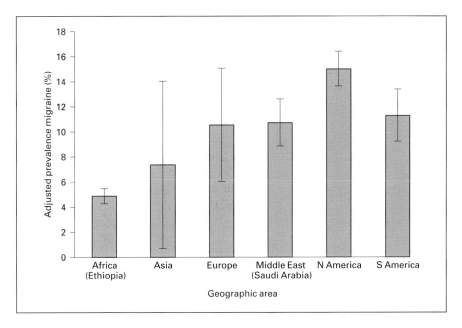

Fig. 2. Prevalence of migraine by geographic area and gender at age 40, based on 21 population-based studies that used International Headache Society (IHS) diagnostic criteria. Estimates are model-based and adjusted for age. Ninety-five percent confidence intervals are shown [20].

pressive illness [34–43] as well as epilepsy [44–47]. In addition, migraine is associated with stroke in women below the age of 45 [48, 49]. Studies have shown that migraineurs have higher health care costs for non-migraine conditions compared to matched non-migraineurs [50–52] (see Economic Impact, below).

Natural History and Transformed Migraine

There are a few longitudinal studies on the natural history of migraine. Bille followed a migrainous cohort for up to 40 years [24, 25, 53]; although 62% were free of migraine as young adults, only 46% were migraine-free after 40 years. An additional 22% who were not migraine-free reported past remissions. Thus, migraine is often a condition of very long duration. Hockaday also reported long-term remissions [54]. Fry [55] and Waters [9, 26], in other longitudinal studies, noted the tendency for attacks to decrease in frequency and severity as patients aged.

Clinic-based studies report on a subgroup of migraineurs who, after years of episodic migraine, experience increasing attack frequency often coupled with decreasing attack severity to the point that daily or near-daily headaches may occur [56–58]. This syndrome has been variously called chronic daily headache evolving from migraine, transformed migraine, drug-induced headache, and malignant migraine. The prevalence of daily headache evolving from migraine in the general population has not been well studied, but is probably about 2% [59–61]. In clinicians, 46–87% of such patients are found to be overusing acute headache medication [62–66] and medication overuse has been hypothesized to be the mechanism by which daily headaches are perpetuated through a rebound cycle [57]. For those patients with medication overuse, drug withdrawal in the absence of any other therapy has been reported to have a success rate of about 60% [67, 68]. Many of these clinic patients (13–54%), however, are not overusing medication. On one population-based study, only 24% of those with chronic daily headache were overusing medication [60]. Thus, there may be a subgroup of migraine sufferers with a progressive condition [62–66].

Economic Impact of Migraine

A number of studies have attempted to quantify the economic costs associated with migraine (see [2, 69–71] for reviews). Although estimates have varied between studies, generally the direct costs of migraine (such as doctor visits, emergency room visits, and medication) are relatively small compared to the cost of missed work or reduced productivity at work. Migraineurs often do not consult physicians for headache [1–3, 15, 50, 72] and treat their attacks primarily with non-prescription medications [73–75], although there are variations by country in these patterns.

Table 2 summarizes some estimates of annual direct costs of migraine treatment. In these studies, the direct costs of migraine (per migraineur) are fairly modest. Two US studies [52, 76] found costs of approximately $100 per year for migraineurs seeking treatment. Another US study found costs ranging from $200 to $800 per year depending on headache severity [77]. Consistent with that finding, another US study found costs of about $800 per year based on participants in a clinical trial, presumably a more severely affected population [78].

It has been estimated that there are 8.7 female and 2.6 million male migraineurs in the United States with moderate to severe disability [28]. If approximately 30% of these migraineurs who currently consult physicians incur costs of $100 per year each, this would result in 339 million dollars

Table 2. Estimates of direct annual costs of migraine

Reference	Country	Year[a]	Expense	Amount	Comment
Clouse [52]	US	1989	Physician/hospital	$127	Based on members of a large managed care
			Excess physician/hospital compared to non-migraineurs	$381	organization. Members with migraine were compared to matched members without migraine. Migraineurs had relatively small expenses coded for migraine ($127) but had higher overall medical expenses.
			Excess pharmacy compared to non-migraneurs	$158	
Hu [76]	US	1994	Physician/hospital/ER/drug	$97	Medstat MarketScan data. Migraine-related claims from employees and dependants from 40 large employers.
Lipton [77]	US	1989	Physician/hospital/ER/drug	$200–$800	Based on members of a large managed care organization. Medical expenses varied depending on the severity of headache.
Osterhaus [78]	US	1986	ER/clinic/hospital	$817	Clinical trial participants.

[a] Year of data collection.

annually being spent on direct costs for migraine. Missing from this amount is the cost of over the counter (OTC) medication as well as the cost of treating complications of medication misuse (i.e. gastritis, ulcers, kidney disease). In addition, there is some evidence that consultation with non-MD practitioners (e.g. chiropractors, herbalists, acupuncturists) is fairly common, although this has not been well studied. A recent US study reported that 24% of those with severe headaches had consulted an alternative practitioner in the last year, most commonly a chiropractor [79]. One Dutch study [51] found that 17% of migraineurs had consulted an alternative practitioner within the last year (compared to about half who had consulted GPs). However, those who had consulted alternative practitioners had more than eight visits per year on average, accounting for more than 80% of all direct costs. In a Danish study [80], 5–8% of the migraineurs had consulted alternative practitioners.

As discussed above, migraineurs are more likely to suffer from other health conditions and have greater expenses for non-migraine conditions than those of the same sex and age. As some of these excess medical expenses may be related to migraine either etiologically (e.g. depression) or iatrogenically (e.g. renal disease as a result of analgesic use), they may be more properly counted as part of the true cost of migraine [77]. These excess costs may be substantial [51] and the effect on a cost-of-disease analysis could be large. One study (table 1) found that excess claims for non-migraine health conditions (compared to non-migraineurs) outweighed the claims for migraine by about 4 to 1 [52]. Another study found that both headache and non-headache medical expenses increased with poor headache outcome [77].

Table 3. Estimates of indirect costs of migraine – annual lost workdays and reduced productivity[a]

Reference	Country	Year[b]	LWD	LWDE[c]	Total (LWD + LWDE)	Comment
Clarke [97]	UK	1994	2.0	5.5	7.5	Hospital employees, 81% female
Cull [87]	UK	1990	1.9	4.4	6.3	
Osterhaus [78]	US	1986	14.8	25.7	40.5	Clinical trial participants
Rasmussen [80]	Denmark	1989				43% had at least 1 absent day
Schwartz [98]	US	1993	3.2	4.9	8.1	
Stewart [81]	US	1989	7.4			'Severe' headache used as screening question
						Includes lost work of homemakers
van Roijen [51]	Netherlands	1992	4.2	8.9	13.1	Population-based 3-month diary study
von Korff [82]	US	1998	2.8	5.6	8.4	

[a] Lost workdays (LWD) and lost workday equivalents (LWDE) were extrapolated to 1 year if not reported annually in the referenced report.
[b] Year of data collection.
[c] LWDE = (Days at work with headache) × (1 – % effectiveness at work with headache).

Table 3 summarizes some estimates of lost workdays due to migraine among employed migraineurs. Included in this table is both lost workdays (LWD), i.e. days of absence from work, and lost workday equivalents (LWDE). LWDE is an estimate of the number of equivalent days lost due to reduced productivity while at work, and is the product of the number of days at work with migraine and percent 'ineffective' (1-effectiveness) while at work with migraine. The estimates of lost workdays are mostly consistent, at about 2–4 days per year. The equivalent of another 4–9 days were lost due to reduced effectiveness while at work. The American Migraine Study estimate of lost work was somewhat higher (7.4 days), perhaps because the screening questions asked about 'severe' headaches. This may have resulted in a bias towards more disabled migraineurs [81]. The study based on participants in a clinical trial [78], not surprisingly, reported the highest rates of missed work since individuals with severe disease are more likely to participate in clinical trials.

Estimating work absence due to migraine retrospectively is limited by the accuracy of recall. It is also difficult to determine whether work loss on a particular day is due to migraine or non-migraine headache. In one study [82], a population-based sample of 122 regularly employed migraineurs completed a diary over a 3-month period. This study found that 4.4 (annualized) days of work (2.8 for migraine, 1.6 for non-migraine headaches) were lost for headache. There were an additional 12.2 days of equivalent work loss due to reduced productivity (5.8 migraine, 6.3 non-migraine headaches). Twenty percent of the respondents accounted for 77% of the lost workdays. This study indicates that non-migraine headaches also account for a substantial amount of work absence and reduced productivity.

Conclusion

Migraine is a very common disorder, with highest prevalence during the peak productive years – between the ages of 25 and 55. The prevalence is greater in females than males after puberty, but the sex ratio varies with age. In the United States, migraine prevalence is higher in those with lower incomes, possibly because migraine interferes with work and schooling.

Most migraineurs do not consult physicians and generally treat their attacks with OTC medication. The direct costs of treating migraine are greatly outweighed by the cost of missed work or reduced productivity at work.

The impact of headache disorders on individuals and society is large and provides an important target for public health interventions. Despite the widespread disability produced by migraine and the increasing availability of effective treatment, the disorder remains under-treated and under-diagnosed.

References

1 Lipton RB, Stewart WF, Simon D: Medical consultation for migraine: Results from the American Migraine Study. Headache 1998;38:87–96.
2 Stang PE, Osterhaus JT, Celentano DD: Migraine. Patterns of healthcare use. [Review] [37 refs]. Neurology 1994;44(suppl 4):S47–S55.
3 Linet MS, Stewart WF, Celentano DD, Ziegler D, Sprecher M: An epidemiologic study of headache among adolescents and young adults. JAMA 1989;261:2211–2216.
4 Headache Classification Committee of the International Headache Society: Classification and diagnostic criteria for headache disorders, cranial neuralgias an facial pain. Cephalalgia 1988;8(suppl 7): 1–96.
5 Olesen J, Lipton RB: Migraine classification and diagnosis. International Headache Society criteria. Neurology 1994;44(suppl 4):S6–S10.
6 Stewart WF, Simon D, Schechter A, Lipton RB: Population variation in migraine prevalence: A meta-analysis. J Clin Epidemiol 1995;48:269–280.
7 Rasmussen BK, Jensen R, Schroll M, Olesen J: Interrelations between migraine and tension-type headache in the general population. Arch Neurol 1992;49:914–948.
8 Ulrich V, Russell MB, Jensen R, Olesen J: A comparison of tension-type headache in migraineurs and in non-migraineurs: A population-based study. Pain 1996;67:501–506.
9 Waters WE: Headache. Littleton, Mass, PSG Pub Co 1986.
10 Featherstone HJ: Migraine and muscle contraction headaches: A continuum. Headache 1985;25: 194–198.
11 Raskin N: Headache. ed 2. New York, Churchill Livingstone, 1988.
12 Rasmussen BK, Jensen R, Olesen J: A population-based analysis of the diagnostic criteria of the International Headache Society. Cephalalgia 1991;11:129–134.
13 Breslau N, Chilcoat HD, Andreski P: Further evidence on the link between migraine and neuroticism. Neurology 1996;47:663–667.

14 Brown NR, Rips LJ, Shevell SK: The subjective dates of natural events in very long-term memory. Cognit Psychol 1985;17:139–177.

15 Rasmussen BK: Epidemiology of headache. Cephalalgia 1995;15:45–68.

16 Stewart WF, Linet MS, Celentano DD, Van NM, Ziegler D: Age- and sex-specific incidence rates of migraine with and without visual aura. Am J Epidemiol 1991;134:1111–1120.

17 Stewart WF, Schechter A, Lipton RB: Migraine heterogeneity: Disability, pain intensity, and attack frequency and duration. Neurology 1994;44(suppl 4):S24–S39.

18 Stewart WF, Shechter A, Rasmussen BK: Migraine prevalence: A review of population-based studies. Neurology 1994;44(suppl 4):S17–S23.

19 Lipton RB, Stewart WF: Prevalence and impact of migraine. Neurologic Clinics 1997;15:1–13.

20 Scher AI, Stewart WF, Lipton RB: Epidemiology of migraine: A meta-analytic review. Forthcoming.

21 Abu-Arefeh I, Russell G: Prevalence of headache and migraine in schoolchildren. Br Med J 1994; 309:765–769.

22 Barea LM, Tannhauser M, Rotta NT: An epidemiologic study of headache among children and adolescents of southern Brazil. Cephalalgia 1996;16:545–549.

23 Raieli V, Raimondo D, Cammalleri R, Camarda R: Migraine headaches in adolescents: A student population-based study in Monreale. Cephalalgia 1995;15:5–12.

24 Bille B: Migraine is schoolchildren. Acta Paediatr Scand 1962;51(suppl):1–151.

25 Bille B: Migraine and other headaches; in Ferrari MD, Lataste Xavier (eds): Migraine in Children: Prevalence, Clinical Features, and a 30-Year Follow-Up. Carnforth, Lancs UK, Park Ridge NJ, USA, Pathenon Publishers, 1989.

26 Waters WE: Migraine: Intelligence, social class and familial prevalence. Br Med J 1971;2:77–81.

27 Stewart WF, Lipton RB, Liberman J: Variation in migraine prevalence by race. Neurology 1996; 47:52–59.

28 Stewart WF, Lipton RB, Celentano DD, Reed ML: Prevalence of migraine headache in the United States. Relation to age, income, race, and other sociodemographic factors. JAMA 1992;267:64–69.

29 Lipton RB, Stewart WF, Celentano DD, Reed ML: Undiagnosed migraine headaches. A comparison of symptom-based and reported physician diagnosis. Arch Intern Med 1992;152:1273–1278.

39 Kryst S, Scherl E: A population-based survey of the social and personal impact of headache. Headache 1994;34:344–350.

31 Rasmussen BK: Migraine and tension-type headache in a general population: Psychosocial factors. Int J Epidemiol 1992;21:1138–1143.

32 Göbel H, Petersen-Braun M, Soyka D: The epidemiology of headache in Germany: A nationwide survey of a representative sample on the basis of the headache classification of the International Headache Society. Cephalalgia 1994;14:97–106.

33 O'Brien B, Goeree R, Streiner D: Prevalence of migraine headache in Canada: A population-based survey. Int J Epidemiol 1994;23:1020–1026.

34 Breslau N, Davis GC, Andreski P: Migraine, psychiatric disorders and suicide attempts: An epidemiologic study of young adults. Psychiatry Research 1991;37:11–23.

35 Silberstein SD, Lipton RB, Breslau N: Migraine: Association with personality characteristics and psychopathology. Cephalalgia 1995;15:358–369.

36 Merikangas KR, Angst J, Isler H: Migraine and psychopathology. Results of the Zurich cohort study of young adults. Arch Gen Psychiatry 1990;47:849–853.

37 Stewart WF, Linet MS, Celentano DD: Migraine headaches and panic attacks. Psychosomatic Medicine 1989;51:559–569.

38 Stewart WF, Shechter A, Liberman J: Physician consultation for headache pain and history of panic: Results from a population-based study. Am J Med 1992:S35–S40.

39 Merikangas KR, Stevens DE, Angst J: Headache and personality: Results of a community sample of young adults. 18th Collegium Internationale Neuro-Psychopharmacologicum Congress: Migraine: The interface between neurology and psychiatry (1991, Nice, France). J Psychiatr Res 1993; 27:187–196.

40 Breslau N: Migraine, suicidal ideation, and suicide attempts. Neurology 1992;42:392–395.

41 Breslau N, Davis GC: Migraine, major depression and panic disorder: A prospective epidemiologic study of young adults. Cephalalgia 1992;12:85–90.

42 Breslau N, Davis GC: Migraine, physical health and psychiatric disorder: A prospective epidemiologic study in young adults. J Psychiat Res 1993;27:211–212.

43 Breslau N, Davis GC, Schultz LR, Peterson EL: Joint 1994 Wolff Award Presentation. Migraine and major depression: A longitudinal study. Headache 1994;34:387–393.

44 Andermann E, Andermann FA: Migraine and epilepsy; in Andermann F, Lugaresi E (eds): Migraine-Epilepsy Relationships: Epidemiological and Genetic Aspects. Boston, Butterworth Publishers, 1987, p 281.

45 Lipton RB, Ottman R, Ehrenberg BL, Hauser WA: Comorbidity of migraine: The connection between migraine and epilepsy. Neurology 1994;44(suppl 7):S28–S32.

46 Ottman R, Lipton RB: Comorbidity of migraine and epilepsy. Neurology 1994;44:2105–2110.

47 Ottman R, Lipton RB: Is the comorbidity of epilepsy and migraine due to a shared genetic susceptibility? Neurology 1996;47:918–924.

48 Tzourio C, Iglesias S, Hubert JB, Visy JM, Alperovitch A, Tehindrazanarivelo A, Biousse V, Woimant F, Bousser MG: Migraine and risk of ischaemic stroke: A case-control study. Br Med J 1993;307: 289–292.

49 Tzourio C, Tehindrazanarivelo A, Iglesias S, Alperovitch A, Chedru F, d'Anglejan-Chatillon J, Bousser MG: Case-control study of migraine and risk of ischaemic stroke in young women. Br Med J 1995;310:830–833.

50 Michel P, Pariente P, Duru G, Dreyfus JP, Chabriat H, Henry P, Dreyfuss JP: MIG ACCESS: A population-based, nationwide, comparative survey of access to care in migraine in France. Cephalalgia 1996;16:50–55.

51 van Roijen L, Essink-Bot M, Koopmanschap MA, Michel BC, Rutten FFH: Societal perspective on the burden of migraine in The Netherlands. PharmacoEconomics 1995;7:170–179.

52 Clouse JC, Osterhaus JT: Healthcare resources use and costs associated with migraine in a managed healthcare setting. Ann Pharmacother 1994;28:659–664.

53 Bille B: A 40-year follow-up of school children with migraine. Cephalalgia 1997;17:488–491.

54 Hockaday JM: Migraine in children and other non-epileptic paroxysmal disorders; in Hockaday JM (ed): Definitions, Clinical Features, and Diagnosis of Childhood Migraine. London/Boston, Butterworths, 1988, p 5.

55 Fry J: Profiles of disease: A study in the natural history of common diseases. Edinburgh/London, Livingstone, 1996.

56 Mathew NT, Reuveni U, Perez F: Transformed or evolutive migraine. Headache 1987;27:102–106.

57 Matthew NT, Stubits E, Nigam MP: Transformation of episodic migraine into daily headache: Analysis of factors. Headache 1982;22:66–68.

58 Silberstein SD, Lipton RB, Solomon S, Mathew NT: Classification of daily and near-daily headaches: Proposed revisions to the IHS criteria. Headache 1994;34:1–7.

59 Scher AI, Stewart WF, Liberman J, Lipton RB: Wolff Award 1998. Prevalence of frequent headache in a population sample. Headache 1998;38:497–506.

60 Castillo J, Munoz P, Guitera V: Epidemiology of chronic daily headache in the general population. Headache 1999;39:190–196.

61 Silberstein SD, Lipton RB, Sliwinski M: Classification of daily and near-daily headaches: Field trial of revised IHS criteria. Neurology 1996;47:871–875.

62 Sandrini G, Manzoni GC, Zanferrari C, Nappi G: An epidemiological approach to the nosography of chronic daily headache. Cephalalgia 1993;13(suppl 12):72–77.

63 Mathew NT: Transformed migraine. Cephalalgia 1993;13(suppl 12):78–83.

64 Manzoni GC, Granella F, Sandrini G, Cavallini A, Zanferrari C, Nappi G: Classification of chronic daily headache by International Headache Society criteria: Limits and new proposals. Cephalalgia 1995;15:37–43.

65 Solomon S, Lipton RB, Newman LC: Clinical features of chronic daily headache. Headache 1992; 32:325–329.

66 von Korff M, Galer BS, Strang P: Chronic use of symptomatic headache medications. Pain 1995; 62:179–186.

67 Diener HC, Dichgans J, Scholz E, Geiselhart S, Gerber WD, Bille A: Analgesic-induced chronic headache: Long-term results of withdrawal therapy. J Neurol 1989;236:9–14.

68 Andersson PG: Ergotamine headache. Headache 1975;15:118–121.
69 de Lissovoy G, Lazarus SS: The economic cost of migraine. Present state of knowledge. Neurology 1994;44(Suppl 4):S56–S62.
70 Solomon GD, Price KL: Burden of migraine: Areview of its socioeconomic impact. Pharmaco-Ecomonomics 1997;11(suppl 1):1–10.
71 Ferrari MD: The economic burden of migraine to society. PharmacoEconomics 1998;13:667–676.
72 Sakai F, Igarashi H: Prevalence of migraine in Japan: A nationwide survey. Cephalalgia 1997;17:15–22.
73 Celentano DD, Stewart WF, Lipton RB, Reed ML: Medication use and disability among migraineurs: A national probability sample survey. Headache 1992;32:223–228.
74 Forward SP, McGrath PJ, MacKinnon D, Brown TL, Swann J, Currie EL: Medication patterns of recurrent headache sufferers: A community study. Cephalalgia 1998;18:146–151.
75 Edmeads J, Findlay H, Tugwell P, Pryse-Phillips W, Nelson RF, Murray TJ: Impact of migraine and tension-type headache on life-style, consulting behaviour, and medication use: A Canadian population survey. Can J Neurol Sci 1993;20:131–137.
76 Hu XH, Markson LE, Lipton RB, Stewart WF, Berger ML: Disability and economic costs of migraine in the United States: A population based approach. Archives of Internal Medicine 1999;159:813–818.
77 Lipton RB, Stewart WF, von Korff M: Burden of migraine: Societal costs and therapeutic opportunities. Neurology 1997;48(suppl 3):S4–S9.
78 Osterhaus JT, Gutterman DL, Plachetka JR: Healthcare resource and lost labour costs of migraine headache in the US. PharmacoEconomics 1992;2:67–76.
79 Paramore LC: Use of alternative therapies: Estimates from the 1994 Robert Wood Johnson Foundation National Access to Care Survey. J Pain Symptom Management 1997;13:83–89.
80 Rasmussen BK, Jensen R, Olesen J: Impact of headache on sickness absence and utilisation of medical services: A Danish population study. J Epidemiol Community Health 1992;46:443–446.
81 Stewart WF, Lipton RB, Simon D: Work-related disability: Results from the American migraine study. Cephalalgia 1996;16:231–238.
82 von Korff M, Stewart WF, Simon DJ, Lipton RB: Migraine and reduced work performance: A population-based diary study. Neurology 1998;50:1741–1745.
83 Al Rajeh S, Awada A, Bademosi O, Ogunniyi A: The prevalence of migraine and tension headache in Saudi Arabia: A community-based study. Eur J Neurol 1997;4:502–506.
84 Alders EE, Hentzen A, Tan CT: A commnity-based prevalence study on headache in Malaysia. Headache 1996;36:379–384.
85 Arregui A, Cabrera J, Leon-Velarde F, Paredes S, Viscarra D, Arbaiza D: High prevalence of migraine in a high-altitude population. Neurology 1991;41:1668–1669.
86 Cruz ME, Cruz I, Preux PM, Schantz P, Dumas M: Headache and cysticercosis in Ecuador, South America. Headache 1995;35:93–97.
87 Cull RE, Wells NEJ, Miocevich ML: The economic cost of migraine. Br J Med Econ 1992;2:103–115.
88 Tekle Haimanot R, Seraw B, Forsgren L, Ekbom K, Ekstedt J: Migraine, chronic tension-type headache, and cluster headache in an Ethiopian rural community. Cephalalgia 1995;15:482–488.
89 Henry P, Michel P, Brochet B, Dartigues JF, Tison S, Salamon R: A nationwide survey of migraine in France: Prevalence and clinical features in adults. GRIM. Cephalalgia 1992;12:229–237.
90 Abdul Jabbar M, Ogunniyi A: Sociodemographic factors and primary headache syndromes in a Saudi community. Neuroepidemiology 1997;16:48–52.
91 Jaillard AS, Mazetti P, Kala E: Prevalence of migraine and headache in a high-altitude town of Peru: A population-based study. Headache 1997;37:95–101.
92 Merikangas KR, Whitaker AE, Angst J: Validation of diagnostic criteria for migraine in the Zurich longitudinal cohort study. Cephalalgia 1993;13(suppl 12):47–53.
93 Rasmussen BK, Jensen R, Schroll M, Olesen J: Epidemiology of headache in a general population – A prevalence study. J Clin Epidemiol 1991;44:1147–1157.
94 Russell MB, Rasmussen BK, Thorvaldsen P, Olesen J: Prevalence and sex-ratio of the subtypes of migraine. Int J Epidemiol 1995;24:612–618.

95   Wang SJ, Liu HC, Fuh JL, Liu CY, Lin KP, Chen HM, Lin CH, Wang PN, Hsu LC, Wang HC, Lin KN: Prevalence of headaches in a Chinese elderly population in Kinmen: Age and gender effect and cross-cultural comparisons. Neurology 1997;49:195–200.
96   Wong TW, Wong KS, Yu TS, Kay R: Prevalence of migraine and other headaches in Hong Kong. Neuroepidemiology 1995;14:82–91.
97   Clarke CE, MacMillan L, Sondhi S, Wells NE: Economic and social impact of migraine. QJM 1996;89:77–84.
98   Schwartz BS, Stewart WF, Lipton RB: Lost workdays and decreased work effectiveness associated with headache in the workplace. J Occup Environ Med 1997;39:320–327.

Richard B. Lipton, MD, Departments of Neurology, Epidemiology and Social Medicine,
Albert Einstein College of Medicine and Headache Unit,
Montefiore Medical Center, Bronx, NY 10467 (USA)
Tel. +1 203 321 1050 × 23, Fax +1 203 321 1044, E-Mail rlipton@imrinc.com

Diener HC (ed): Drug Treatment of Migraine and Other Headaches.
Monogr Clin Neurosci. Basel, Karger, 2000, vol 17, pp 16–23

....
Classification and Symptoms

Birthe Krogh Rasmussen[a], *Jes Olesen*[b]

Departments of Neurology
[a] Hillerød Hospital, Hillerød, and
[b] Glostrup Hospital, University of Copenhagen, Glostrup, Denmark

In the past, several classifications of headache syndromes have been used, but they have all lacked precision, included ambiguous expressions, and were non-operational, which resulted in vague criteria [1–3]. In 1985 the International Headache Society (IHS) appointed a headache classification committee and in 1988, the first international headache classification including operational diagnostic criteria for all headache disorders was published [4]. That classification was endorsed by all the national headache societies represented in the International Headache Society and very quickly also by the World Federation of Neurology. The World Health Organization accepted the major principles of the new classification which have been used in a simplified form for the classification of these disorders in the tenth revision of the international classification of diseases (ICD 10) [5] and more detail was included in the ICD 10's neurological adaptation [6]. The ICD 10 and especially its neurological adaptation [5, 6] closely follow the IHS classification and a so-called fascicle on headache provides a crosswalk between these two coding systems and brings the operational diagnostic criteria of the IHS together with the ICD 10 code numbers. Most recently, WHO decided to publish a separate booklet containing even more extensive details of the IHS classification: the ICD 10 Guide for Headaches [7]. The complete international headache classification has already been translated into more than 12 languages and has been widely accepted. It has been used in the great majority of drug trials carried out since 1988 and the diagnostic criteria of the IHS Classification must be regarded as indispensible in both clinical and research work with patients suffering from headaches.

The Headache Classification Committee of the IHS created a standardized nomenclature and new terms when necessary. Common migraine became mi-

Table 1. International Headache Society classification of migraine

1 *Migraine*
   1.1 Migraine without aura
   1.2 Migraine with aura
      1.2.1 Migraine with typical aura
      1.2.2 Migraine with prolonged aura
      1.2.3 Familial hemiplegic migraine
      1.2.4 Basilar migraine
      1.2.5 Migraine aura without headache
      1.2.6 Migraine with acute onset aura
   1.3 Ophthalmoplegic migraine
   1.4 Retinal migraine
   1.5 Childhood periodic syndromes that may be precursors to or associated with migraine
      1.5.1 Benign paroxysmal vertigo of childhood
      1.5.2 Alternating hemiplegia of childhood
   1.6 Complications of migraine
      1.6.1 Status migrainosus
      1.6.2 Migrainous infarction
   1.7 Migrainous disorder not fulfilling above criteria

graine without aura, and classic/classical migraine became migraine with aura. The latter now includes the following previously used terms: migraine accompagné, hemiplegic, complicated, ophthalmic, hemisensory, aphasic, basilar and confusional migraine.

The IHS classification is hierarchically constructed. It contains 13 diagnostic groups which are subdivided to allow for coding up to a four-digit level. Thus, it is possible to use the classification at different levels of sophistication. Doctors in general practice can code just to one or two digits, whereas specialists and research centers can also code the third and fourth digit. Table 1 gives the subgroupings of migraine according to the IHS classification.

Classification of Migraine

The subtypes of migraine are classified according to their clinical features and current concepts of pathophysiology. Migraine without aura is characterized by normal cerebral blood flow and absence of neurological symptoms, whereas migraine with aura is associated with typical changes in regional cerebral blood flow. Migraine with aura encompasses all forms of migraine with preceding neurological symptoms originating from brain or brainstem.

Migraine with aura is subgrouped in six types: migraine with typical aura, migraine with prolonged aura, familial hemiplegic migraine, basilar migraine, migraine aura without headache, and migraine with acute onset aura (table 1). Ophthalmoplegic migraine is recognized as a separate form of migraine because of a quite different clinical picture and pathophysiology, possibly caused by retro-orbital granulomatous inflammation. Retinal migraine is also regarded as separate due to its presumed origin in retina. Good studies to substantiate its existence are lacking. Finally, a mixed group of conditions of childhood periodic syndromes which may be precursors to or associated with migraine and complications of migraine are recognized. In order to make the classification exhaustive, the condition 1.7: Migrainous disorder not fulfilling above criteria is included.

Operational Diagnostic Criteria

The difficulty with an operational headache diagnosis is the lack of abnormalities of routine laboratory investigations. The headache diagnoses must be made exclusively on the basis of information provided by the patient. During this century various sophisticated measurement techniques such as regional cerebral blood flow and transcranial doppler have been developed. However, these tests mainly show changes during attacks and they are not generally accessible for diagnostic use. The criteria of the International Headache Society, therefore, largely depend on the headache history and the exclusion of organicity by physical and neurological examinations and necessary laboratory tests. The operational diagnostic criteria for migraine with and without aura are given in table 2. Each set of criteria consists of a number of letter headings A, B, C etc. The requirements under each of these letter headings has to be fulfilled in order to make a diagnosis of for example, migraine without aura. Each letter heading may consist of several characteristics not all of which need to be fulfilled. Features present only in possibly 50% of patients can thus be included. This pertains for instance to the characteristics of both headache and associated symptoms. Note that under C it is only required that pain characteristics fulfill two out of the four criteria. All neurologists have seen typical migraine patients who's pain was bilateral and not pulsating. Such patients have migraine according to the IHS classification as long as the two other features of criterion C are fulfilled. A similar thing is true of criterion D. Although most patients have nausea and/or vomiting during migraine attacks, an occasional patient will have absolutely typical migraine but without gastrointestinal symptoms. This is accepted if they have photophobia as well as phonophobia. The purpose of criterion E is to rule out intracranial disease.

Table 2. Diagnostic criteria for migraine without aura and migraine with aura

---

Migraine without aura

A At least 5 attacks fulfilling B–D

B Headache attacks lasting 4–72 h (untreated or unsuccessfully treated)

C Headache has at least two of the following characteristics:
  (1) Unilateral location
  (2) Pulsating quality
  (3) Moderate or severe intensity (inhibits or prohibits daily activities)
  (4) Aggravation by walking stairs or similar routine physical activity

D During headache at least one of the following:
  (1) Nausea and/or vomiting
  (2) Photophobia and phonophobia

E At least one of the following:
  (1) History, physical and neurological examinations do not suggest one of the disorders listed in groups 5–11
  (2) History and/or physical and/or neurological examinations do suggest such disorder, but it is ruled out by appropriate investigations
  (3) Such disorder is present, but migraine attacks do not occur for the first time in close temporal relation to the disorder

Migraine with aura

A At least 2 attacks fulfilling B

B At least 3 of the following 4 characteristics:
  (1) One or more fully reversible aura symptoms indicating focal cerebral cortical – and/or brainstem dysfunction
  (2) At least one aura symptom develops gradually over more than 4 min or, 2 or more symptoms occur in succession
  (3) No aura symptom lasts more than 60 min. If more than one aura symptom is present, accepted duration is proportionally increased
  (4) Headache follows aura with a free interval of less than 60 min (it may also begin before or simultaneously with the aura)

C At least one of the following:
  (1) History, physical and neurological examinations do not suggest one of the disorders listed in groups 5–11
  (2) History and/or physical and/or neurological examinations do suggest such disorder, but it is ruled out by appropriate investigations
  (3) Such disorder is present, but migraine attacks do not occur for the first time in close temporal relation to the disorder

---

It is rather lengthy but this is so because it serves to protect patients from over-investigation. It specifies that laboratory investigations are not necessary to rule out organic disorder in the great majority of headache patients.

The operational diagnostic criteria constitute the most important part of the headache classification. However, short descriptions of the disorders in a normal language are also given. The short description of migraine without aura, for example, is as follows: 'Idiopathic, recurring headache disorder manifesting in attacks lasting 4–72 hours. Typical characteristics of headache are unilateral location, pulsating quality, moderate or severe intention, aggravation by routine physical activity, and association with nausea, photo- and phonophobia.'

How to Use the International Headache Society Classification

The fact that one patient frequently has more than one type of headache has not been realized in most previous classification systems, where patients have been categorized as having for example either migraine or tension-type headache. In the IHS classification system, however, patients receive a diagnosis for each distinct headache form.

However, difficulties may arise from this coexistence of different types of headache in the individual patient and from changes in headache diagnoses of individual patients over time. Each discrete form of headache in a person must be diagnosed. Some patients indicate that they have many different forms of headache, even if they are all varieties of a single diagnosis according to the IHS classification. Other patients believe that their different forms of headache are just variations of the same diagnosis. Careful history taking must clarify how many different forms of headache the patient has and which criteria they fulfill. The terms 'mixed headache' or 'combination headache' have been abandoned. These patients should now receive at least two diagnoses, i.e. migraine and tension-type headache. Subforms of tension-type headache and cluster headache are mutually exclusive but subforms of migraine are not. A patient can thus have more than one migraine diagnosis e.g. migraine without aura and migraine with aura. If a patient gets two diagnoses, which one is then the more important? And how do we get an impression of the severity of the headache disorder? It is recommended to add the estimated number of headache days per year in brackets after each diagnosis thereby providing the quantitative aspect of headache diagnosis. Not all headache episodes in a patient can or should be diagnosed. Atypical episodes are frequent because of early treatment, lack of ability to remember symptoms exactly and other factors. The patient should be asked to describe typical untreated or unsuccessfully treated episodes. It should be decided which set of diagnostic criteria these episodes fulfill and if the required number of episodes have been experienced. Then the number of days per year with this type of headache should be estimated, adding also treated attacks and less typical attacks believed to be of the same type. Considering the severity of the headache, the classification distinguishes between a mild, a moderate, and a severe pain intensity. A mild pain is not inhibiting daily activities, a moderate pain is inhibiting, but not preventing daily activities, and a severe pain is suspending daily activities.

In unclear cases it is recommended to ask the patient to keep a diagnostic headache diary [8]. Prospective recording of symptoms will usually make the diagnosis more precise. If a particular form of headache fulfills two sets of criteria, the diagnosis mentioned first in the classification should be coded for.

Scientific Evaluation of the IHS Headache Classification

The primary headaches constitute disease entities characterized by a clustering of specific combinations of symptoms. It is intuitively evident that the explicit diagnostic criteria for all headache disorders of the International Headache Society (IHS) [4] represent a substantial improvement over previous diagnostic systems. Nevertheless, the criteria require systematic field testing. There are some fundamental requirements of a classification and one is that it should be generalizable which means that it should be applicable in diverse settings (headache clinics, general practices, general populations etc.). The IHS criteria are derived from expert consensus. As such they are mostly based on the experience with highly selected migraine patients. Thus, the criteria may be expected to be most relevant in a specialist practice or in a hospital setting. However, in recent years the IHS criteria have been used in several epidemiological studies from the general population and have been found to be highly applicable [9–11]. Other basic requirements to the ideal classification are that of exhaustiveness, reliability and validity. These aspects of the classification have been addressed in a number of field studies [10–17]. *Exhaustiveness* indicates that it is possible to classify all headaches according to its diagnostic criteria [10, 14]. This was shown to be the case in a large Danish population-based study [10]. *Reliability* encompasses low interobserver variability and repeatability, which have been found to be quite good [8, 12, 13]. *Validity*, which means that the diagnosis reflects the underlying biological disorder. However, it is very difficult to evaluate the validity since no gold standard exists. Nonetheless, different approaches have been used to study the validity of the classification. Some have compared the IHS diagnoses with the diagnoses of expert clinicians [14, 15]. Others [11, 17] have validated the criteria by comparison to diagnoses obtained using the former Ad Hoc Committee Classification of Headache [1]. Somewhat divergating results are reported mainly due to various methodological limitations in some of these studies.

In recent years, the IHS criteria have been used worldwide in several large, multicenter, multinational double-blind drug trials [18–24]. These studies have shown remarkably consistent response rates to the triptanes, reflecting the homogeneity of the defined migraine group. The validity is also reflected in consistent epidemiological profiles and homogenous nosologic entities of the various headache types which have been found in several epidemiologic studies all employing the IHS diagnostic criteria [9, 14, 25–30].

With the aim of assessing and improving the reliability and validity of the IHS criteria future work should focus on continued field testing in various settings. More precise operationalization including more explicit behavior-oriented criteria to define each individual feature may possibly improve reliability, sensitivity and specificity of the IHS diagnostic criteria.

References

1   Ad hoc committee on classification of headache: Classification of headache. JAMA 1962;179: 717–718.
2   Friedman AP, von Storch TJC, Merritt HH: Migraine and tension headaches: A clinical study of two thousand cases. Neurology 1954;4:773–778.
3   World Federation of Neurology: Definition of migraine; in Cochrane AL (ed): Background to Migraine: Third Migraine Symposium. Heinemann, London, 1970, pp 181–182.
4   Headache Classification Committee of the International Headache Society: Classification and diagnostic criteria for headache disorders, cranial neuralgias and facial pain. Cephalalgia 1988;8(suppl 7): 1–96.
5   World Health Organization: The International Statistical Classification of Diseases and Related Health Problems. Tenth Revision, vol 1. Tabular List, vol 2. Instruction Manual, vol 3. Index. Geneva, World Health Organization, 1992–1994.
6   World Health Organization: Application of the International Classification of Diseases to Neurology, ed 2. Geneva, World Health Organization, 1997.
7   World Health Organization and International Headache Society: ICD-10 Guide for Headaches. Cephalalgia 1997;17(suppl 19):1–82.
8   Russell MB, Rasmussen BK, Brennum J, Iversen HK, Jensen R, Olesen J: Presentation of a new instrument: The diagnostic headache diary. Cephalalgia 1992;12:369–374.
9   Rasmussen BK, Jensen R, Schroll M, Olesen J: Epidemiology of headache in a general population – A prevalence study. J Clin Epidemiol 1991;44:1147–1157.
10   Rasmussen BK, Jensen R, Olesen J: A population-based analysis of the diagnostic criteria of the International Headache Society. Cephalalgia 1991;11:129–134.
11   Merikangas KR, Whitaker AE, Angst J: Validation of diagnostic criteria for migraine in the Zürich longitudinal cohort study. Cephalalgia 1993;13(suppl 12):47–53.
12   Granella F, D'Alessandro R, Manzoni GC, Cerbo R, Colucci D'Amato C, Pini LA, Savi L, Zanferrari C, Nappi G: International Headache Society classification: Interobserver reliability in the diagnosis of primary headaches. Cephalalgia 1994;14:16–20.
13   Leone M, Filippini G, D'Amico D, Farinotti M, Bussone G: Assessment of International Headache Society diagnostic criteria: A reliability study. Cephalalgia 1994;14:280–284.
14   Henry P, Michel P, Brochet B, Dartigues JF, Tison S, Salamon R and the GRIM: A nationwide survey of migraine in France: Prevalence and clinical features in adult. Cephalalgia 1992;12:229–237.
15   Michel P, Dartigues JF, Henry P, Tison S, Auriacombe S, Brochet B, Vivares C, Salamon R and the GRIM: Validity of the International Headache Society Criteria for Migraine. Neuroepidemiology 1993;12:51–57.

16   Rasmussen BK, Jensen R, Olesen J: Questionnaire versus clinical interview in the diagnosis of headache. Headache 1991;31:290–295.

17   Iversen HK, Langemark M, Andersson PG, Hansen PE, Olesen J: Clinical characteristics of migraine and episodic tension-type headache in relation to old and new diagnostic criteria. Headache 1990; 30:514–519.

18   Cady RK, Wendt JK, Kirchner JR, Sargent JD, Rothrock JF, Skaggs H: Treatment of acute migraine with subcutaneous sumatriptan. JAMA 1991;265:2831–2835.

19   The Subcutaneous Sumatriptan International Study Group: Treatment of migraine attacks with sumatriptan. N Eng J Med 1991;325:316–321.

20   The Oral Sumatriptan Dose-Defining Study Group: Sumatriptan – An oral dose-defining study. Eur Neurol 1991;31:300–305.

21   Dahlöf C, Diener HC, Goadsby PJ, Massiou H, Olesen J, Schoenen J, Wilkinson M, Sweet RM, Klein KB: A multinational, double-blind, placebo-controlled, dose range finding study to investigate the efficacy and safety of oral doses of 311C90 in the acute treatment of migraine. Headache 1995; 35:292.

22   Visser WH, Klein KB, Cox RC, Marks SJ, Ferrari MD: 311C90, a new central and peripherally acting 5-HT$_{1D}$ receptor agonist in the acute treatment of migraine: A double-blind, placebo-controlled, dose-ranging study. Neurology 1996;46:1–5.

23   Mathew N, Asgharnejad M, Reykamian M, Laurenza A: Naratriptan is effective and well tolerated in the acute treatment of migraine. Results of a double-blind, placebo-controlled, crossover study. Neurology 1997;49:1485–1490.

24   Kramer MS, Matzura-Wolfe D, Polis A, Getson A, Amaraneni PG, Solbach MP, McHugh W, Feighner J, Silberstein SD, Reines SA: A placebo-controlled crossover study of rizatriptan in the treatment of multiple migraine attacks. Neurology 1998;51:773–781.

25   Stewart WF, Lipton R, Celentano DD, Reed ML: Prevalence of migraine headache in the United States. JAMA 1992;267:64–69.

26   Breslau N, Davis GC, Andreski P: Migraine, psychiatric disorders, and suicide attempts: An epidemiologic study of young adults. Psychiatry Research 1991;37:11–23.

27   Edmeads J, Findlay H, Tugwell P, Pryse-Philips W, Nelson RF, Murray TJ: Impact of migraine and tension-type headache on life-style, consulting behaviour, and medication use: A Canadian population survey. Can J Neurol Sci 1993;20:131–137.

28   Michel P, Pariente P, Duru G, Dreyfuss J-P, Chabriat H, Henry P: Mig Access: A population-based, nationwide, comparative survey of access to care in migraine in France. Cephalalgia 1996; 16:50–55.

29   Russell MB, Rasmussen BK, Thorvaldsen P, Olesen J: Prevalence and sex-ratio of the subtypes of migraine. Int J Epidemiol 1995;24:612–618.

30   Stewart WF, Lipton RB, Liberman J: Variation in migraine prevalence by race. Neurology 1996; 47:52–59.

Dr. Birthe Krogh Rasmussen, Department of Neurology, Hilleroed Hospital,
DK–3400 Hilleroed (Denmark)
Tel. +45 4829 42 45, Fax +45 4829 4253, E-Mail bira@fa.dk

Diener HC (ed): Drug Treatment of Migraine and Other Headaches.
Monogr Clin Neurosci. Basel, Karger, 2000, vol 17, pp 24–29

....

Conduct of Clinical Trials in Acute Migraine Treatment and Their Interpretation

Peer Tfelt-Hansen [a], *Berit H. Rasmussen* [b]

[a] Department of Neurology, Glostrup Hospital, Glostrup, and
[b] Department of Neurology, Gentofte Hospital, Hellerup, Denmark

Randomized controlled clinical trials (RCTs) are the only way to demonstrate convincingly the efficacy of a drug. A RCT in acute migraine treatment should be regarded as a scientific experiment in which a relevant question is answered.

Firstly, it should be demonstrated in randomized, double-blind, placebo-controlled, clinical trials that a drug is more effective than placebo. Then the dose-response curve should be established; and the optimum dose (taking both efficacy and tolerability into account) and minimum effective dose should be determined. The drug should then in the optimum dose be compared to currently established treatment for efficacy and tolerability.

The following mini-review is based on the recommendation of the Drug Trial Committee of the International Headache Society (IHS) from 1991 [1], the published literature on mainly triptans [2] and our personal experiences with conducting RCTs in acute migraine treatment. Finally, a short checklist to assist with the evaluation of a RCT in migraine is presented.

Selection of Patients

Migraine Definition. The operational diagnostic criteria of the IHS [3] should be strictly adhered to. It is well recognized that there are in clinical practice, patients who do not conform to the IHS criteria but, nevertheless, are diagnosed as having migraine, treated accordingly and responding appropriately. For clinical drug trials, however, requirements are more rigid than in clinical practice. Relatively few people will be excluded by requiring IHS criteria.

Regarding the separation of migraine without aura and tension-type headache, consult the IHS criteria.

Interval Headaches. Interval headaches are permitted if they are well recognized by the patient. The patient should be able to differentiate migraine from an interval headache by the quality of pain (one-sided, pulsating, moderate or severe intensity) and/or by associated symptoms (nausea, discomfort to light or sound, visual symptoms or other aura).

Frequency of Attacks. Attacks of migraine should occur one to six times per month. The frequency of interval headaches should be no more than 6 days per month. There should be at least 24 h of freedom from headache between treated attacks of migraine.

Duration Since Onset. Migraine attacks should have been present for more than one year.

Age at Onset. The age at onset of migraine should be less than 50 years. Migraine beginning after the age of 50 is atypical and headache onset in these years is often due to underlying organic disease that sometimes mimics migraine. Few patients will be excluded by this limitation.

Concomitant Drug Use. Other concomitant therapy is undesirable. In early trials of safety and efficacy, the patient should not take any other drugs. In later trials contraceptive drugs and other drugs not taken for migraine are not contraindicated if there are no important side effects or interactions and the dose has been stable for 6 months.

Trial Design

Blinding. Controlled trials concerning acute treatment should be double-blind.

Placebo Control. Drugs used for the acute treatment of migraine should be compared with placebo. When two presumably active drugs are compared, placebo control should also be included in order to test the reactivity of the patient sample. That two presumably active drugs are not significantly different in a trial is no proof of efficacy or comparability. To refer to a previously found efficacy of the established drug is a use of historical controls, a method largely discouraged in medicine. Both drugs should also be shown to be superior to placebo in the current trial.

Crossover/Parallel Group Comparison. Both the crossover and the parallel group comparison designs can be used. There is probably no risk of a carryover effect in acute treatment, but a period effect using the crossover design has been observed in some trials.

The parallel group comparison design has dominated the recent trial programs for the triptans [2]. One advantage of the crossover design is that it allows assessments by the patients of the benefit:risk ratio by asking for preference [4]. In addition, the crossover design can be used to evaluate consistency of response [5, 6].

Dosage. The dose-response curve should be established by testing a wider range of doses in RCTs. In addition, the minimum effective dose should be defined in RCTs. In comparative RCTs the dose recommended for clinical use should be used.

Rescue Medication. Rescue medication should be allowed after ≥ 2 h. In some cases with parenteral drug administration, rescue medication could be used after, say 60 min, but in most cases with oral administration it is preferable to wait 2 h before rescue medication is allowed. In our opinion, to ask patients to wait 4 h [7] before escape medication is allowed is not acceptable in placebo-controlled RCTs.

Evaluation of Results

Number of Attacks Resolved Within 2 Hours. Number of migraine attacks resolved within 2 h, before any rescue medication, should usually be the primary parameter of efficacy (pain free).

This parameter is clinically relevant, simple and not affected by rescue medication. This parameter is suggested as the primary but not the only one for efficacy. With parental administration a drug may be quickly effective and the time point for resolution of the attack can be less than 2 h.

Headache Relief. In most of current and recent RCTs a success is defined as a decrease in headache from severe or moderate, to none or mild, the so-called 'Glaxo criterion' [8]. This criterion is more powerful than the IHS' criterion [9], but by using this criterion one gets the problem that a drug may succeed easily on moderate headaches, where only a decrease from moderate to mild is required. In addition, a decrease from moderate to mild headache is generally not judged as clinically relevant by the patients [10].

This criterion of a success should, however, be a secondary efficacy parameter in order to allow comparison with new results in RCTs with the results obtained in previous RCTs with triptans.

Severity of Headache. The severity of headache should be noted by the patient just before the drug intake and up to 2 h later, before any rescue medication, on a verbal scale: 0 = no headache; 1 = mild headache; 2 = moderate headache; 3 = severe headache. Speed of onset of effect can be evaluated by comparing headache response for active drugs with placebo at early time points (e.g. 30 min after oral administration). Alternatively, visual analogue scales can be used.

Rescue Medication. The use of rescue medication 2 h (or before) after the intake of the test drug can be used as an efficacy parameter. This parameter seems well correlated with the patient's judgement of the efficacy of the test drug. It is, however, less sensitive than the main parameter, resolution within 2 h.

Global Evaluation of Medication. A simple verbal scale should be used by the patient: nil, moderate, good, excellent. This criterion may be one of most clinically relevant, taking into account both efficacy and tolerance; the latter excluding its use as the primary measure. It is probably best used in later trials.

Presence of Nausea and/or Vomiting. The presence of nausea and/or vomiting should be recorded at time of intake of test medication and after 2 h.

Statistics and Presentation of Results

The recommended primary parameter of proportion of attacks resolved within 2 h per patient (and per treatment if crossover) can with standard statistical methods be used in calculations of sample size. The investigator thus needs to estimate the placebo response and define the difference to be detected.

Standard statistical methods can also be used for analysis of assessment parameters in both crossover and parallel group comparison trials.

Confidence intervals for differences among two drugs [11] are recommended in order to inform the reader fully of the results of the trial. A statement that two drugs are comparable without giving confidence intervals is unacceptable. Because of the very variable success rates reported (e.g. 56% to 88% for subcutaneous sumatriptan), most likely due to the variable placebo response in different clinical settings [12] calculation of therapeutic gain (proportion of patients responding to active drug minus proportion of patients responding to placebo) is often a suitable way to present results.

Evaluation of Randomized Clinical Trials (see table 1)

The Aim of the Study. Often the aim of the study is stated vaguely, for example, 'we wanted to compare A and B'. If a new drug is compared with placebo, then the aim of the study is clearly to demonstrate superiority with regard to efficacy and/or safety over placebo. When a new drug is compared with a standard drug and placebo is included, then the aim is probably to demonstrate that both 'active' drugs are comparable in efficacy (and/or safety) and superior to placebo. If placebo is not included, there is no way of knowing,

Table 1. Checklist to assist with the evaluation of a controlled trial in migraine

---

1 Aim of the study
   a New drug better than placebo?
   b New drug better than standard drug?
   c New drug comparable to standard drug?
2 Design of the study
   a Double-blind?
   b Placebo controlled?
   c Parallel or crossover comparison?
3 Efficacy parameters
   a Simple efficacy parameter?
   b 'Glaxo criterion' or headache resolved within 2 h?
   c Side effects?
4 Presentation of results?
   a Confidence intervals?
   b Therapeutic gain?

---

unless explicitly stated, whether the investigator intended to demonstrate superiority of the new drug over the standard drug or comparability which, in any case, needs the inclusion of placebo.

The Design of the Study. The subjective nature of the response measured in migraine trials and the variable and sometimes high placebo response, necessitate the use of the double-blind technique. A placebo control is needed.

Either crossover or parallel group comparisons can be used in drug trials in acute migraine treatment. Opinion is divided as to their relative merits and the practical consequences of the drawbacks, such as carryover effect, problems with blinding etc., of the crossover trial [1]. The main advantage of the crossover trial is its power, the probability of detecting a certain difference between treatments having regard to the likely variability in response to treatment within the population sample. Furthermore, this design is often more powerful in detecting significant differences in adverse events and one can ask for patients preference with this design. The trend in acute treatment trials has, however, been to use parallel group comparison [2, 12], but this design demands inclusion of several hundreds of patients in each treatment group if comparability is to be demonstrated with narrow confidence limits.

Efficacy Parameters. Simple efficacy parameters such as the proportion of headaches resolved within 2 h of taking the drug [1] or a clinically relevant decrease of headache on a simple verbal scale after say, 2 h [8] should be used. Only then can the clinician judge whether a clinically relevant effect has been

---

observed. If no more side effects are observed with active drug than with placebo, then the trial is probably not powerful enough (it has too few patients).

Presentation of Results and Statistics. Preferably, the results of all the objectives stated in the study protocol should be presented in a subsequent publication. The most fair and informative way of presenting the results is to give confidence intervals, usually a 95% interval [11]. The reader can then judge, whether what he or she considers to be a clinically relevant effect falls within the confidence interval. Furthermore, when comparability of two active drugs is claimed, this should be evidenced by narrow confidence intervals.

References

1   International Headache Society Committee on Clinical Trials in Migraine: Guidelines for controlled trials of drugs in migraine, ed 1. Cephalalgia 1991;11:1–12.
2   Saxena PR, Tfelt-Hansen P: Triptans, 5-HT$_{1B/1D}$ receptor agonists, in the acute treatment of migraine; in Olesen J, Tfelt-Hansen P, Welch KMA (eds): The Headaches, ed 2. New York, Lippincott, Williams & Wilkins, in press.
3   Headache Classification Committee of the International Headache Society: Classification and diagnostic criteria for headache disorders, cranial neuralgias and facial pain. Cephalalgia 1988;8(suppl 7): 1–96.
4   The S2BM11 Study Group: Patients preference between 25, 50 and 100 mg oral doses of sumatriptan. Eur J Neurol 1996;3(suppl 3):86.
5   Kramer MS, Matzura-Wolfe D, Polis A, Getson A, Amaraneni PG, Solbach MP, McHugh W, Feighner J, Silberstein SD, Reines SA and the Rizatriptan Multiple Attack Study Group: A placebo-controlled crossover study of rizatriptan in the treatment of multiple attacks. Neurology 1998;51: 773–781.
6   Rederich G, Rapoport A, Cutler N, Hazelrigg R, Jamerson B: Oral sumatriptan for the long-term treatment of migraine: Clinical findings. Neurology 1995;45(suppl 7):S15–S20.
7   Mathew NT, Asgharnejad M, Peykamian M, Laurenza A, on behalf on the Naratriptan S2Wa3003 Study Group: Naratriptan is effective and well tolerated in the acute treatment of migraine. Results of a double-blind, placebo-controlled crossover study. Neurology 1997;49:1485–1490.
8   Pilgrim AJ: Methodology of clinical trials of sumatriptan in migraine and cluster headache. Eur Neurol 1991;31:295–299.
9   Tfelt-Hansen P: Complete relief (IHS' criterion) or no or mild pain ('Glaxo criterion')? Estimation of relative power in placebo-controlled clinical trials of sumatriptan; in Olesen J, Tfelt-Hansen P (eds): 6th International Headache Research Seminar. Headache Treatment. Trial Methodology and New Drugs. New York, Lippincott-Raven, 1997, pp 157–160.
10   Massiou H, Tzourio C, El Amrani M, Bousser MG: Verbal scales in the acute treatment of migraine: Semantic categories and clinical relevance. Cephalalgia 1997;17:37–39.
11   Gardner MJ, Altman DG: Confidence intervals rather than P values: estimation rather than hypothesis testing. Br Med J 1986;292:746–750.
12   Tfelt-Hansen P: Efficacy and adverse events of subcutaneous, oral, and intranasal sumatriptan used for migraine treatment: A systematic review based on number needed to treat. Cephalalgia 1998; 18:532–538.

P. Tfelt-Hansen, Department of Neurology, Glostrup Hospital,
DK–2600 Glostrup (Denmark)
Tel. +45 43 23 30 50, Fax +45 43 23 39 26, E-Mail tfelt@inet.uni2.dk

Diener HC (ed): Drug Treatment of Migraine and Other Headaches.
Monogr Clin Neurosci. Basel, Karger, 2000, vol 17, pp 30–43

....

Analgesics

Volker Limmroth, Saskia Przywara

Department of Neurology, University of Essen, Germany

In classical Greek civilization, Hippocrates unwittingly used the chemical precursor of acetylsalicylic acid (ASA) to treat pain – the extract from willow bark, now known to contain salicylic acid. Thus, analgesics from the family of the non-steroidal anti-inflammatory drugs (NSAIDs) have probably been used for more than 2,000 years. Following its development in 1897 by Felix Hoffman, acetylsalicylic acid soon became the prototype analgesic, and despite a lack of controlled clinical studies, in the 1900s ASA became an established treatment for pain and migraine [1]. The oral treatment of acute migraine attacks, however, was not thought to be effective, hence, other routes of administration were recommended [2]. This belief was enhanced by the widespread use of ergot alkaloids, the 'classic' anti-migraine medication, in non-oral preparations. This began to change when it could be shown that oral medication's lack of effectiveness could be attributed to the reduced gastrointestinal absorption during migraine attacks. It could further be proven that stomach motility is dramatically reduced during migraine attacks; this affected all analgesics, but ASA in particular, since it is mainly absorbed in the duodenum. This corresponds to pharmaco-kinetic studies showing that ASA, even in migraine patients, reaches its t-max much faster during the headache free interval [3].

The detection of the main mechanism of ASA's clinical effects by John R. Vane's group 1972 [4], who received the Nobel Prize for Medicine in 1982 for his discovery of the prostaglandin synthesis inhibition, gave new and persistent drive into the development of other chemically different NSAIDs. Until now many clinical trials followed, suggesting that NSAIDs can be even as effective as the new triptans when smartly used. It became clear that their efficacy in the acute treatment of migraine attacks depends on a few simple factors:

- Sufficient dosage (e.g. 500 mg of ASA is too low, 1,000 mg should be the minimal oral dosage).
- All NSAIDs should be combined with an antiemetic drug in order to improve the absorption.
- Oral drugs should be taken as effervescent formulation to further improve the absorption.

Pharmacological Background

ASA as well as the newer NSAIDs are weak organic acids. They all share at least one mechanism of action: the inhibition of prostaglandin synthesis from arachidonic acid. Other mechanisms may play an important role as well, such as the inhibition of free radical synthesis and superoxide and the interaction with adenylyl cyclase, which alters the cellular concentration of cAMP. Clinically these drugs exhibit anti-inflammatory, analgesic and antipyretic effects and, partly, inhibit platelet aggregation secondary to the inhibition of thromboxane A2, a potent aggregating agent. ASA attaches its acetyl group to cyclooxygenase in a covalent bond, resulting in an irreversible blockage [5, 6]. Cells lacking a nucleus, such as thrombocytes, cannot synthesize new enzymes, so the effects of the blockade are permanent. In endothelial cells, although cyclooxygenase is irreversibly blocked, new, fully functional enzymes can still be synthesized. While classical studies of ASA's mechanisms have focused overwhelmingly on biochemical effects and the interaction between ASA and arachidonic acid, new results suggest ASA may act on the molecular level e.g. inhibiting gene expression of cyclooxygenase, and, additionally, that ASA is likely to inhibit other signal transduction factors, such as nFκb [7, 8]. For the biochemical details of particular NSAIDs the reader is referred to pharmacological reviews. Table 1 gives an overview over the different NSAIDs.

Possible Mode of Action in Migraine

Not every NSAID is effective in the treatment of acute migraine attacks. The exact mechanism by which ASA or other NSAID function in the treatment of headache remains a matter of controversial discussion. On the one hand, ASA seems to act peripherally upon cyclooxygenase at the vessel site (especially the endothelium), blocking the painful (aseptic) inflammatory process, which is caused by the release of vasoactive neuropeptides from free c-fiber endings. This hypothesis has been substantiated by in vivo experiments [9]. Recent in

Table 1. NSAIDs and their chemical groups

Salicylic acids	Aspirin
	Benorylate
Acetic acids	Indomethacin (indole acetic acid)
	Diclofenac (phenylacetic acid)
	Fenclofenac (phenylacetic acid)
Propionic acids	Fenoprofen
	Flurbiprofen
	Ibuprofen
	Indoprofen
	Ketoprofen
	Naproxen
	Pirprofen
Anthranilic acid	Meclofenamic acid
	Mefenamic acid
	Tolfenamic acid
Pyrazolones	Phenylbutazone
	Azapropazone
Oxicams	Piroxicam
	Tenoxicam

vitro investigations have further shown that ASA can reduce *de novo* protein synthesis of nitric oxide, a free radical thought to play a key role in the pathophysiology of migraine [10]. On the other hand, central mechanisms of action may also play a role in ASA's efficacy. Autoradiographic studies have shown that ASA binds with high affinity to nociceptive structures such as the dorsal horn and certain brain-stem nucleii, suggesting that central effects occur when the substance reaches these structures [11]. Furthermore, in animal models, ASA inhibits the activity of central brain-stem nuclei following the stimulation of the sagittal superior sinus [12]. Taken together, these studies suggest that ASA's efficacy is achieved through a combination of central and peripheral mechanisms.

Clinical Trials on Analgesics

Acetylsalicylic acid (table 2): ASA, as the classical NSAID has been evaluated extensively in clinical trials for the treatment of migraine attacks (for a review see [13]). In the early 1970s, two developments occurred that increased the clinical efficacy of ASA: its use as an effervescent and its combination with anti-emetics [3, 14]. This observation was later confirmed to be the same for other NSAID as well [15, 16]. In the following years a variety of clinical trials were conducted to evaluate oral anti-migraine drugs, ASA in particular. With or without anti-emetic drugs, both tablet and effervescent forms of ASA have repeatedly proven superior to placebo in the treatment of migraine attacks [17]. Unfortunately, most clinical trials have evaluated ASA in (pure) tablet form and not in its ideal formulation as an effervescent combined with anti-emetics. Furthermore, trials have typically involved varying dosages (between 500 and 1,000 mg), rendering impossible firm comparative conclusions. As a (plain) tablet, 1,000 mg ASA was shown to be as effective as 1,000 mg acetaminophen [18]. Later, however, it was shown that acetaminophen's efficacy could also be improved by combining it with an anti-emetic drug [16]. In the few controlled trials in which ASA tablets were compared to other oral anti-migraine preparations (ASA vs. acetaminophen plus codeine), efficacies were comparable [19]. In comparison to other substances which were not administered orally, such as ergot alkaloids, standard ASA tablets were less effective [20]. Overall, the various study results remain comparatively inconclusive. Recently, two multicenter trials using fixed combinations of ASA, paracetamol with caffeine or codeine confirmed again that these combinations perform better than placebo in the treatment of migraine attacks [21, 22]. Since the combination of different analgesics with caffeine or codeine clearly increases the risk to develop drug induced headache, these type of combinations can not be recommended.

Standardized headache trial designs were first established in the early 1990s in conjunction with sumatriptan's clinical evaluation. In a multicenter trial with 382 patients, a 100 mg dose of oral sumatriptan was compared with 900 mg ASA plus 10 mg metclopramide (MCP) (ASA was used as a tablet, not in effervescent form). Three consecutive attacks were treated and evaluated: a significant improvement in headache was reported by 56% of patients who took sumatriptan and by 45% who took ASA and MCP. This difference, however, was not statistically significant. For attacks 2 and 3, headache relief was achieved in 58 vs. 36% and 65 vs. 34% of patients, respectively. Autonomic symptoms improved in an identical corresponding fashion. Recurrence rates (reincidence of headache 24–48 h after successful therapy) were higher in the sumatriptan group [23]. In another randomized double-blind multicenter trial, water-soluble lysine-acetylsalicylic acid (LAS 1,620 mg = 900 mg ASS) plus 10 mg MCP was compared to placebo [24]. The primary aim of this study was the attenuation of headache intensity by 2 to 3 steps on a 4-step scale (none, mild, moderate, severe). Two hours after drug administration, 56% of

Table 2. Clinical trials with acetylsalicylic acid (ASA), lysine – acetylsalicylic acid (LAS) or injectable lysine – acetylsalicylic (iLAS) in the treatment of acute migraine attacks

N	Design (drug, dosage, study design)	Primary outcome criterion	Results	Comment	Author
20/160 attacks	ASA 500 mg vs. Erg 1 mg vs. Tolfenamic acid 200 mg vs. Pla/Co	Duration of attack, Intensity, Working ability, Subjective evaluation	Duration: Tolfenamic acid < Erg = ASA < Pla; Sub. Evaluation: Tolfenamic acid, Erg, ASA >> Pla	Small number of patients	Hakkarainen et al. 1980 [20]
254/435	ASA 1,000 mg vs. Para 1,000 mg/Pa	Discharge condition, Supplem. treatment	Equal potency for all parameters	Not double-blind	Tfelt-Hansen and Oleson 1980 [18]
85	ASA 650 mg vs. ASA 650 mg + MCP 10 mg vs. Pla/DB – Co	Escape medication, Effect on pain	ASA + MCP = ASA > Pla	ASA + MCP was given as an effervescent tablet	Tfelt-Hansen and Oleson 1984 [17]
358	ASA 900 + MCP 10 mg vs. Sumatriptan 100 mg/DB – Pa	% patients with 2-step improvement on 4-step scale in 3 attacks after 2 h, Rescue medication	1. attack Sumatriptan = ASA + MCP, 2. and 3. Attack Sumatriptan > ASA + MCP	ASA was not used in an effervescent formulation. Third Attack: significantly more recurrence headache in the SUM group	The oral Sumatriptan and Aspirin plus Metoc. Compar. Study Group 1992 [23]
198	ASA 1,000 mg vs. Para 400 mg + Cod 25 mg/DB – Co	Pain free after 2 h, Differences in pain intensity	ASA = Para + Cod > Pla for all parameters	Criterion 'pain free' included 'almost' pain free. No difference between groups after 2 when the term 'pain free' was rigidly used	Boureau et al. 1994 [19]
266	LAS 1,620 mg + MCP vs. Pla/DB – Pa	% patients with 2-step improvement on 4-step scale after 2 h, % patients pain free after 2 h	LAS + MCP >> Pla for all parameters	Not compared to other drugs	Chabriat et al. 1994 [24]

Table 2 (continued)

N	Design (drug, dosage, study design)	Primary outcome criterion	Results	Comment	Author
421	LAS 1,620 mg + MCP vs. Sumatriptan 100 mg vs. Pla/DB – Pa	% patients with 2-step improvement on 4-step scale in 2 attacks after 2 h	LAS + MCP = Sumatriptan ≫ Pla	Both drugs were equally effective, LAS + MCP was superior for the treatment of nausea and caused significantly less side effects than SUM	Tfelt-Hansen et al. 1995 [21, 25]
1357 (1220)	Para or ASA and caffeine (2 Tbl) vs. Pla/Pa	Pain intensity difference from baseline; Percentage of patients with pain reduced to mild or none	Para or ASA and caffeine > Pl; Para or ASA and caffeine (59.3%) > Pl (32.8%) after 2 h and 79% > 52% after 6 h		Lipton et al. (1998) [21]
1220	Para + ASA + caffeine (AAC) vs. Pla/Pa	Proportion of patients with reduction of pain intensity to mild or none at 0.5, 1, 2, 3, 4, 6 h	AAC > Pl in menstrual migraine and not menstrual-related migraine	Side effect AAC > Pl; vomiting: AAC > Pl	Silberstein et al.(1999) [22]
		Lysine – acetylsalicylic acid in non-oral formulation			
40	iLAS 1,000 mg vs. Pla iv DB	Mean pain reduction on VAS	iLAS ≫ Pla	Side effects/adverse events: iLAS = Pla	Taneri & Petersen Braun 1995 [27]
56	iLAS 1,000 mg vs. Erg 0.5 mg s.c./Co	Reduction of pain intensity on VAS	iLAS = Erg	iLAS caused significantly less side effects/adverse events than Erg	Limmroth et al. 1999 [28]
275	iLAS 1,000 mg vs. Sumatriptan 6 mg s.c.	% patients with 2-step improvement on 4-step scale in two attacks after 2 h	Sumatriptan >iLAS	iLAS caused significantly less side effects/adverse events than SUM	Diener et al. 1999 [29]

Co = Crossover, Pa = parallel, Cod = codeine, Erg = ergotamine, Para = paracetamol (acetaminophen), Pla = placebo.
* LAS 1,620 mg equals ASA 1,000 mg.

the LAS + MCP patients and only 28% of placebo patients reported significant reduction in headache pain. One year later, Tfelt-Hansen et al. [25] presented a multicenter trial of 421 patients comparing LAS (1,620 mg = 900 mg ASA) plus 10 mg MCP with 100 mg of oral sumatriptan. The study was again intended to measure the improvement of headache pain intensity by 2 to 3 steps on a 4-step scale. In two consecutive attacks, both preparations were equally effective. The combination of LAS and MCP was more effective than sumatriptan in improving autonomic symptoms such as nausea and vomiting and caused significantly less side effects. Further clinical trials comparing formulations of ASA with second generation triptans have not yet been performed. Taken together, the results of clinical trials conducted over the last 20 years suggest the following conclusions: the efficacy of oral ASA can be improved by the usage of effervescent tablets combined with anti-emetics. In this preparation, ASA appears to be almost as effective as ergotamine derivatives or oral sumatriptan and to have fewer side effects.

Injectable Lysine Acetylsalic Acid in the Acute Treatment of Migraine

As early as the mid-1970s, an injectible form of LAS (iLAS = Aspisol®) was available for the treatment of post-surgical, traumatic, tumor and rheumatic pain conditions. It would be years before iLAS was 'discovered' for treatment of acute migraine attacks. Case reports appeared in the 1980s describing iLAS's positive performance in migraine attack treatment [26]. Its evaluation in clinical trials did not take place until the mid-1990s [27, 28]. In these trials, iLAS proved superior to placebo and at least as effective as non-oral ergotamine derivatives. Recently in a double-blind multicenter trial including 278 patients, iLAS was compared to subcutaneous sumatriptan and placebo. Both drugs were superior to placebo. After 2 h 76.3, 43.7 and 14.3% of the patients following the administration of sumatriptan, iLAS and placebo, respectively, were pain-free. ILAS, however was significantly better tolerated than sumatriptan: adverse events with iLAS were observed in 7.6%, with sumatriptan in 37.8% of the patients [29]. Table 2 summarizes the clinical trials with ASA, LAS and iLAS in the acute treatment of migraine.

Other NSAIDs in Treatment of Migraine

Aside the group of the indole acetic acids, the pyrazolones and the oxicams all other groups of NSAIDs were shown to be effective in the treatment of acute migraine attacks. The reasons for these differences are not clear. Most

Table 3. Clinical trials with NSAIDs in the treatment of acute migraine attacks

N	Drug, dosage (mg)/study design	Primary endpoint	Results	Comments	Reference
20	Tolfenamic acid 200 vs. Erg 1 vs. ASA 500 vs. Pla/Co	Mean duration of attacks (h)	Tolfenamic acid (3.2) = Erg (3.8) = ASA (4.2) > Pla (7.1)	Small number of patients	Hakkarainen et al. (1979) [30]
49	Tolfenamic acid 200 (400) vs. Pla/Co	Duration of attacks (h)	Tolfenamic acid (5.6) > Pla (7.5)	Only duration of attacks evaluated	Tokola et al. (1984) [15]
58	Tolfenamic acid 200 or tolfenamic acid 400 Para 500 or Para 1,000 Co	Severity of headache after 2 h	Both tolfenamic acid dose (1.63) > Para (1.75); Escape medication: tolfenamic acid (26%) > Para (35%)	No dose response relationship	Larsen et al. (1990) [31]
22	Mefenamic acid 500 vs. Para 500 Co	Mean reduction in headache intensity on VAS scale	Mefenamic acid (36%) vs. Para (27%), NS	The only trial on mefenamic acid	Peatfield et al. (1983) [32]
32	Naproxen 750 vs. Pla/Co	Headache severity	Naproxen (2.1) > Pla (2.3); Naproxen > Pla for overall rating	Escape medication: Naproxen (24%) > Pla (46%)	Nestvold et al. (1985) [34]
32	Naproxen 750 vs. Pla/Co	Headache severity after 2 h	Naproxen (2.0) > Pla (2.2); headache severity for whole: Naproxen (2.2) vs. Pla (2.2), NS		Andersson et al. (1989) [35]
24	Naproxen Sodium 825 vs. Pla/Pa	Change in headache severity	Naproxen Sodium (3.8) > Pla (5.0)	Small number of patients, escape medication: Naproxen Sodium (44%) > Pla (67%)	Johnson et al. (1985) [36]
95	Naproxen Sodium 825 vs. Erg 2/Pa	For test drug taken within 2 h	Naproxen Sodium > Erg for headache relief; later intake of test drug, NS		Pradalier et al. (1985) [37]
122	Naproxen Sodium 825 vs. Erg 2/Pa	Relief of headache at 1 h	Naproxen Sodium > Pla, Erg = Pla; overall efficacy: Erg > Pla, Naproxen Sodium = Pla		Sargent et al. (1988) [38]

Table 3 (continued)

N	Drug, dosage (mg)/study design	Primary endpoint	Results	Comments	Reference
42	Naproxen Sodium *vs.* Erg 2/Pa	Overall efficacy rated by patients	Naproxen Sodium > Erg, reducing severity and duration of headache: Naproxen Sodium = Erg	Less rescue medication in naproxen Sodium group	Treves et al. (1992) [39]
63	Naproxen (550) + Met (10) + Erg (1) + Caffeine (100)/open	Pain relief; side effects; judgment to prior medication	Complete in 84%; minor side effects in 40%; 87% superior to all prior medication	Combination of drug and purpose of trial questionable	Saadah et al. (1992) [40]
19	Flurbiprofen 100 vs. Pla/Pa	Relief score	Flur (3.2) > Pla (0.7)	Small number of patients	Awidi (1982) [41]
22	Ibuprofen 400 vs. Para 900/Co	Severity and duration	Ibuprofen > Para: preference: Ibuprofen (13%) > Para (2%)	Small number of patients	Pearce et al. (1983) [42]
27	Ibuprofen 800 vs. Pla/Co	Duration of attacks	Ibuprofen (5 h) > Pla (11 h); mild attacks: Ibuprofen (33%) > Pla (7%)	Small number of patients	Havanka-Kanniainen (1989) [43]
25	Ibuprofen 1,200 vs. Pla/Co	Headache severity	Ibuprofen (1.78%) > Pla (2.33%); migraine index: Ibuprofen (25) > Pla (46)	Small number of patients	Kloster et al. (1992) [44]
40	Ibuprofen-arginin 400 vs. Pla/Co	Pain relief	Significant improvement after 30 min, 1, 2, 4 and 6 h with ibuprofen-arginine compared with Pla		Sandrini et al. (1998) [45]
88	Para (15 mg/kg) vs. Ibuprofen (10 mg/kg) vs. Pla/Co	Reduction in severe or moderate headache on a scale of 1–5 by 2 grades after 2 h	Three times as often with Ibuprofen, two times as often with Para as with Pla	Only children (4–16 years)	Hamalainen et al. (1997) [46]
50	Ketoprofen 100 rectally vs. Erg 2/Co	Median change in pain on VAS scale	Ketoprofen (15%) > Pla (7%), Ketoprofen = Erg (12%)	Working ability: Keto > Erg = Pla	Kangasneimi and Kaaja (1992) [47]

Table 3 (continued)

N	Drug, dosage (mg)/study design	Primary endpoint	Results	Comments	Reference
64	Ketoprofen (100) i.m. Para (30) i.m./Co	Partial or complete pain relief (min); complete pain relief after 30–40 min (percentage of patients)	Ketoprofen (15-20) > Para (35); Ketoprofen (82.5%) > Para (17.5%)		Karabetsos et al. (1997) [48]
55	Pirprofen 200 vs. Erg 2 vs. Pla/Co	Escape medication	Pirprofen (18/58) = Erg (18/59) > Pla (32/60); duration of attacks in h: Erg (6.5) > Pla (10.5) but vs. Pirprofen NS	For most parameters Pirprofen vs. Erg, NS	Kinnunen et al. (1988) [49]
20	Pirprofen 600 rectally vs. Pla/Co	Escape medication	Pirprofen (58%) > Pla (98%)	Small number of patients	Guidotti et al. (1989) [50]
32	Diclofenac 75 i.m. vs. Pla/Co	Response to treatment	Diclofenac (3.4) > Pla (1.7)	Preference: Diclofenac (21) ≫ Pla (1)	Del Bene et al. (1987) [51]
91	Diclofenac 50 vs. Pla/Co	Attack aborted within 2 h	Diclofenac (27%) > Pla (19%)	Escape medication: Diclofenac (54%) > Pla (66%)	Massiou et al. (1991) [52]
84	Diclofenac 75 i.m. vs. Para 500 i.m./Pa	Complete relief after 30 min	Diclofenac (40/46) > Para (7/40)	Diclofenac-result impressive, but para-dosage low	Karachalios et al. (1992) [53]
72	Diclofenac 50 vs. Pla/Co	Change in pain intensity on a 100 mm Visual Analogue Scale	Diclofenac 50 (100) > Pla		Dahlöf et al. (1993) [54]

Co = Crossover; Pa = parallel; Cod = codeine; Erg = ergotamine; Para = paracetamol (acetaminophen); Pla = placebo; i.m. = intramuscular; Met = metoclopramide.

of the NSAIDs were already established in the treatment of rheumatoid arthritis before their introduction into headache treatment. In the late seventies, tolfenamic was the first (of the new) NSAIDs to be evaluated for this indication [30]. It was shown to be superior to placebo [15] and paracetamol [31] and to be as effective as ASA or ergotamine [30]. A difference between 200 mg and 400 mg was not shown [31]. Mefenamic acid, another member of the anthranilic acids, was not superior to paracetamol in a single trial [32]. The entire group of anthranilic acids, however, lost its importance in the late 1980s due to the high frequency of adverse events (e.g. allergic reactions, high incidence of exanthems). Very recently, however, a rapid release form of tolfenamic acid 200 mg was evaluated against oral sumatriptan 100 mg. Both drugs were shown to be equally effective [33].

The large group of propionic acids is, still today, well established in treatment of various types of pain and headache in particular. Naproxen, and naproxen sodium, a formulation with a faster absorption kinetics, were later extensively investigated as well. Naproxen was clearly superior to placebo [34–36] and possibly even superior to ergotamine derivatives [37–39]. Due to its low profile of adverse events, naproxen became an established alternative for short-time prophylaxis in menstrual migraine. Fixed combinations of naproxen with other other analgesics, caffeine, or codeine and clinical trial to evaluate these combinations cannot be justified [40]. Other members of this group such as flurbiprofen, ibuprofen, ketoprofen or pirprofen were successfully tested as well and mostly shown to be superior to placebo and paracetamol, or even superior to ergotamine [39–50]. Within the group of acetic acids only diclofenac, which unlike indomethacin is a phenylacetic acid, was shown to be superior to placebo and paracetamol [51–54] and available in non-oral formulations. It was, however, not tested against other NSAIDs or ergotamine (details are shown in table 3).

Current Status and Significance of NSAIDs in the Treatment of Migraine

The efficacy of NSAIDs in the treatment of acute attacks has been shown in many trials and cannot be called into question. When given orally it was shown by several trials as well that the combination with anti-emetic acting drugs improves their clinical efficacy. Recently, a few trials evaluated NSAIDs against modern triptans. Surprisingly, NSAIDs in adequate dosages and in combination with an anti-emetic drug, can be as effective as the treatment with triptans. It is clearly justified to put further efforts in the development of improved NSAIDs, e.g. in formulations that enable faster absorption and a higher serum level within the first 30 min after administration. More than ever before, NSAIDs deserve to be considered first-line drugs in the treatment of acute migraine attacks.

References

1   Curschmann H: Erkrankungen des Nervensystems; in Mohr L, Staehlin R (eds): Handbuch der Inneren Medizin Bd 5, Berlin, Springer, 1912.
2   Heyck H, Krayenbühl H: Der Kopfschmerz. Stuttgart, Thieme, 1958.
3   Volans GN: The absorption of effervesent aspirin in migraine. Br Med J 1974;4:265–268.
4   Vane JR: Inhibition of prostaglandin synthesis as a mechanism of action for aspirin-like drugs. Nature 1971;231:232–234.
5   Roth GJ, Stanford N, Majerus PW: Acetylation of prostaglandin synthesis by aspirin. Proc Natl Acad Sci 1975;72:3073–3075.
6   Roth GJ, Siok CJ: Acetylation of the NH_2-terminal serine of prostaglandin sythetase by aspirin. J Biol Chem 1978;253:3782.
7   Wu KK, Sanduja R, Tsai AL, Ferhanoglu B, Loose-Mitchell DS: Aspirin inhibits interleukin-1 induced prostaglandin H synthase expression in cultured endothelial cells. Proc Natl Acad Sci USA 1991;88:2384–2386.
8   Kwon G, Hill JR, Corbett JA, McDaniel ML: Effects of aspirin on nitric oxide formation and de novo protein synthesis by RINm5F cells and rat islets. Mol Pharmacol 1997;52:398–405.
9   Buzzi MG, Sakas DE, Moskowitz MA: Indomethacin and acetylsalicylic acid block neurogenic plasma protein extravasation in rat dura mater. Eur J Pharmacol 1989;165:251–258.
10 Oleson J, Thomsen LL, Iversen H: Nitric oxide is a key molecule in migraine and other vascular headaches. TIPS 1994;15:149–153.
11 Goadsby PJ, Hoskin KL, Kaube H: Autoradiographic evaluation of acetylsalicylic acid distribution in the brain-stem of the cat; in Rose FC (ed): New Advances in Headache Research: 4. London, Smith-Gordon, 1994, pp 151–153.
12 Kaube H, Hoskin KL, Goadsby PJ: Acetylsalicylic acid inhibits cerebral cortical vasodilatation caused by superior sagittal sinus stimulation in the cat. Eur J Neurol 1994;1:141–146.
13 Limmroth V, Kazarawa S, Diener HC: Acetylsalicylic acid in the treatment of migraine and other headche – A historical and current overview. Cephalalgia 1999;19:545–551.
14 Volans GN: The effect of metoclopramide on the absorption of effervescent aspirin in migraine. Br J Clin Pharmacol 1975;2:75–63.
15 Tokola RA, Kangasneimi P, Neuvonen PJ, Tokola O: Tolfenamic acid, metoclopramide, caffeine and their combinations in the treatment of migraine attacks. Cephalalgia 1984;4:253–263.
16 MacGregor EA, Wilkinson M, Bancroft K: Domperidone plus paracetamol in the treatment of migraine. Cephalalgia 1993;13:124–127.
17 Tfelt-Hansen P, Olesen J: Effervescent metoclopramide and aspirin (Migravess) versus effervescent aspirin or placebo for migraine attacks: A double-blind study. Cephalalgia 1984;4:107–111.
18 Tfelt-Hansen, Olesen J: Paracetamol (acetaminophen) versus acetylsalicylic acid in migraine. Eur Neurol 1980;19:163–165.
19 Boureau F, Joubert JM, Lasserre V, Prum B, Delecoeuillerie G: Double-blind comparison of an acetaminophen 400 mg-codeine 25 mg combination versus aspirin 1,000 mg and placebo in acute migraine attack. Cephalalgia 1994;14:156–161.
20 Hakkarainen H, Quiding H, Stockman O: Mild analgesics as an alternative to ergotamine in migraine. A comparative trial with acetylsalicylic acid, ergotamine tartrate, and dextropropoxyphene compound. J Clin Pharmacol 1980;20:590–595.
21 Lipton RB, Stewart WF, Ryan RE Jr, Saper J, Silberstein SD, Sheftell F: Efficacy and safety of acetaminophen, aspirin, and caffeine in alleviating migraine headache pain: Three double-blind, randomized, placebo-controlled trials. Arch Neurol 1998;55:210–217.

22 Silberstein SD, Armellino JJ, Hoffman HD, Battikha JP, Hamelsky SW, Stewart WF, Lipton RB: Treatment of menstruation-associated migraine with the nonprescription combination of acetaminophen, aspirin, and caffeine: Results from three randomized, placebo-controlled studies. Clin Ther 1999;21:475–491.

23 The Oral Sumatriptan and Aspirin plus Metoclopramide Comparative Study Group: A study to compare oral sumatriptan with oral aspirin plus oral metoclopramide in the acute treatment of migraine. Eur Neurol 1992;32:177–184.

24 Chabriat H, Joire JE, Danchot J, Grippon P, Bousser MG: Combined oral lysine acetylsalicylate and metoclopromide in the acute treatment of migraine: A multicentre double-blind placebo-controlled study. Cephalalgia 1994;14:297–300.

25 Tfelt-Hansen P, Henry P, Mulder LJ, Scheidewaert RG, Schoenen J, Chazot G: The effectiveness of combined oral lysine acetylsalicylate and metoclopramide compared with oral sumatriptan for migraine. Lancet 1995;346:923–926.

26 Noda S, Itoh H, Umezaki H, Fukuda Y: Successful treatment of migraine attacks with intravenous injection of aspirin. J Neurol Neurosurg Psychiat 1985;48:1187–1188.

27 Taneri Z, Petersen-Braun M: Therapie des akuten Migräneanfalls mit intravenös applizierter Acetylsalicylsäure. Eine placebokontrollierte Doppelblindstudie. Der Schmerz 1995;9:124–129.

28 Limmroth V, May A, Diener HC: Lysine-acetylsalicylic acid in acute migraine attacks. Eur Neurol 1999;41:88–93.

29 Diener HC for the ASASUMAMIG Study Group: The efficacy and safety of acetylsalicylic acid lysinate compared to subcutaneous sumatriptan and parenteral placebo in the acute treatment of migraine. A double-blind, double-dummy, randomized multicenter, parallel group study. Cephalalgia 1999;19:581–589.

30 Hakkarainen H, Vapaatalo H, Gothoni G, Parantainen J: Tolfenamic acid is as effective as ergotamine during migraine attacks. Lancet 1979;2:326–327.

31 Larsen BH, Christiansen LV, Andersen B, Olesen J: Randomized double-blind comparison of tolfenamic acid and paracetamol in migraine. Acta Neurol Scand 1990;81:464–467.

32 Peatfield RC, Petty RG, Rose FC: Double blind comparison of mefenamic acid and acetaminophen (paracetamol) in migraine. Cephalalgia 1983;3:129–134.

33 Myllylä VV, Havanka H, Herrala L, Kangasniemi P, Rautakorpi I, Turkka J, Vapaatalo H, Eskerod O: Tolfenamic acid rapid release versus sumatriptan in the acute treatment of migraine: Comparable effect in a double-blind, randomized, controlled, parallel-group study. Headache 1998;38:201–207.

34 Nestvold K, Kloster R, Partinen M, Sulkava R: Treatment of acute migraine attack: Naproxen and placebo compared. Cephalalgia 1985;5:115–119.

35 Andersson PG, Hinge HH, Johansen O, Andersen CU, Lademann A, Gotzke PC: Double-blind study of naproxen vs placebo in the treatment of acute migraine attacks. Cephalalgia 1989;9:29–32.

36 Johnson ES, Ratcliffe DM, Wilkinson M: Naproxen sodium in the treatment of migraine. Cephalalgia 1985;5:5–10.

37 Pradalier A, Rancural G, Dordain G, Verdure L, Rascol A, Dry J: Acute migraine attack therapy: Comparison of naproxen sodium and an ergotamine tartrate compound. Cephalalgia 1985;5:107–113.

38 Sargent JD, Baumel B, Peters K, Diamond S, Saper JR, Eisner LS, Solbach P: Aborting a migraine attack: Naproxen sodium vs. ergotamine plus caffeine. Headache 1988;28:263–266.

39 Treves TA, Streiffler M, Korczyn AD: Naproxen sodium versus ergotamine tartrate in the treatment of acute migraine attacks. Headache 1992;32:280–282.

40 Saadah HA: Abortive migraine therapy with oral naproxen sodium plus metoclopramide plus ergotamine tartrate with caffeine. Headache 1992;32:95–97.

41 Awidi AS: Efficacy of flurbiprofen in the treatment of acute migraine attacks: A double blind cross-over study. Curr Ther Res 1982;32:492–497.

42 Pearce I, Frank GJ, Pearce JMS: Ibuprofen compared with paracetamol in migraine. Practitioner 1983;227:465–467.

43 Havanka-Kanniainen H: Treatment of acute migraine attack: Ibuprofen and placebo compared. Headache 1989;29:507–509.

44 Kloster R, Nestvold K, Vilming ST: A double-blind study of ibuprofen versus placebo in the treatment of acute migraine attacks. Cephalalgia 1992;12:169–171.

45 Sandrini G, Franchini S, Lanfranchi S, Granella F, Manzoni GC, Nappi G: Effectiveness of ibuprofen-arginine in the treatment of acute migraine attacks. Int J Clin Pharmacol Res 1998;18:145–150.

46 Hamalainen ML, Hoppu K, Valkeila E, Santavuori P: Ibuprofen or acetaminophen for the acute treatment of migraine in children: A double-blind, randomized, placebo-controlled, crossover study. Neurology 1997;48:103–107.

47 Kangasneimi P, Kaaja R: Ketoprofen and ergotamine in acute migraine. J Intern Med 1992;231: 551–554.

48 Karabetsos A, Karachalios G, Bourlinou P, Reppa A, Koutri R, Fotiadou A: Ketoprofen versus paracetamol in the treatment of acute migraine. Headache 1997;37:12–14.

49 Kinnunen E, Erkinjuntti T, Färkkilä M, Palomaki H, Porras J, Teirmaa H, Freudenthal Y, Andersson P: Placebo-controlled double-blind trial of pirprofen and an ergotamine tartrate compound in migraine attacks. Cephalalgia 1988;8:175–179.

50 Guidotti M, Zanasi S, Garagiola U: Pirprofen in the treatment of migraine and episodic headache attacks; a placebo-controlled crossover clinical trial. J Intern Med Res 1989;17:48–54.

51 Del Bene E, Poggioni M, Garagiola U, Maresca V: Intramuscular treatment of migraine attacks using diclofenac sodium: A crossover clinical trial. J Intern Med Res 1987;15:44–48.

52 Massiou H, Serrurier D, Lassere O, Bousser M-G: Effectiveness of oral diclofenac in the acute treatment of common migraine attacks; a double-blind study versus placebo. Cephalalgia 1991;11: 59–63.

53 Karachalios GN, Fotiadou A, Chrisikos N, Karabetsos A, Kehagioglou K: Treatment of acute migraine attack with diclofenac sodium: A double-blind study. Headache 1992;32:98–100.

54 Dahlöf C, Bjorkman R: Diclofenac-K (50 and 100 mg) and placebo in the acute treatment of migraine. Cephalalgia 1993;13:117–123.

Dr. Volker Limmroth, Department of Neurology, University of Essen,
Hufelandstrasse 55, D–45122 Essen (Germany)
Tel. +49 201 723 2495, Fax +49 201 723 5901, E-Mail volker.limmroth@t-online.de

Diener HC (ed): Drug Treatment of Migraine and Other Headaches.
Monogr Clin Neurosci. Basel, Karger, 2000, vol 17, pp 44–51

....

Anti-Emetics

E. Anne MacGregor

The City of London Migraine Clinic, London, UK

Migraine is frequently associated with nausea and vomiting and in some cases these symptoms are more distressing than headache. Therefore, it is not surprising that combined with analgesics, anti-emetics have a prominent role in the management of migraine. Prokinetic anti-emetics such as metoclopramide and domperidone have the added effect of reversing gastric stasis during migraine, which can otherwise impair intestinal absorption of analgesics. In addition, several anti-emetics have been used as single-agent therapies in migraine, with varying reports of success.

Neurological Control of Nausea and Vomiting

Central control of vomiting involves the chemoreceptor trigger zone (CTZ) situated in the floor of the fourth ventricle and the vomiting centre (VC) in the brain stem (fig. 1). The CTZ is rich in dopamine receptors and lies outside the blood-brain barrier. It is the site at which toxins and many drugs, such as opioids, act to induce vomiting, the effects of which are blocked by dopamine receptor antagonists. The VC co-ordinates afferent impulses from the CTZ, higher cortical centres, the vestibular apparatus, viscera and the upper gastrointestinal tract. It is rich in muscarinic cholinergic and histamine H-1 receptors and is consequently the site of action of anticholinergic and antihistamine anti-emetics.

Anti-Emetics Used in Migraine

The majority of effective anti-emetic drugs used in migraine are dopamine-receptor antagonists including domperidone, metoclopramide and the phenothiazines.

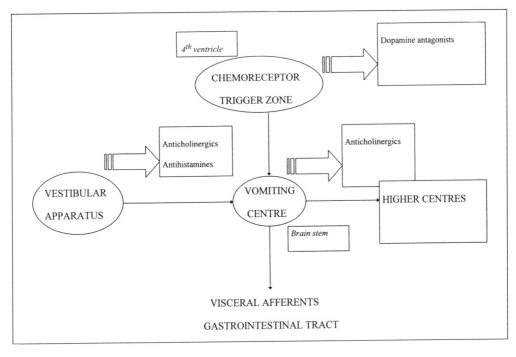

Fig. 1. Neurological control of nausea and vomiting.

Metoclopramide

Metoclopramide is a dopamine- and 5HT3-receptor antagonist with some 5HT4-receptor agonist properties. It is rapidly absorbed after oral administration and readily crosses the blood-brain barrier. In addition to its anti-emetic action on the CTZ, metoclopramide has a prokinetic effect, accelerating gastric-emptying. Bioavailability is reduced to 75% due to hepatic first-pass metabolism. The half-life of metoclopramide is 4–6 h.

Clinical Trials

Radiological examinations taken during migraine attacks have demonstrated gastric stasis and prolongation of gastric emptying time, whilst repeat observations on the same patients when headache free showed normal gut function [1]. It was later shown that this may account for therapeutic failure of oral medication in migraine due to delayed drug absorption [2]. This effect could be reversed, and efficacy improved, by the addition of intramuscular metoclopramide 10 mg [3]. Despite these results, there is little other evidence to support the use of metoclopramide combined with oral analgesics for migraine. In a double-blind randomized study, rectal metoclopramide 20 mg followed 30 min later by oral effervescent paracetamol 1,000 mg in water did not affect peak concentration or time to peak concentration of paracetamol compared to the administration of paracetamol alone [4]. A double-blind cross-over study of effervescent aspirin 650 mg vs. an effervescent preparation of aspirin 650 mg and metoclopramide 10 mg vs. placebo showed that the active treatments were more effective than placebo but there was no significant difference between aspirin alone and aspirin plus metoclopramide with regard to analgesic efficacy (p = 0.330) or antinauseant effect (p = 0.18) [5]. Certainly, there is no question regarding the efficacy of the combination as a recent double-blind randomized parallel group study has shown that oral aspirin 900 mg with oral metoclopramide 10 mg is as effective as oral sumatriptan 100 mg in the treatment of migraine and better tolerated [6]. The efficacy of the combination can be improved by repeated doses [7]. However, is not known if aspirin alone is as effective as no comparative clinical trials have been undertaken or, indeed, are in progress. Clinical trial data do not support additional efficacy from oral metoclopramide combined with ergotamine over ergotamine alone [8].

Based on these results, it would seem unlikely that metoclopramide would be effective in migraine as a single-agent therapy. Results from several clinical trials using intramuscular and intravenous metoclopramide are conflicting [9–12].

Dosage and Administration

The usual adult dose of metoclopramide is 10 to 20 mg orally, 20 mg rectally, or 10 mg intravenously or intramuscularly at 8-h intervals.

Side Effects, Contraindications and Interactions

Extrapyramidal side effects including akathisia, dystonic reactions and oculogyric crisis are more common in women and children. Sedation can be useful in migraine as sleep can aid recovery [13].

Hyperprolactinaemia, secondary to blockade of endogenous dopamine in the pituitary, can result in mastalgia, galactorrhoea, gynaecomastia and menstrual irregularities. These usually only occur with chronic use and are unlikely with intermittent treatment of migraine.

Special precautions include phaeochromocytoma, epilepsy and renal or hepatic impairment. Interactions include anticholinergics, phenothiazines and butyrophenones.

Domperidone

Domperidone has similar properties to those of metoclopramide, including increased gastric emptying and stimulation of prolactin release, but does not readily cross the blood-brain barrier. Peak plasma levels are attained at 10 to 30 min after intramuscular injection, within an hour of oral administration and at 1 to 2 h after rectal administration [14]. Bioavailability of oral domperidone is 13 to 17% due to hepatic first-pass and gut wall metabolism [14]. The elimination half-life of domperidone is 12 to 16 h [14].

Clinical Trials

Clinical trials confirm the therapeutic benefit of oral domperidone 20 mg combined with oral paracetamol 1,000 mg over oral paracetamol 1,000 mg alone for treatment of headache and associated symptoms, shortening the duration of the attack with few associated side effects [15].

Clinical trials have shown that single-agent treatment with domperidone 30 mg can prevent the development of headache and associated symptoms when taken during the prodromal phase of migraine [16]. No such effect was seen with cisapride, a gastrokinetic drug devoid of dopamine-receptor anatagonist properties [17].

Dosage and Administration

The usual recommended adult dose of domperidone is 20 mg orally or 30 to 60 mg rectally at 4- to 8-h intervals.

Side Effects, Contraindications and Interactions

Domperidone is better tolerated than metoclopramide with a low incidence of side effects [14]. Unlike metoclopramide, it does not cross the blood-brain barrier, so sedation and extrapyramidal reactions are unlikely. Chronic use, which is not indicated for migraine, can result in mastalgia, galactorrhoea, gynaecomastia and menstrual irregularities from hyperprolactinaemia. Cardiac dysrhythmias can occur following intravenous domperidone.

Phenothiazines

Phenothiazines have varying degrees of antagonist activity at alpha-adrenergic-, cholinergic-, dopaminergic-, and tryptaminergic-receptors, in addition to antihistamine properties. Chlorpromazine, prochlorperazine and thiethylperazine have been used for migraine although clinical trial data is scarce. Other drugs in this class are more commonly used in the treatment of psychosis.

Clinical Trials

Trials have used phenothiazines combined with anti-emetics. Thiethylperazine 10 mg given intramuscularly will suppress gastrointestinal symptoms in migraine but will not promote the absorption of an analgesic [18]. Rectal prochlorperazine 25 mg has a minor delaying effect on oral effervescent paracetamol 1,000 mg absorption but there is no difference in peak concentration or time to reach the peak compared to paracetamol alone during acute migraine attacks [4].

Trials with single-agent prochlorperazine have shown varied results. One trial showed efficacy of intravenous prochlorperazine 10 mg over intravenous metoclopramide 10 mg [11] and another, of rectal prochlorperazine 25 mg over placebo [19]. Intramuscular prochlorperazine 10 mg was more effective than intramuscular metoclopramide 10 mg in relieving symptoms, but neither was sufficiently effective for the authors to recommend either drug for acute migraine [12].

Single-agent trials with chlorpromazine show evidence of efficacy in migraine. Following treatment with intravenous metoclopramide 10 mg and saline 1,000 ml given over one hour, intravenous chlorpromazine 12.5 to 37.5 mg was equivalent to the efficacy of intramuscular sumatriptan 6 mg [20]. Intravenous chlorpromazine 25 mg was as effective as intramuscular ketorolac troinethamine 60 mg [21]. Intravenous chlorpromazine 12.5 to 37.5 mg has also been shown to be more effective than intravenous dihydroergotamine 1 to 2 mg [22] and equal to intravenous metoclopramide 0.1 mg kg^{-1} [10].

Dosage and Administration

The usual adult doses of chlorpromazine are 25 mg orally, 50 to 100 mg rectally, and 25 mg intramuscularly or intravenously; prochlorperazine 10 mg orally, 25 mg rectally, 10 mg intramuscularly; thiethylperazine 10 mg orally, rectally, or intramuscularly.

Side Effects, Contraindications and Interactions

Side effects include extrapyramidal reactions, sedation, postural hypotension, and ECG irregularities. Contraindications include liver or renal dysfunction, phaeochromocytoma, epilepsy and hypothyroidism. Interactions include CNS depressants, alcohol, antihypertensives, antidepressants and anticonvulsants.

Butyrophenones
Butyrophenones, including droperidol, are antipsychotics with dopamine-receptor antagonist activity. They are weak antihistamines and almost completely lack anticholinergic and alpha-adrenolytic activity in therapeutic doses.

Clinical Trials

Preliminary data suggest that intravenous droperidol 2.5 to 7.5 mg may be effective as single-agent therapy for status migrainosus and refractory migraine [23, 24].

Dosage and Administration

The usual adult dose of droperidol is 5 to 15 mg intravenously four to six hourly.

Side Effects, Contraindications and Interactions

Side effects include extrapyramidal reactions but fewer autonomic symptoms than phenothiazines. Contraindications and interactions are similar to the phenothiazines.

Other Anti-Emetics
Buclizine is a piperazine derivative with anti-histamine properties, given mainly for its anti-emetic action. It is used for the treatment of migraine combined with paracetamol and codeine, which appear to act synergistically with buclizine. It induces mild hypoglycaemia, which may result in appetite stimulation and weight gain. Its sedative effects are less pronounced than promethazine but the antihistamine effects are prolonged for more than 12 h. A double-blind, randomized crossover trial of 34 patients confirmed efficacy

over placebo of a combined preparation of oral buclizine 12.5 mg, paracetamol 1,000 mg and codeine 16 mg [25]. This is the usual recommended dose in 24 hours. Buclizine is well tolerated but may produce sedative, antihistaminic (drowsiness and fatigue) and anticholinergic (dry mouth and palpitations) side effects. Contraindications include previous sensitivity and caution is indicated in those with a history of renal disease.

Several other antihistamines, including cinnarizine, cyclizine and promethazine, have anti-emetic properties but their use in migraine is not established.

Practical Advice

Given the limited clinical trial data, an empirical approach to the use of anti-emetics in migraine is necessary. Oral anti-emetics with prokinetic properties, such as metoclopramide and domperidone, are recommended early in the attack in combination with oral simple analgesics, regardless of associated nausea. If nausea or vomiting precludes oral medication, rectal analgesic/anti-emetic combinations should be used. Intramuscular chlorpromazine or metoclopramide can be considered for emergency treatment when attacks have not responded to more standard migraine therapies and have the added advantage of promoting sleep. Migraineurs who can identify prodromal symptoms could try domperidone at this stage of the attack.

References

1   Kaufman J, Levine I: Acute gastric dilatation of the stomach during attack of migraine. Radiology 1936;27:301–302.
2   Volans GN: Absorption of effervescent aspirin during migraine. Br Med J 1974;4:265–269.
3   Volans GN: The effect of metoclopramide on the absorption of effervescent aspirin in migraine. Br J Clin Pharmacol 1975;2:57–63.
4   Tokola RA: The effect of metoclopramide and prochlorperazine on the absorption of effervescent paracetamol in migraine. Cephalalgia 1988;8:139–147.
5   Tfelt-Hansen P, Olesen J: Effervescent metoclopramide and aspirin (Migravess) versus effervescent aspirin or placebo for migraine attacks: A double-blind study. Cephalalgia 1984;4:107–111.
6   Tfelt-Hansen P, Henry P, Mulder LJ, Scheldewaert RG, Schoenen J, Chazot G: The effectiveness of combined oral lysine acetylsalicylate and metoclopramide compared with oral sumatriptan for migraine. Lancet 1995;346:923–926.
7   Hugues FC, Lacoste JP, Danchot J, Joire JE: Repeated doses of combined oral lysine acetylsalicylate and metoclopramide in the acute treatment of migraine. Headache 1997;37:452–454.
8   Hakkarainen H, Allonen H: Ergotamine vs. metoclopramide vs. their combination in acute migraine attacks. Headache 1982;22:10–12.
9   Ellis GL, Delaney J, DeHart DA, Owens A: The efficacy of metoclopramide in the treatment of migraine headache. Ann Emerg Med 1993;22:191–195.
10 Cameron JD, Lane PL, Speechley M: Intravenous chlorpromazine vs intravenous metoclopramide. Acad Emerg Med 1995;2:597–602.

11   Coppola M, Yealy DM, Leibold RA: Randomized placebo-controlled evaluation of prochlorperazine versus metoclopramide for emergency department treatment of migraine headache. Ann Emerg Med 1996;27:529–530.

12   Jones J, Pack S, Chun E: Intramuscular prochlorperazine versus metoclopramide as single-agent therapy for the treatment of acute migraine headache. Am J Emerg Med 1996;14:262–264.

13   Wilkinson M, Williams K, Leyton M: Observations on the treatment of an acute attack of migraine. Res Clin Stud Headache 1978;6:141–146.

14   Brogden RN, Carmine AA, Heel RC, Speight TM, Avery GS: Domperidone: A review of its pharmacological activity, pharmacokinetics and therapeutic efficacy in the symptomatic treatment of chronic dyspepsia and as an anti-emetic. Drugs (updated in January 1988) 1982;24:360–400.

15   MacGregor EA, Wilkinson M, Bancroft K: Domperidone plus paracetamol in the treatment of migraine. Cephalalgia 1993;13:124–127.

16   Waelkens J: Warning symptoms in migraine: Characteristics and therapeutic implications. Cephalalgia 1985;5:223–228.

17   Reyntjens A, Verlinden M, De Coster R, Janish HD, Smout A, De Cree J, Leempoels J, Verhaegen H: Clinical pharmacological evidence for cisapride's lack of antidopaminergic or direct cholinergic properties. Curr Ther Res 1984;36:1045–1051.

18   Wainscott G, Kaspi T, Volans GN: The influence of thiethylperazine on the absorption of effervescent aspirin in migraine. Br J Clin Pharmacol 1976;3:1015–1021.

19   Jones EB, Gonzalez ER, Boggs JG, Grillo JA, Elswick RK Jr: Safety and efficacy of rectal prochlorperazine for the treatment of migraine in the emergency department. Ann Emerg Med 1994;24:237–241.

20   Kelly AM, Ardagh M, Curry C, D'Antonio J, Zebic S: Intravenous chlorpromazine versus intramuscular sumatriptan for acute migraine. J Accid Emerg Med 1997;14:209–211.

21   Shrestha M, Singh R, Moreden J, Hayes JE: Ketorolac vs chlorpromazine in the treatment of acute migraine without aura. A prospective, randomized, double-blind trial. Arch Intern Med 1996;156:1725–1728.

22   Bell R, Montoya D, Shuaib A, Lee MA: A comparative trial of three agents in the treatment of acute migraine headache. Ann Emerg Med 1990;19:1079–1082.

23   Rothrock JF: Treatment of acute migraine with intravenous droperidol. Headache 1997;37:256–257.

24   Wang SJ, Silberstein SD, Young WB: Droperidol treatment of status migrainosus and refractory migraine. Headache 1997;37:377–382.

25   Adam EI: A treatment for the acute migraine attack. J Int Med Res 1987;15:71–75.

E. Anne MacGregor, The City of London Migraine Clinic,
22 Charterhouse Square, London EC1M 6DX (UK)
Tel. +44 207 251 3322, Fax +44 207 490 2183

Diener HC (ed): Drug Treatment of Migraine and Other Headaches.
Monogr Clin Neurosci. Basel, Karger, 2000, vol 17, pp 52–65

The History and Pharmacology of Ergotamine and Dihydroergotamine

Stephen D. Silberstein[a], *Richard J. Hargreaves*[b]

[a] Jefferson Headache Center, Thomas Jefferson University, Philadelphia, Pa., and
[b] Merck Research Laboratories, West Point, Pa., USA

Over the last century preclinical and clinical studies of the actions of
ergotamine have been important for the progressive development of hypotheses
on the pathophysiology of migraine. Ergotamine (E) and dihydroergotamine
(DHE) share structural similarities with the neurotransmitters of the adrenergic, dopaminergic, and, particularly, the serotonergic systems. As a result,
they exert wide-ranging effects on physiologic processes mediated by these
receptor systems. E and DHE are highly potent at the anti-migraine 5-HT1B
and 5-HT1D receptors and as a consequence the plasma concentrations of
these substances necessary to produce the appropriate therapeutic and physiologic effects are very low. The broad spectrum of activity at other monoamine
receptors (5-HT1A, 5-HT2A, adrenergic and dopamine) is responsible for
their side effect profile (dysphoria, nausea, emesis, unwanted vascular effects).
Both E and DHE have sustained vasoconstrictor actions.

Ergot has been a treasure house to pharmacologists. The chemical diversity of the ergot alkaloids is paralleled by their wide range of pharmacological
effects that result from their interactions with multiple monoamine (serotonin,
norepinephrine, dopamine) receptor subtypes. The ergots have highly varied
receptor affinity and efficacy such that in some systems they appear to have
agonist properties whilst in others antagonism can be demonstrated. Ergotamine tartrate (ET) was one of the first ergot alkaloids to be isolated and
used in the treatment of migraine. DHE was synthesized by reducing an
unsaturated bond in E. This simple chemical modification resulted in an
ergot derivative with greater alpha-adrenergic antagonist activity and reduced
vasoconstrictor and emetic potential. DHE has been extensively used in the

treatment of migraine. Both E and DHE have pronounced activity at monoaminergic (serotonergic, adrenergic and dopaminergic) receptors. Of particular relevance to their anti-migraine efficacy is their agonist activity at 5-HT1B, 5-HT1D, and 5-HT1F receptors. Their agonist activity at 5-HT1A, 5-HT2A, and dopamine D2 receptors may contribute to their side effect profiles. It is noteworthy that although the ergot alkaloids have many pharmacological actions, specificity can be achieved in their effects if their dose and plasma concentrations are carefully controlled.

The vasoconstrictor action of ergot compounds such as E and DHE was for a long time believed to be the basis of their clinical effects. However, recent advances in the understanding of the pathophysiology and pharmacology of migraine suggest that their inhibitory effects on trigeminal nerves (blocking neurogenic inflammation in peripheral meningeal tissues and nociceptive neuronal transmission centrally in the trigeminal nucleus caudalis) may also contribute to their anti-migraine efficacy. This chapter reviews the history of E and DHE, their receptor pharmacology and anti-migraine mechanisms of action. The pharmacology of the ergot alkaloids was reviewed previously by Berde and Sturmer [1] and Silberstein [2].

Historical Exploration of the Clinical Potential of Ergot Alkaloids

The earliest reports in the medical literature on the use of ergot in the treatment of migraine were those of von Eulenburg of Germany in 1883 [3], Thomson of the United States in 1894 [4], and Campbell from England in 1894 [5].

The first pure ergot alkaloid, ergotamine (trade name Gynergen), was isolated by Stoll in 1920 [5]. Gynergen was used primarily in obstetrics and gynecology to control postpartum hemorrhage but in 1925, when Rothlin [6] successfully treated a case of severe and intractable migraine by subcutaneous injection of ET, E became the cornerstone of migraine treatment for several decades. The migraine indication was pursued vigorously by various researchers over the following decades [7, 8] and, due to its potent vasoconstrictor properties, reinforced the belief in a vascular origin for migraine [9, 10]. Lennox in Boston and others independently conducted the first controlled studies of ET in 1934 [9]. Graham and Wolff in 1937 demonstrated the vasoconstrictor effects of ET on blood vessels giving support to the hypothesis that migraine was the result of an abnormal distension of pain-producing intracranial blood vessels [10]. Lennox showed that injected E was better than oral confirming the poor oral bioavailability of these compounds [11].

Dihydroergotamine was synthesized (using hydrogenation (reduction) of the double bond at the 9–10 position of the ergoline ring of ergotamine) by Stoll and Hofmann in 1943. DHE was originally envisaged as a treatment for blood pressure but it was later shown to be highly effective in the treatment of migraine. DHE was first used to treat migraine in 1945 by Horton, Peters, and Blumenthal at the Mayo Clinic [12]. Its use for migraine was low and the use and assessment of E in migraine continued [13–15]. In 1986 Raskin reconfirmed the effectiveness of DHE for both intermittent and intractable migraine [16, 17]. In 1997 a nasal spray version was approved for use in migraine [18]. The use of DHE was reviewed by Scott in 1992 [18].

Whilst both DHE and ET are effective for the acute treatment of migraine, DHE has appreciably fewer side effects. Most notably DHE is much less nauseant and emetic than E (a considerable advantage when considered on top of the nausea and vomiting associated with migraine) and has considerably less vasoconstrictor effects. DHE also appears to be relatively free of the risk for chronic rebound headaches that is associated with E usage. Indeed since DHE is much less constrictor than E but retaining comparable anti-migraine efficacy, it has been suggested that there must be other mechanisms involved in its anti-migraine effects [20, 21].

Table 1 gives a chronology of the development of migraine usage for ergotamine and dihydroergotamine.

It is interesting to note that ergotamine has been very important for the development of pathophysiological hypotheses for migraine. Indeed Dale in 1906 showed that ergotamine could reverse the effects of adrenaline and then Maier introduced E as a sympatholytic drug. Subsequently the elegant studies of Graham and Wolff showed that ergotamine was a potent long-lasting vasoconstrictor giving rise to the vascular hypothesis of migraine. In 1972, Saxena showed that ergotamine could reduce blood flow in carotid arterio-venous anatomoses and he identified an atypical receptor using methysergide, another ergot derivative. This discovery was the start of the pharmacological development of the 5-HT1B/1D selective agonist (Triptan) drugs that have found wide use today in the treatment of migraine. In 1988 Moskowitz took the theory one step further when he developed a trigeminovascular hypothesis for migraine postulating that headache pain arose from sterile inflammation in the meninges as a result of trigeminal sensory nerve activation. Most recently the studies from the Goadsby group have clearly shown that DHE has central effects in inhibiting trigeminal pain signal transmission showing that these drugs also have central sites of action. Current theories suggest that all three of these mechanisms could be in play during the use of the ergots to treat migraine (see below for discussion)

Table 1. History of the use of ergotamine and dihydroergotamine for the treatment of migraine

Year	Investigator	Notes
Middle Ages (France/Germany)	Ergotism	Gangrenous or convulsive
1883	Eulenberg (Germany)	Used s.c. injections of ergotinin (tantret) extract for headache
1894	Thompson (USA)	Used oral fluid extract of ergot and proposed rectal use to reverse migraine if patients vomiting
1894	Campbell (England)	Anti-migraine effects of ergot in medical textbook
1920	Stoll (Switzerland)	Isolated ergotamine (gynergen) used first for obstetrics and gynecology
1925	Rothlin (Switzerland)	Used s.c. injections of ET for migraine
1926	Maier (Switzerland)	Sympatholytic use of ET for migraine reported
1928	Tzanck (France)	Reported on ET in migraine for 101 patients
1928	Trautman (Germany)	Compared oral ET successfully with placebo
1934	Lennox, Brock, O'Sullivan, Young, Logan and Allen (USA)	First 3 US reports of controlled trials with ET
1938	Graham and Wolff (USA)	Scientific clinical studies show E was a vasoconstrictor
1938	Lennox (USA)	Injection (89%) better than oral (41%) E
1943	Stoll and Hoffman (Switzerland)	Synthesis of DHE
1945	Horton, Peters and Blumenthal (USA)	First report of DHE use in migraine
1951	Friedman and von Storch	E plus caffeine (86%) as effective as injection (81%)
1957	Brazil and Friedman (USA)	Clinical craniovascular studies on E
1961	Ostfeld (USA)	First randomized double-blind trial of oral E
1986	Raskin (USA)	Repeated i.v. DHE for intractable migraine
1996	Multiple investigators	Intranasal DHE formulation

Pharmacokinetics of Ergotamine and Dihydroergotamine

The ergot compounds have an intrinsically low bioavailability and are subject to substantial (greater than 90%) first pass metabolism by the liver following oral administration; as a result very little of the unchanged parent drug ultimately reaches the systemic circulation. [22–25]. However, several of the metabolites of E and DHE have biologic activity similar to that of the parent drug, and these metabolites are often present in concentrations that may be several times higher than that of the parent compound [26, 27]. E and DHE are strongly sequestered by tissues, which could contribute to the persistence of biologic effects well after the parent drug or metabolites can no

Table 2. Pharmacokinetics of erogotamine tartrate and dihydroergotamine in healthy volunteers

	Ergotamine tartrate		Dihydroergotamine	
	Oral	Rectal	IM	IV
Dose, mg	2	2	1	1
C_{max}, ng/ml	0.02	0.45	2.88	>10
T_{max}, min	69	50	24	1–2
$t_{1/2}$, min[1]	NA	10.5	59	NA
$t_{1/2}$, h[2]	NA	3.35	10–13	10–13

[1] Initial.
[2] Terminal.

longer be detected in plasma [22, 28]. Table 2 summarizes the pharmacokinetic parameters of E and DHE obtained in studies with normal volunteers.

Ergotamine tartrate is rapidly but incompletely and variably absorbed after oral (~1%), rectal (1–2%), or intramuscular (47%) administration [23, 24, 29]. Peak plasma levels are attained approximately 1 h after oral or rectal administration [24, 30]. Plasma levels are highest following rectal administration [30]. Caffeine enhances the absorption of ET following oral administration [31].

Little is known about the tissue distribution of E in humans. The drug is apparently distributed into the cerebrospinal fluid [32]. Following oral or intravenous (IV) administration in rats, E is distributed in high concentrations in the liver and lung and in lower concentrations in the kidney, heart, and brain [33]. Ergotamine is extensively metabolized by the liver. Following oral administration, it is rapidly cleared from the blood by first-pass hepatic metabolism. Ergotamine and its metabolites are excreted principally in the feces via biliary elimination (greater than 90%) [32]. Only a small amount of unchanged drug is excreted in the urine [35]. In some studies, a second peak plasma concentration has been observed after about 48 h, which suggests enterohepatic recirculation [25]. Elimination of E follows a biphasic pattern, with mean half-lives of approximately 10 min and approximately 3.4 h [30].

Dihydroergotamine mesylate has a very low oral bioavailability (<1%), less than that of ET [36] due to incomplete drug passage across the gastrointestinal mucosa and a high first-pass metabolism. The absolute bioavailability of intramuscular (IM) DHE is 100% [37]. The absolute bioavailability of DHE following intranasal (IN) administration is approximately 40% [37, 38]. Peak plasma levels occur approximately 1 to 2 min after IV administration, 24 min after IM administration, and 30 to 60 min after IN administration. Intranasal administration of DHE which avoids first-pass hepatic metabolism, delivers adequate plasma concentrations of the drug and eliminates the need for parenteral administration.

Little is known about the tissue distribution of DHE in humans. Following oral or IV administration in rats, DHE is distributed in high concentrations in the liver, lung and kidney and in lower concentrations in the stomach, intestines and brain [33].

Like E, DHE is rapidly and extensively metabolized in the liver. Only 6 to 7% of an IM dose is excreted in the urine. The major route of elimination is the feces following biliary excretion of unchanged drug and metabolites. DHE has many metabolites; only those that retain the essential ring structures of the ergot alkaloids (the ergoline ring and the peptide side chain) are active. The major metabolite is 8′-OH DHE which is present at a concentration five to seven times greater than that of DHE. The pharmacologic effects of the active metabolites are qualitatively similar to those of the parent compound [26]. Dihydroergotamine is eliminated in a biphasic manner, with mean half-lives of approximately 0.7 to 1 and 10 to 13 h [37, 38]. The long half-life may account for the low rate of headache recurrence observed with DHE. The pharmacokinetics of DHE are summarized in table 2.

Receptor Pharmacology of Ergotamine and Dihydroergotamine

There are multiple 5-HT receptors with varied biologic effects [24]. At least seven classes and 14 5-HT receptor subtypes exist. All 5-HT receptors are linked to G proteins, except for the 5-HT3 receptor, which is linked to an ion channel. E and DHE have affinity for the 5-HT1A, 5-HT1B, 5-HT1D, 5-HT1E and 5-HT1F, 5-HT2A 5-HT2C, and 5-HT3 receptor subtypes. In addition they bind to receptors in the adrenergic and dopaminergic systems.

Table 3 shows the affinity of ergotamine and DHE at monoaminergic receptors. It is likely that the beneficial effects of E and DHE arise from their agonist properties at 5-HT1B, 5-HT1D, and perhaps 5-HT1F receptors that lead to meningeal vasoconstriction and trigeminal inhibition (see mechanism section below).

The unwanted side effects of E and DHE arise most probably from actions at central 5-HT1A receptors that will be pro-nauseant and dysphoric and dopamine D2 receptors that will also be nauseant and pro-emetic. E produces a much greater incidence of dizziness, acroparesthesia, nausea, and emesis than does DHE [20, 21].

Table 3. Pharmacological activity of dihydroergotamine and ergotamine at human monoaminergic receptors (except where specified)

	5-HT1A	5-HT1B	5-HT1D	5-HT1E	5-HT1F	5-HT2A	5-HT2C	r5-HT3	gp5-HT4		
DHE	0.4	0.7	0.5	1100	180	9.0	1.3	>3700	60		
E	0.3	1.0	0.8	840	170	n.d.	n.d.	>3700	65		

	α1a	α1b	α2a	α2b	α2c	β1	β2	β3	D2	D3	D4
DHE	6.6	8.3	1.9	3.3	1.4	3100	2700	271	1.2	6.4	8.7
E	15	12	n.d.	n.d.	n.d.	n.d.	n.d.	n.d.	4	3.2	12

Top rows are 5-HT receptors, r is rat 5-HT3 receptors and gp 4 is guinea pig 5-HT4 receptors. Second row are alpha α (α1 rat liver, α2 human prostate) and cloned β beta adrenergic receptors and cloned dopamine D receptors. All values are affinity IC50 nM. n.d. = Not determined.

E and DHE have complex inhibitory or excitatory actions at adrenergic receptors in the vasculature and have agonist activity at constrictor 5-HT2A receptors. These actions are likely to underlie the unwanted peripheral vasoconstrictor effects of the ergots. Both DHE and E can cause vasoconstriction by stimulating alpha-adrenergic and 5-HT2A receptors, although E is a much more potent vasoconstrictor than DHE [see 38, 39]. Both can inhibit the actions of norepinephrine (NE) and 5-HT [40]. Both are venoconstrictors via their action on alpha-adrenoceptors [41, 42]. The interactions between NE and E or DHE are complex and depend critically upon receptor reserve and vasomotor tone such that they show both agonist and antagonist effects in different vascular beds [43, 44].

The peripheral vascular effects of E are pronounced relative to the 5-HT1B/1D receptor selective serotonin agonist anti-migraine agents since these newer agents lack activity at adrenergic and 5-HT2A receptors. Figure 1 demonstrates the consequences of this increased selectivity using clinical data from a peripheral hemodynamic study using rizatriptan and E alone and in combination. It can be seen that rizatriptan 10 mg orally, the recommended therapeutic dose for migraine treatment, has only a small transient effect on peripheral arteries when given alone. Further, rizatriptan exerts no additional effects on the pronounced constriction produced by ergotamine (0.25 mg i.v.) since it lacks activity at the receptors producing the ergotamine effect. The long-lasting peripheral vasoconstrictor effect of ergotamine (>8 h) can be clearly seen [45]. These pronounced effects may contribute to the biological effectiveness of the ergot alkaloids and to their problems in chronic use [46, 47].

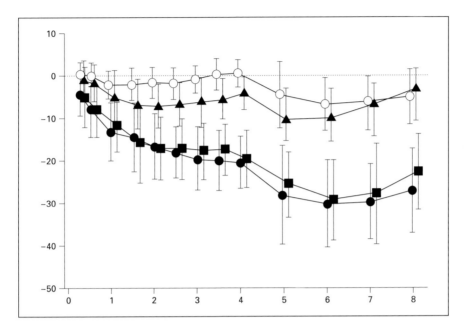

Fig. 1. The effects of rizatriptan and ergotamine on peripheral arteries in man measured using toe arm systolic blood pressure gradients. Changes are expressed on the ordinate as change in mmHg against time in hours on the abscissa. Rizatriptan was dose orally 10 mg and ergotamine i.v. 0.25 mg. ○ = Ergotamine placebo i.v., ▲ = rizatriptan 10 mg, ■ = ergotamine 0.25 mg, ● = rizatriptan 10 mg plus ergotamine 0.25 mg. (Data are from Seidelin Tfelt-Hansen, Mendel and Stepanavage 1994.)

Antimigraine Actions of Ergotamine and Dihydroergotamine

The putative anti-migraine mechanism of action proposed for the ergot alkaloids has changed as understanding of the pathophysiology of migraine has developed. Many mechanisms have been proposed: constriction of large capacitance arteries, closure of arteriovenous anastomoses (AVAs), inhibition of neurogenic inflammation, and blockade of transmission in the trigeminal nucleus caudalis [48–50].

Vascular Mechanisms of Action

An initial hypothesis was that E and DHE targeted the cerebral vasculature, based on the belief that migraine was a vascular disorder. Lauritzen and Olesen measured serial cerebral blood flow (CBF) during migraine utilizing Xenon-133 with single photon emission computed tomography (SPECT) [51]. They found that CBF decreases during migraine with aura but does not change in migraine without aura. While the aura developed, CBF progressively decreased as a wave of spreading oligemia, which began in the occipital cortex, moved forward at a rate of 2 to 3 mm/min. These blood-flow changes are consistent with a primary neuronal event causing secondary vascular changes. No change in CBF occurs after administration of ET or DHE [52, 53]. While particular vascular beds may be idiosyncratically affected, the consensus is that overall CBF is not significantly altered by ET or DHE and their effect in migraine is independent of any change in CBF [52–54].

It has been suggested that the headache of migraine could result from dilatation of the large pain-producing conductance intracranial arteries and its relief from their constriction. Since the resistance vessels would not be affected, there is no marked change in CBF (see above). While balloon inflation of the middle cerebral artery (MCA) produces focal headache, the relevance of this painful experimental vasodilatation to migraine is uncertain. Indeed dilatation of the MCA during a migraine attack is not a consistent finding using transcranial laser Doppler techniques and migraine is not relieved by all vasoconstrictors active in middle meningeal vessels (e.g. norepinephrine). Nonetheless, the 5-HT1 agonists such as E and DHE (and the triptan class of drugs) constrict meningeal blood vessels through their agonist activity at 5-HT1B receptors that are preferentially expressed in intracranial extracerebral arteries and this could contribute to their pharmacological action by decreasing activation of perivascular trigeminal sensory nerves [55].

Cardiovascular Safety Profile

E and DHE have the potential to produce vasconstriction of coronary blood vessels through actions at 5-HT1B and 5-HT2A receptors that are present on coronary artery smooth muscle. 5-HT1B receptors are present in much lower abundance in coronary than in meningeal arteries that are the target for the antimigraine effects and so the ergots retain selectivity for cranial over coronary blood vessels. The affinity of the ergots at constrictor 5-HT2A receptors is at least 20-fold lower than affinity at anti-migraine 5-HT1B and 5-HT1D receptors giving a therapeutic window (see table 3). Recent studies from Maassen Van Den Brink et al. [56] have shown that all current and prospective serotonin 5-HT1 agonist antimigraine drugs including E and DHE contract coronary artery ring segments in vitro but that all are partial agonists compared to the endogenous ligand serotonin and all have similar minimal effects at clinically relevant concentrations. However, it was noteworthy that in these studies the contractile response to E and DHE was prolonged relative to the newer 5-HT1B/1D receptor selective anti-migraine agents ('triptans') suggesting a possible disadvantage in reduced reversibility of an unwanted effect with these older ergot agents [56]. This sustained effect is consistent with the slow diffusion of the ergots from the receptor biophase and the clinical situation where the effects of E and DHE appear to be maintained much longer than is to be expected from their plasma concentration profiles. It should be remembered however that all the serotonin agonist anti-migraine drugs without exception are contraindicated in patients with coronary artery disease and require risk assessment prior to use in those individuals with cardiovascular disease risk factors.

Inhibition of Neurogenic Inflammation

The trigeminal nerve innervates the cranial blood vessels. The trigeminal sensory C-fibers contain the neurokinins substance P (SP), neurokinin A (NKA), and calcitonin gene-related peptide (CGRP). Experimental stimulation of the trigeminal nerve causes release of SP, CGRP, and NKA from the sensory C-fibers and Aδ-fibers resulting in neurogenic inflammation and meningeal vasodilation [57]. The released neuropeptides interact with mast cells (further releasing histamine) and with the blood vessel wall, producing dilatation, plasma extravasation, platelet activation, and sterile inflammation. This sterile inflammatory process is believed to sensitize nerve fibers to respond to previously innocuous stimuli such as blood vessel pulsations.

The ergot alkaloids are 5-HT1 receptor agonists that inhibit the trigeminal sensory nerves through prejunctional 5-HT1D receptors thereby blocking the release of vasoactive neuropeptide mediators (SP, GCRP) that could produce or exacerbate the pain and vasodilatation of migraine [58]. Administration of DHE, prevents substance P mediated neurogenic plasma protein extravasation in the dura mater [58], CGRP-mediated neurogenic vasodilation in the meningeal arteries (D. Williamson pers. commun.). Inhibition of these effects is due to inhibition of trigeminal C- and Aδ-fibers respectively. The latter of these observations has clear relevance to migraine, since elevated CGRP levels have consistently been found in human jugular blood during a migraine attack and 5-HT1 agonists such as DHE and sumatriptan abort the headache and reduce CGRP to control levels [59].

Inhibition of Transmission in the Trigeminal Pathway

In cats, DHE has been shown to distribute into the nuclei in the brain stem and spinal cord that are closely involved with pain transmission and modulation [60]. DHE blocks electrical and metabolic activation of second order trigeminal sensory relay neurons resulting from trigeminal nerve stimulation [61]. In this protocol, no blood vessels are involved indicating a direct inhibitory action, probably at 5-HT1D receptors, that blocks sensory neurotransmitter release from trigeminal nerves thereby reducing activation of the central pain relay neurons in the trigeminal nucleus caudalis.

The anti-migraine action of ergot alkaloids, including E and DHE, may also involve effects on other receptors and nuclei within the central nervous system since the headache recurrence rates appear to be lower with these older agents compared to the newer 5-HT1B/1D receptor selective triptan drugs. The receptor basis for this effect is not known but could involve inhibitory actions in brainstem monoaminergic nuclei that are thought to be activated during a migraine attack and may be involved in the pathophysiology of the disease as central migraine 'generator' regions.

Summary

E and DHE share structural similarities with the neurotransmitters of the adrenergic, dopaminergic, and, particularly, the serotonergic systems. As a result, they exert wide-ranging effects on physiologic processes mediated by these receptor systems. E and DHE are highly potent at the anti-migraine 5-HT1B and 5-HT1D receptors and as a consequence the plasma concentrations of these substances necessary to produce the appropriate therapeutic and physiologic effects are very low. The broad spectrum of activity at other monoamine receptors (5-HT1A, 5-HT2A, adrenergic and dopamine) is responsible for their side effect profile (dysphoria, nausea, emesis, unnecessary vascular effects)

Migraine is now thought of as a neurovascular disorder. Migraine may begin centrally and affect blood vessels secondarily. When activated the trigeminal vascular system may generate or enhance pain and produce secondary increases in the blood vessel caliber. The acute antimigraine mechanisms of action of ergot derivatives principally involves constriction of pain-producing intracranial extracerebral blood vessels at 5-HT1B receptors and inhibition of trigeminal neurotransmission by actions at 5-HT1D receptors.

References

1 Berde B, Sturmer E: Introduction to the pharmacology of ergot alkaloids and related compounds as a basis of their therapeutic application; in Berde B, Schild HO (eds): Ergot Alkaloids and Related Compounds. New York, Springer-Verlag, 1978, pp 1–28.

2 Silberstein SD: The pharmacology of ergotamine and dihydroergotamine. Headache 1997;37(suppl 1):S15–S25.

3 Eulenburg A: Subcutane Injectionen von Ergotinin- (Tantret): Ergotinum citricum solutum (Gehe). Dtsch med Wochenschr 1883;9:637.

4 Thomson WH: Ergot in the treatment of periodic neuralgias. J Nerv Ment Dis 1894;21:124.

5 Stoll A: Zur Kenntniss der Mutterkornalkaloide. Verhandl Schweiz Naturf Gesellsch 1920;101:190.

6 B. Rothlin E: Historical development of the ergot therapy of migraine. Int Arch Allergy 1955;7: 205–209.

7 Maier HW: L'ergotamine inhibitteur du sympathique étudié en clinique, comme moyen d'exploration et comme agent thérapeutique. Rev Neurol 1926;33:1104–1108.

8 Tzanck A. Le traitement des migraines par le tartrate d'ergotamine. Bull et mém Soc méd d'hop de Paris 1928;52:1057.

9 Lennox WG: Use of ergotamine tartrate in migraine. N Engl J Med 1934;210:1061.

10 Graham JR, Wolff HG: Mechanism of migraine headache and action of ergotamine. Arch Neurol Psychiatr 1938;39:737–763.

11 Lennox WG: Ergonovine versus ergotamine as a terminator of migraine headaches. Am J Med Sci 1938;195:458–468.

12 Horton ST, Peters GA, Blumenthal LS: A new product in the treatment of migraine: A preliminary report. Mayo Clin Proc 1945;20:241–248.

13 Friedman AP, von Storch TJC: Recent advances in the treatment of migraine. JAMA 1951;145: 1325–1327.

14 Brazil P, Friedman AP: Further observations in craniovascular studies. Neurology 1957;7:52–55.

15 Ostfeld AM: A study of migraine pharmacotherapy. Am J Med Sci 1961;241:192–198.

16 Callaham M, Raskin N: A controlled study of dihydroergotamine in the treatment of acute migraine headache. Headache 1986;26:168–171.

17 Raskin NH: Repetitive intravenous dihydroergotamine as therapy for intractable migraine. Neurology 1986;36:995–997.

18 Scott AIK. Dihydroergotamine: A review of its use in the treatment of migraine and other headaches. Clin Neuropharmacol 1992;15:289–296.

19 Ziegler D, Ford R, Kriegler J, Gallagher RM, Peroutka S, Hammerstad J, Saper J, Hoffert M, Vogel B, Holtz N: Dihydroergotamine nasal spray for the acute treatment of migraine. Neurology 1994;44:447–453.

20 Lipton R: Ergotamine tartrate and dihydroergotamine mesylate: Safety profiles. Headache 1997;37 (suppl 1):S33–S41.

21 Silberstein SD, Young WB: Safety and efficacy of ergotamine tartrate and dihydroergotamine in the treatment of migraine and status migrainosus. Neurology 1995;45:577–584.

22 Tfelt-Hansen P: Clinical pharmacology of ergotamines. An overview; in Diener H-C, Wilkinson M (eds): Drug-Induced Headache. Berlin, Springer-Verlag, 1988, pp 105–116.

23 Ibraheem JJ, Paalzow L, Tfelt-Hansen P: Kinetics of ergotamine after intravenous and intramuscular administration to migraine sufferers. Eur J Clin Pharmacol 1982;23:235–240.

24 Ibraheem JJ, Paalzow L, Tfelt-Hansen P: Low bioavailability of ergotamine tartrate after oral and rectal administration in migraine sufferers. Or J Clin Pharmacol 1983;16:695–699.

25 Ala-Hurula V, Myllyli VV, Arvela P, Heikkild J, Kfirki N, Hokkanen E: Systemic availability of ergotamine tartrate after oral, rectal and intramuscular administration. Eur J Clin Pharmacol 1979; 15:51–55.

26 Müller-Schweinitzer E: Pharmacological actions of the main metabolites of dihydroergotamine. Eur J Clin Pharmacol 1984;26:699–705.

27 Maurer G, Frick W: Elucidation of the structure and receptor binding studies of the major primary, metabolite of dihydroergotamine in man. Eur J Clin Pharmacol 1984;26:463–470.

28 Müller-Schweinitzer E, Rosenthaler J: Dihydroergotamine: pharmacokinetics, pharmacodynamics, and mechanism of venoconstrictor action in beagle dogs. J Cardiovasc Pharmacol 1987;9:686–693.

29 Ekbom K, Krabbe AE, Paalzow G, Paalzow L, Tfelt-Hansen P, Waldenlind E: Optimal routes of administration of ergotamine tartrate in cluster headache patients: A pharmacokinetic study. Cephalalgia 1983;3:15–20.

30 Sanders SW, Haering N, Mosborg H, Jaeger H: Pharmacokinetics of ergotamine in healthy volunteers following oral and rectal dosing. Eur J Clin Pharmacol 1986;30:331–334.

31 Schmidt R, Fanchamps A: Effect of caffeine on intestinal absorption of ergotamine in man. Eur J Clin Pharmacol 1974;7:213–216.

32 Perrin VL: Clinical pharmacokinetics of ergotamine in migraine and cluster headache. Clin Pharmacokinet 1985;10:334–352.

33 Eckert H, Kiechel JR, Rosenthalor J, Schmidt R, Schreier E, Biopharmaceutical aspects. Analytical methods, pharmacokinetics, metabolism and bioavailability; in Berde B, Schild HO (eds): Ergot Alkaloids and Related Compounds. New York, Springer-Verlag, 1978, pp 719–803.

34 Perrin VL: Clinical pharmacokinetics of ergotamine in migraine and cluster headache. Clin Phormsookiner 1985;10:334–352.

35 Aellig WH, Nuesch E: Comparative pharmacokinetic investigations with tritium labelled ergot alkaloids after oral and intravenous administration in man. Int J Clin Pharmacol 1977;15:106–112.

36 Little PJ, Jennings GL, Skews H, Bobik A: Bioavailability of dihydroergotamine in man. Br J Clin Pharmacol 1982;13:785–790.

37 Sandoz Pharmaceuticals Corporation, East Hanover, NJ. Data on file.

38 Tfelt-Hansen P, Lipton RS. Dihydroergotamine; in Olesen J, Tfelt-Hansen P, Welch KMA (eds): The Headaches. New York, Raven Press, 1993, pp 323–327.

39 Tfelt-Hansen P, Johnson ES. Ergotamine; in Olesen J, Tfelt-Hansen P, Welch KMA (eds): The Headaches, New York, Raven Press, 1993, pp 313–322.

40 Melancier S, Nordenfelt 1: Comparative effects of dihydroergotamine and noradrenaline on resistance, exchange and capacitance functions in the peripheral circulation. Clin Sci 1970;39:183–201.

41 de Maribes H, Welzol D, de Mardes A, Klotz U, T'iedjon KU, Knaiup G: Relationship between the venoconstrictor activity of dihydroergotamine and its pharmacokinetics during acute and chronic oral dosing. Eur J Clin Pharmacol 1986;30:685–689.

42 Aellig WH, Rosenthaler J: Venoconstrictor effects of dihydroergotamine after intranasal and intramuscular administration. Eur J Clin Pharmacol 1986;30:581–584.

43 Müller-Schweinitzer E, Weidmann H: Basic pharmacological properties; in Borde B, Schild HO (eds): Ergot Alkaloids and Related Compounds. New York, Springer Verlag, 1978, pp 87–232.

44 Clark BJ, Chu D, Aellig WH: Actions an the heart and circulation; in Berde B, Schild HO (eds): Ergot Alkaloids and Related Compounds. New York, Springer Verlag, 1978, pp 321–420.

45 Seidelin KN, Tfelt-Hansen P, Mendel CN, Stepanavage M: Peripheral hemodynamics study of MK-462 (rizatriptan) and ergotamine and their combination in man. Poster Presentation, IHS Toronto, 1995.

46 Tfelt-Hansen P, Eickhoff JH, Olesen J: The effect of single dose ergotamine tartrate on peripheral arteries in migraine patients: Methodological aspects and time effect curve. Acta Pharmacol Toxicol 1980;47:151–156.

47 Tfelt-Hansen P, Eickhoff JH, Olesen J: Duration of the biological effect of ergotamine tartrate. Adv Neurol 1982;33:315–319.

48 De Vries P, Villalon CM, Saxena PR: Pharmacological aspects of experimental headache models in relation to acute anti-migraine therapy. Eur J Pharmacol 1999;375:61–74.

49 Hargreaves RJ: Receptor pharmacology in the trigeminal nervous system: A window to understanding migraine mechanisms and treatment. Seminars in headache management. Migraine Pathophysiology Part 1. 1999;4:10–15.

50 Silberstein SD: Serotonin (5-HT) and migraine. Headache 1994;34:408–417.

51 Lauritzen M, Olesen J: Regional cerebral blood flow during migraine attacks by xenon-133 inhalation and emission tomography. Brain 1984;107:447–461.

52 Andersen AR, Tfelt-Hansen P, Lassen NA: The effect of ergotamine and dihydroergotamine on cerebral blood flow in man. Stroke 1987;18:120–123.

53 Hachinski V, Norris JW, Edmeads J, Cooper PW: Ergotamine and cerebral blood flow. Stroke 1978; 9:594–596.

54 Diener HC, Peters C, Rudzio M, Noe A, Dichgans J, Haux R, Ehrmann R, Tfelt-Hansen P: Ergotamine, flunarizine and sumatriptan do not change cerebral blood flow velocity in normal subjects and migraineurs. J Neurol 1991;238:245–250.

55 Longmore J, Shaw D, Smith D, Hopkins R, McAllister G, Pickard JD, Sirinathsinghji DJ, Butler AJ, Hill RG: Differential distribution of 5-HT1D and 5-HT1B immunoreactivity within the human trigemino-cerebrovascular system: implications for the discovery of new antimigraine drugs. Cephalalgia 1997;17:833–842.

56 Maassen Van Den Brink A, Reekers M, Bax W, Ferrari MD, Saxena PR: Coronary side-effect potential of current and prospective anti-migraine drugs. Circulation 1998;98:25–30.

57 Moskowitz MA: Basic mechanisms in vascular headache. Neurol Clin 1990;8:801–815.

58 Saito K, Markowtiz S, Moskowitz MA: Ergot alkaloids block neurogenic extravasation in dura mater: Proposed action in vascular headaches. Ann Neurol 1988;24:732–737.

59 Goadsby PJ, Edvinsson L: The trigeminovascular system in migraine: Studies characterising cerebrovascular and neuropeptide changes seen in humans and cats. Ann Neurol 1993;33:48–56.

60 Goadsby PJ, Gundlach AL. Localization of 3H-dihydroergotamine-binding sites in the cat central nervous system: Relevance to migraine. Ann Neurol 1991;29:91–94.

61 Hoskin, K, Kaube H, Goadsby PJ: Central activation of the trigeminovascular pathway in the cat is inhibited by dihydroergotamine: A c-fos and electrophysiological study. Brain 1996;119:249–256.

Stephen D. Silberstein, MD, FACP, Professor of Neurology, Director Jefferson Headache Center, Thomas Jefferson University, Philadelphia, PA 19107 (USA)
Tel. +1 215 955 7734, Fax +1 215 955 6682, E-Mail Stephen.Silberstein@mail.tju.edu

Diener HC (ed): Drug Treatment of Migraine and Other Headaches.
Monogr Clin Neurosci. Basel, Karger, 2000, vol 17, pp 66–82

Ergots – Therapy

Carl Dahlöf [a], *Peter J. Goadsby* [b]

[a] Gothenburg Migraine Clinic, Sociala Huset, Gothenburg, Sweden
[b] Institute of Neurology, National Hospital for Neurology and Neurosurgery,
Queen Square, London, UK

Medical use of ergot extract had begun by the 16th century and consisted of quickening childbirth and controlling postpartum hemorrhage [1, 2]. Stoll isolated the first pure ergot alkaloid, ergotamine (ET) in 1918 [3]. Due to its remarkable uterotonic and vasoconstrictor effects, ET (Gynergen®) was used primarily in obstetrics and gynecology until 1925 [2, 4]. ET has been used in the acute treatment of migraine from 1926 with no alternative specific acute anti-migraine treatment for some decades [5, 6]. Dihydroergotamine (DHE) which is a dihydro-derivative of ET was formed by reduction of a double-bond of the ergoline ring of ergotamine in 1943 [7, 8]. ET tartrate and DHE mesylate have now been widely used in the treatment of migraine for many decades, although relatively few randomized, controlled clinical trials have been conducted with these compounds [9–12]. Despite the limited number of studies of ET and DHE using contemporary methodology, there is some evidence for the efficacy of ET and DHE in the literature [11, 13, 14]. Considerable uncertainty exists, however, regarding the appropriate use and dose limitations for ET tartrate in the acute treatment of migraine. A more detailed account of ET and a consensus of its use can be found in a recent publication [15].

Pharmacodynamics of Ergots

The ergot alkaloids have a complex mode of action that involves interaction with a variety of receptors [16–21]. Indeed, both ET and DHE have affinities for 5-hydroxytryptamine (5-HT), dopamine and noradrenaline receptors. In lower therapeutically relevant concentrations, ET and DHE act as agonists at α-adrenoceptors, 5-HT (particularly 5-HT$_{1B/1D}$) and dopamine D2 receptors [22–26]. In addition, there is evidence that both ET and DHE can activate novel, not yet characterized receptors [22].

The most important and conspicuous pharmacological effect of ergot alkaloids is undeniably the vasoconstrictor action [23, 24]. Extensive studies in animals show that this vasoconstrictor effect is particularly marked within the carotid vascular bed. The selectivity extends to the arteriovenous anastomotic part; blood flow to a number of tissues, including that to the brain are little affected [22, 27]. In humans, ET and DHE can constrict several isolated blood vessels, including the pulmonary, cerebral, temporal and coronary arteries [24, 28–30]. The drugs seem to be more active on large arteries (conducting vessels) than on arterioles (resistance vessels). Basal cerebral or myocardial blood flow may not change, although ET and DHE do affect coronary vasodilator reserve [31–33]. Arterial blood pressure is moderately increased in therapeutic doses [32, 34]. An important feature of ET and DHE is that their effects in isolated human coronary arteries are resistant to repeated wash [30]. This appears to be mainly due to slow diffusion from the receptor biophase and, therefore, their effects last far longer than can be expected from prevailing plasma concentrations [34].

ET and DHE have been reported to inhibit dural plasma extravasation after stimulation of the trigeminal ganglion in rat [35, 36]. In addition, as has been demonstrated for DHE, ET may block the trigeminovascular pathway centrally [37, 38].

Pharmacokinetics of Ergots

Oral absorption of ET is 60–70% and the concurrent administration of caffeine improves both the rate and extent of absorption. However, due to high first-pass metabolism ET has a very low oral and rectal bioavailability. If compared with its intravenous (i.v.) bioavailability (100%), oral bioavailability of ET is <1%, rectal bioavailability of ET is 1–3% and intramuscular bioavailability of ET is 47% [13, 39, 40]. ET is metabolized in the liver by largely undefined pathways, and 90% of the metabolites are excreted in the bile [13]. The elimination half-life of ET is 2 h. DHE mesylate has also a very low oral bioavailability (less than 1%), due to incomplete drug passage across the gastrointestinal mucosa and a high first-pass metabolism [14, 41]. The absolute bioavailability of intramuscular (i.m.) DHE is 100%. The absolute bioavailability of DHE following intranasal (i.n.) administration, which avoids first-pass hepatic metabolism, is approximately 40%. Peak plasma levels occur approximately 1 to 2 min after i.v. administration, 24 min after i.m. administration, and 30 to 60 min after i.n. administration [42–44]. Like ET, DHE is rapidly and extensively metabolized in the liver. Only 6% to 7% of an i.m. dose is excreted in the urine [44]. The major route of elimination is the feces following biliary excretion of unchanged drug and metabolites. DHE has many metabolites; only those that retain the essential ring structures of the ergot alkaloids (the ergoline ring and the peptide side chain) are active [14, 44]. The major metabolite is 8′-OH DHE which is present at a concentration five to seven times greater than that of DHE. The pharmacological effects of the active metabolites are qualitatively similar to those of the parent compound. DHE is eliminated in a biphasic manner, with mean half-lives of approximately 0.7 to 1 and 10 to 13 h [14, 44].

An interaction with erythromycin may dramatically increase the oral bioavailability of ET and DHE [45–48]. Since the same cytochrome P450 enzyme CYP3A4 metabolizes a number of other drugs, including bromocriptine, dexamethasone, ethinyloestradiol, ketoconazole, nifedipine, omeprazole and verapamil, this interaction may extend to these drugs as well [49].

Due to slow diffusion from the receptor biophase the effects of ET, as well as DHE, last far longer than can be expected from plasma concentrations. For this reason, the pharmacokinetic data of ET and DHE available cannot be used to predict the biological response [13, 14, 30, 44].

Clinical Trials with Ergotamine

Because of its age, ET did not undergo the controlled clinical trial program that would be expected of a new drug. Accordingly, the number of good clinical trials incorporating this widely used drug is rather small. Nevertheless, oral ET has been used over the past 30 years as the standard comparative drug in controlled trials of other medicines [13]. In a review in press, a summary of 18 controlled double-blind trials of oral ET, or oral ET plus caffeine were presented; in 10 trials ET was compared with placebo, whereas ET served as the standard comparative drug in eight other trials without placebo-control [15]. The initial dose of ET varied from 1 to 5 mg, and in several trials repeated intake of test drugs were used. The reported parameters for efficacy were not all validated and varied considerably from benefit based on a clinical interview to use of changes on a verbal headache scale. Other methodological flaws in these trials include the lack of clearly stated inclusion criteria, no reporting of baseline criteria and the randomization procedure, unusual design of some of the crossover trials with a variable number of attacks per patient, and superiority claims without appropriate statistics [15]. Despite the limited number of studies with contemporary methodology that involve ET there is evidence for the efficacy of ET in the literature, and this is summarized briefly below.

ET (1–5 mg) was superior to placebo for some parameters in seven trials and no better than placebo in three studies using a dose of 2 to 3 mg [50–59]. In two comparative trials ET was superior to aspirin (500 mg), and was inferior to an isometheptene compound in one trial and superior to it in another trial [60–63]. In two recent comparative trials, there was no significant differences in measures of pain relief at 2 h between oral ET (Cafergot®, 2 mg ET tartrate and 200 mg caffeine) and oral diclofenac-potassium 50 or 100 mg [59]. However, diclofenac-potassium reduced pain more effectively than ET plus caffeine at 1 h after treatment and, in contrast to the comparator, was also significantly different compared with placebo [59]. Drugs, such as ergocristine, tolfenamic acid, dextropropoxyphene, naproxen sodium, pirprofen, were generally found comparable to ET. An exception is the combination of calcium carbasalate (equivalent to 900 mg aspirin) plus metoclopramide (10 mg) which was superior to a rather small dose of 1 mg ET plus 100 mg caffeine [64]. Similarily, the combination of lysin-acetylsalicylate (equivalent to 900 mg aspirin) plus metoclopramide (10 mg) was superior to the combination of ET and caffeine (2 mg ET and 200 mg caffeine) for most of the outcome parameters assessed [65]. Early use of ergotamine has been tried in two of the trials in which the drugs were administered as soon as the patients felt the onset of an attack [60, 61]. The use of escape medication is a clinically relevant efficacy parameter, and 31%, 44% and 46% of patients treated with ergotamine used this [51, 53, 66].

Ergotamine vs. Triptans Orally

The effect of oral ET in acute treatment of migraine has been compared to that of triptans orally in randomized controlled clinical trials. The concern is that despite several direct comparative trials that have been performed between ET and different triptans only few have been or are going to be published. In a former trial performed without placebo, the efficacy and tolerability of oral sumatriptan as a 100-mg dispersible tablet was compared with oral ET (Cafergot®, 2 mg ET tartrate and 200 mg caffeine) in a multicentre, randomized, double-blind, double-dummy, parallel-group trial [66]. In the trial, 580 patients were treated from 47 investigating centres in nine European countries. Sumatriptan was significantly more effective than Cafergot at reducing the intensity of headache from severe or moderate to mild or none; 66% (145/220) of those treated with sumatriptan improved in this way by 2 h, compared with 48% (118/246) of those treated with Cafergot (p < 0.001). The onset of headache resolution was more rapid with sumatriptan, whereas recurrence of migraine headache within 48 h was lower with Cafergot. Sumatriptan was also significantly more effective at reducing the incidence of photophobia/phonophobia ($p < 0.001$), nausea ($p < 0.001$) and vomiting ($p < 0.01$) 2 h after treatment, and fewer patients on sumatriptan (24%) than on Cafergot (44%, $p < 0.001$) required other medication after 2 h [66]. The overall incidence of patients reporting adverse events was 45% after sumatriptan and 39% after Cafergot; the difference was not significant. The most commonly reported events in the sumatriptan-treated patients were malaise or fatigue and bad taste; these were generally mild and transient. A greater proportion of Cafergot-treated patients reported nausea, vomiting, or both, abdominal discomfort, and dizziness or vertigo. It was concluded that oral sumatriptan was well tolerated and was more effective than Cafergot in the acute treatment for migraine.

In more recent studies, the efficacy and tolerability of oral ET was recently compared with that of eletriptan, a selective 5-HT$_{1B/1D}$ agonist, in the acute treatment of migraine [56]. In a double-blind, parallel group, randomized placebo-controlled trial, patients (n = 773) took up to two doses of study medication to treat an acute migraine attack. The patients were randomized to receive 40 mg eletriptan, 80 mg eletriptan, ET (Cafergot®, 2 mg ET tartrate and 200 mg caffeine) or placebo (in the ratio 2:2:2:1) for the first dose. The onset of headache relief was more rapid in eletriptan groups, with response rates at 1 h of 29% and 39% for 40 mg and 80 mg eletriptan, compared to 13% for Cafergot and placebo ($p < 0.002$). Both doses of eletriptan were significantly more effective than Cafergot in terms of headache response (54% and 68% vs. 33%; $p < 0.0001$) and pain-free response (28% and 38% vs. 10%; $p < 0.0001$) at 2 h after treatment [56]. Eletriptan was also significantly superior ($p < 0.005$) to Cafergot in terms of functional response and the incidence of accompanying symptoms at 2 h. The incidence of treatment-related adverse events for patients based on the first dose of study medication was 32, 43, 34 and 34% in the eletriptan 40 mg, 80 mg, Cafergot and placebo groups, respectively.

Non-Oral Routes of Administration

Other routes of administration of ergotamine, which from a kinetic point of view should be more efficacious, have scarcely been investigated. In one trial, inhaled ergotamine (maximum dose of 1.8 mg) was found to be superior to sublingual ergotamine (maximum dose of 2 mg), and sublingual ergotamine was not better than sublingual placebo [67]. In one single-centre, double-blind, placebo-controlled, crossover comparison of a single dose a suppository of ergotamine (2 mg) was no better than placebo, whereas ketoprofen (100 mg as a suppository) was superior to placebo in the treatment of acute migraine attacks [68]. Fifty patients were included in the statistical evaluation and ketoprofen was found more efficient than ET and placebo in reducing the severity of pain. In a recent randomized, crossover, double-blind trial including 251 patients, published so far only on the Internet, ergotamine + caffeine suppositories (2 mg + 100 mg) were superior to 25 mg sumatriptan suppositories with response rates of 73% and 63% after 2 h, respectively [69]. Headache recurrence, see below, occurred more frequently in sumatriptan (22%) than in ergotamine (11%) treated patients.

Randomized Controlled Clinical Trials with DHE

The safety and efficacy of an intranasal spray formulation of DHE mesylate in the acute treatment of migraine has been addressed in four double-blind, placebo-controlled trials in patients with migraine [70–73]. Patients self-administered either 2 mg of DHE mesylate (0.5 mg per nostril, repeated after 15 min) or a placebo for each of two moderate to severe migraine headaches using a nasal spray apparatus. Patients rated pain severity, functional ability, headache pain relief (severe/moderate to mild/no pain), incidence and severity of nausea, and the incidence of vomiting, photophobia, and phonophobia prior to treatment (base-line) and again at 0.5, 1, 2, 3 and 4 hours after treatment. Recurrences of headache pain within 24 h were also noted. Self-administration of DHE resulted in significant increases in headache pain relief and functional ability, and significant decreases in pain intensity and nausea compared with the placebo. In one of these four placebo-controlled studies, 27% of patients treated with 2 mg of DHE mesylate obtained headache pain relief (i.e. no pain or mild pain) as early as 30 min after treatment [73]. By 4 h after treatment, 70% of these patients' headaches obtained pain relief. Headache pain returned within 24 h in only 14% of patients who have had a headache response at 2 h [73]. In general, no serious adverse effects of DHE treatment were observed, and the majority of adverse events reported by the DHE-treated patients were nasopharyngeal, primarily related to the route of administration [70–73]. The results of these four placebo-controlled studies demonstrate that DHE nasal spray as monotherapy is significantly more effective than placebo at 2 h in the acute treatment of migraine attacks for most of the parameters evaluated.

A randomized, double-blind, two-attack, crossover study design was used to compare the efficacy of sumatriptan nasal spray 20 mg with a 1-mg dose of dihydroergotamine (DHE) nasal spray [74, 75]. After 30 min, if headache was not completely relieved, the DHE patients had the option of taking an additional 1-mg dose and the sumatriptan-treated patients could take an optional placebo dose. (The recommended dose of DHE is 1 mg to start, followed by another 1 mg in 15 min.) The second dose of dihydroergotamine was taken by 81% of patients after initial treatment with dihydroergotamine, and an optional second dose of placebo was taken by 76% of patients after initial treatment with sumatriptan nasal spray 20 mg. A significantly greater percentage of patients reported headache relief after treatment with sumatriptan nasal spray 20 mg than after DHE 1 mg (or 1 mg plus 1 mg) beginning at 45 min after treatment and continuing through 2 h after treatment [75]. Complete elimination of headache pain, normal functioning or only mild clinical disability, and freedom from associated symptoms did not differ between sumatriptan-treated and DHE-treated patients at 2 h. The incidence of headache recurrence was greater in the sumatriptan group (23%) than in the DHE group (13%) [75].

The efficacy and tolerability of subcutaneous (SC) sumatriptan (6 mg) has been compared with that of DHE nasal spray (1 mg plus optional 1 mg) in the acute treatment of migraine [76]. Two hundred and sixty-six adult migraineurs (International Headache Society criteria) completed a multicentre, double-blind, double-dummy, crossover study. Patients took SC sumatriptan for one attack and DHE nasal spray for the other in random order. Data from both treatment periods show that at all time points from 15 min, SC sumatriptan was significantly better than DHE nasal spray at providing both headache relief (moderate/severe headache improving to mild/none) and resolution of headache [76]. Similarly, SC sumatriptan was superior to DHE nasal spray for the other efficacy endpoints assessed in the study. Patients reported that both treatments were well tolerated. Adverse events were reported by 43% of patients taking SC sumatriptan and 22% of patients taking DHE nasal spray. These were usually mild and transient. It was concluded that subcutaneous sumatriptan has a faster onset of action than DHE nasal spray and provides greater relief of acute migraine symptoms.

The efficacy and tolerability of subcutaneous DHE mesylate has also been compared with that of SC sumatriptan succinate for the acute treatment of migraine with or without aura in a double-blind, randomized trial with parallel treatment arms [77]. Patients with moderate or severe head pain were randomized to receive either 1 mg of SC DHE mesylate or 6 mg of SC sumatriptan succinate. Patients rated head pain, functional ability, nausea, and vomiting at baseline and at 0.5, 1, 2, 4 and 24 h after the injection. If pain persisted after 2 h, a second injection of the same study medication was allowed, and self-ratings were repeated 30 and 60 min later. Follow-up data were collected at 24 h. There were 295 evaluable patients. At 2 h, 73% of the patients treated with DHE and 85% of those treated with sumatriptan had relief (p = 0.002). There was no statistical difference in headache relief between the groups at 3 or 4 h. Headache relief was achieved by 85% of those treated with DHE and by 83% of those treated with sumatriptan by 4 h [77]. By 24 h 90% of DHE-treated patients and 77% of sumatriptan-treated patients had relief (p = 0.004). Headache recurred within 24 h after treatment in 45% of the sumatriptan-treated patients and in 18% of the DHE-treated patients (p < or = 0.001). It was concluded that both SC sumatriptan and SC DHE are effective in aborting migraine headaches but that headache recurrence is two and a half times as likely with sumatriptan as with DHE.

Based on the results from a prospective, double-blind trial of a sample of emergency departments, patients randomly assigned to receive either 1 mg DHE or 1.5 mg/kg meperidine (MEP) by intramuscular injection [78]. The anti-nauseant hydroxyzine was co-administered in both treatment groups. The conclusion was made that DHE and MEP were comparable therapies in the acute treatment of migraine headache. The use of DHE, however, appears to avoid several problems associated with opioid analgesia, including dizziness.

In a randomized double-blind, double-dummy study the efficacy of intra-venously administered dihydroergotamine (1 mg) and metoclopramide (10 mg) was compared to that of the intramuscularly injected combination of meper-idine (75 mg) and hydroxyzine (75 mg) in the treatment of severe migraine headaches [79]. Both treatment groups experienced improvement in headache severity but improvement in pain scale score tended to be greater for the combination dihydroergotamine (1 mg) and metoclopramide (10 mg) [79].

Tolerability and Safety of Ergots

ET has been found to be reasonably well tolerated and safe in the acute treatment of migraine as long as recommended dosages are not exceeded and high-risk patients such as those with uncontrolled hypertension, coronary or peripheral artery disease, thyrotoxicosis, or sepsis do not receive these compounds [13, 15, 80, 81]. ET affects a number of receptor types, which increases the risk of experiencing a drug-induced side effect. In addition, most formulations include in addition to ET one to three ingredients, which may further increase the risk for having side effects. Weakness in legs is commonly reported, and occasionally severe muscle pains, may occur in the extremities [15, 81]. Numbness and tingling of the fingers and toes are other reminders of the ergotism that this alkaloid may cause. In doses used in the treatment of migraine, the rectal administration of ET produces little change in blood pressure but does cause a slowly progressing increase in peripheral vessel constriction that persists for up to 24 h [34]. ET often causes nausea and vomiting in a migraine sufferer which are major clinical disadvantages given the high prevalence of these symptoms during the migraine attack. Nausea and vomiting occur in approximately 10% of patients after oral administration of ET and in about twice that number after parenteral administration. Nausea is most likely caused by a direct effect on CNS emetic centres.

A number of severe side effects associated with ET usage has been reported in the literature, including myocardial infarction, ischaemia of limb extremities, and fibrotic changes [15, 81]. Diffuse abdominal pain, nausea and vomiting due to retroperitoneal fibrosis: a rare but often missed diagnosis [82]. Vascular stasis, thrombosis, and gangrene result and are prominent features of ergot poisoning. The propensity of ET to cause gangrene appears to parallel its vasoconstrictor activity [83]. Ergot toxicity, which can result in severe vasospasm, does not spare the fetus or mother and ET should not be considered without risk [15, 81]. ET should be avoided in pregnancy, and the counselling of the woman with an exposed fetus should focus on possible toxic exposure.

Significant pharmacodynamic differences exist between ET and DHE [14, 44, 83]. DHE mesylate is a less potent arterial vasoconstrictor than ET, although nearly equipotent as a venoconstrictor. It is a more potent alpha-adrenergic antagonist, but is much less emetic, has less effect on the uterus, and is not associated with rebound headache [81, 84]. Reports of serious adverse effects following recommended doses of DHE are rare [81, 85]. As with most antimigraine drugs, the most frequent adverse effect with i.v. DHE is nausea; however, following i.m. or i.n. administration, the incidence of nausea is low and concomitant administration of an antiemetic is not needed [81, 84]. The side effects most commonly observed with DHE are abdominal discomfort, muscle pain, diarrhea and anxiety [14, 81].

Interactions

ET and DHE are extensively metabolized by the cytochrome P450 CYP3A4 hepatic enzyme in man. Potent inhibitors of CYP3A4 have the potential to attenuate the metabolism of ET and DHE [86]. Accordingly, caution should be advised in the clinical use of ET when other drugs are also administered inhibit P450 CYP3A4, such as antibiotics of the macrolides class [49, 87]. Propranolol, a known mild inhibitor of CYP3A4 and CYP2D6 metabolism, is assumed to produce a small reduction in the clearance of ET, which is unlikely to cause clinically important changes in therapeutic effect.

Contraindications

ET and DHE are contraindicated in women who are or may become pregnant since the drugs may cause fetal harm. ET and DHE are also contra-indicated in patients with peripheral vascular disease, coronary heart disease, uncontrolled hypertension, stroke, impaired hepatic or renal function, and sepsis [12–15, 81, 84, 85]. ET and DHE should not be taken within 6 h of the use of triptans, based on the theoretical additive pharmacological effects of the drugs, and similarly that triptans should not be administered within 24 h of ET or DHE. It is also recommended that ET is not used in complicated migraine or migraine with prolonged aura.

ET Misuse and Drug-Induced Daily Headache

The general impression among migraine sufferers is that ET has no effect or is less effective when taken late in the migraine attack. The most likely explanation for this notion is that ET, due to its very low and variable oral bioavailability, is more susceptible to the consequences of migraine induced gastric stasis. The apparent characteristics of ET with a slow onset of response may be responsible for the frequent and inadequate usage of ET in clinical practice [15]. It is very common that the migraine patients initiate treatment with ET when they anticipate a migraine attack or as a prophylactic the night before in order to avoid a debilitating migraine attack. If this form of use of ET becomes too frequent the patient risks development of drug-induced daily headache, addiction to ET and other constituents in the formulation, as well as severe side effects [88]. Once the effect of previous doses of ET wanes, the headache may escalate until the next dose of ET is taken, thus ET-rebound headache [89, 90]. These patients show an increasing pattern of ET usage, and weekly total usage frequently exceeds safety limitations. This patient category once represented a significant proportion of the headache patients attending specialist headache clinics [91]. If these patients discontinue ET, this invariably results in a predictable, protracted and extremely debilitating headache accompanied by nausea, vomiting and at times diarrhoea, as well as other physical and mental complaints [92]. This withdrawal headache usually begins within 3 days following discontinuation of the drug and may last for another three or more days once the headache starts. Spontaneous improvement is common after the medication is discontinued. When ET is discontinued, the prophylactic medications that have previously been largely without benefit, become more effective.

Misuse and/or drug-induced daily headache is rarely seen with DHE.

Discussion

Although oral ET alone or in combination with caffeine is widely used for the acute treatment of migraine, there is limited but clear evidence that it is significantly more effective than placebo [15]. No evidence-based rationale for dosing recommendations exists, and its long-term tolerability can be questioned [11]. In addition, no clinical trial data are available on subject consistency, which from pharmacokinetics and clinical practice is probably poor when compared to triptans. The overuse of ET in some instances has been associated with physical and psychological dependence resulting in rebound headaches, and subsequent severe withdrawal symptoms, including nausea, upon discontinuance of ET. Most formulations of ET are not very useful due to an inappropriate amount of ET or compounding with other drugs, such as caffeine, chlorcyclizine or meprobamate. ET is marketed as aerosol, oral and suppository formulations. In some countries, ET can be used alone in an oral formulation, or particularly in the inhalational form, but most often the suppository formulation is compounded and contains 1–2 mg ET with 100–200 mg caffeine.

An expert group from Europe met and reviewed the preclinical and clinical data on ET as it relates to the treatment of migraine. From this review, specific suggestions for the patient groups and appropriate use of ET have been agreed [15]. In essence, ET, from a medical perspective, is the drug of choice in a limited number of migraine sufferers who have infrequent or long duration headaches and are likely to comply with dosing restrictions. When ET is ineffective, a repeated dosing within half an hour is sometimes recommended, but this group of authors does not support this recommendation. Partly due to the reason that one simply cannot expect onset of efficacy within this short time frame and thus, this approach increases the risk for drug-induced side effects. ET should therefore be dosed at one time as early as practicable in the attack, at a dose that produces a response with as few side effects as possible. It is useful to test this dose for tolerability for nausea between attacks. A single dose of 0.5 to 2 mg per attack and a frequency of dosing about 1/week or 6/month are generally recommended [15]. Although still useful orally, ergotamine is generally better used, provided it is acceptable to the patient, by the rectal route because of improved absorption. Where it is available, the ergotamine puffer is preferred to the oral route for the same reasons.

The recent introduction of the more selective 5-HT$_{1B/1D}$ agonists (triptans) has challenged the place of ET in migraine therapy. Many patients who would have received ET in the pre-triptan era are probably now better off not being prescribed the drug. There is, however, no immediate need for switching patients established on ET to a triptan who are responding satisfactorily, with no contraindications to its use and with no signs of dose escalation.

DHE mesylate has also been used in the treatment of migraine for many decades. Although there is limited evidence from double-blind clinical trials, DHE does appear to be effective in the acute treatment of migraine attacks. This appears to be particularly true for intranasal and parenteral administrations [72, 73, 75–78, 93]. Indirect comparisons suggest that DHE causes nausea and vomiting less frequently than ET but the sustained vascular contraction by ET and DHE seems to be an important disadvantage compared with triptans [15, 81, 84]. The side effects most commonly observed with DHE are local irritation, abdominal discomfort, muscle pain, diarrhea and anxiety. DHE offers, however, several benefits compared to ET, including a lower incidence of nausea and vomiting and headache recurrence, and a lack of rebound headache [81, 84]. DHE mesylate is readily soluble in water, but to ensure stability, DHE must be contained within a glass ampoule. DHE is marketed as an injection, nasal spray and oral tablet formulations. The oral tablet is, however, not likely to be effective in the acute treatment of migraine due to its poor bioavailability.

Intranasal administration is probably the most convenient, particularly since the device has recently been improved. In addition, intranasal administration of DHE avoids first-pass hepatic metabolism, delivers adequate plasma concentrations of the drug and diminishes the need for parenteral administration. Dosing of i.n. DHE is one spray (0.5 mg) into each nostril at the first sign of migraine headache followed 15 min later by an additional spray into each nostril [94]. The total dose administered is 2 mg in four sprays. The maximum recommended dose is 4 mg per attack.

DHE may be administered i.m. in an office setting as well as at home. The patient will need training to self-administer DHE by i.m. injection starting with a single i.m. injection of DHE 1 ml (1 mg) which may be repeated if needed, after 60 min. With some experience, patients may find that they need less than 1 mg to obtain the desired relief. In any case, the maximum recommended daily dose for an individual attack is 3 ml (3 mg). Administration of DHE by the i.m. route provides a relative freedom from nausea and therefore minimal need for antiemetic medication compared with i.v. dosing.

Status migrainosus can be managed according to a modification of Raskin's protocol [95]. The patient who has had continuous headache with nausea and vomiting for more than 48 h is usually dehydrated and should receive i.v. metoclopramide 10 mg in 50 ml of dextrose 5% infusion administered over 30 min. A 0.5-mg test dose of intravenous DHE is then administered over 1 min. Signs of intolerance to DHE include increased blood pressure or chest pain; the few patients who experience these reactions should not continue on DHE. The majority of patients will tolerate the DHE test dose and will be able to continue. Patients reporting improvement can continue to receive 0.5 mg

DHE every 8 h [84]. For those whose headaches improve, but who experience severe nausea, the dose of metoclopramide can be increased to 20 mg, or the next dose of DHE decreased to 0.25 mg. For patients with persistent headache but no nausea, the next DHE dose can be increased to 1 mg 60 min after the test dose [84]. All patients continuing on therapy should receive DHE every 8 h until the headache is eliminated, then switched to a 12-hourly schedule for an additional two or three doses, with metoclopramide as needed. The usual recommended period of repetitive intravenous DHE treatment is 72 h.

Conclusions

Clinical trials performed with ET, some of them placebo-controlled, suggest that oral ET is effective in the acute treatment of migraine. Putting aside financial considerations, however, a triptan appears generally to be a better option than ET for most migraine sufferers requiring a specific anti-migraine treatment, from both efficacy and side effect perspectives.

The place of DHE in treatment is in cases where simple analgesics alone or in combination with other agents fail to provide relief. Further studies are, however, necessary to compare DHE with more triptans in the acute treatment of migraine attacks in order to determine its future role in acute migraine therapy.

References

1   Thoms H: John Stearns and pulvis parturiens. Am J Obstet Gynecol 1931;2:418–423.
2   Hofmann A: Historical view on ergot alkaloids. Pharmacology 1978;16(suppl 1):1–11.
3   Stoll A: Zur Kenntnis der Mutterkornalkaloide. Verh Naturf Ges (Basel) 1920;101:190–1.
4   Moir JC: Ergot: From 'St. Anthony's Fire' to the isolation of its active principle, ergometrine (ergonovine). Am J Obstet Gynecol 1974;120:291–296.
5   Maier HW: L'ergotamine inhibiteur du sympathique étudié en clinque, comme moyen d'exploration et comme agent thérapeutique. Revue Neurologie 1926;33:1104–1108.
6   Rothlin E: Historical development of the ergot therapy of migraine. Int Arch Allergy 1955;7:205–209.
7   Hofmann A: Historical view on ergot alkaloids. Pharmacology 1978;16(suppl 1):1–11.
8   Hofmann A: Die Mutterkornalkaloide. Stuttgart, F Enke Verlag, 1964.
9   Saxena VK, De Deyn PP: Ergotamine: its use in the treatment of migraine and its complications. Acta Neurol (Napoli) 1992;14:140–146.
10 Moskowitz MA, Cutrer FM: Sumatriptan: A receptor-targeted treatment for migraine. Annu Rev Med 1993;44:145–154.
11 Dahlöf C: Placebo-controlled clinical trials with ergotamine in the acute treatment of migraine. Cephalalgia 1993;13:166–171.
12 Young WB: Appropriate use of ergotamine tartrate and dihydroergotamine in the treatment of migraine: Current perspectives. Headache 1997;37(suppl 1):S42–S45.
13 Tfelt-Hansen P, Johnson ES: Ergotamine; in Olesen J, Tfelt-Hansen P, Welch KMA (eds): The Headaches. New York, Raven Press, 1993, pp 313–322.

14   Tfelt-Hansen P, Lipton RB: Dihydroergotamine; in Olesen J, Tfelt-Hansen P, Welch KMA (eds): The Headaches. New York, Raven Press, 1993, pp 323–327.

15   Tfelt-Hansen P, Saxena PR, Dahlöf C, Pascual P, Lainez M, Henry P, Diener H.-C, Schoenen J, Ferrari MD, Goadsby PJ: Ergotamine in the acute treatment of migraine – A review and European consensus. Brain 2000;123:in press.

16   Adham N, Bard JA, Zgombick JM, Durkin MM, Kucharewicz S, Weinshank RL, Branchek TA: Cloning and characterization of the guinea pig 5-HT1F receptor subtype: A comparison of the pharmacological profile to the human species homolog. Neuropharmacology 1997;36:569–576.

17   Glusa E, Roos A: Endothelial 5-HT receptors mediate relaxation of porcine pulmonary arteries in response to ergotamine and dihydroergotamine. Br J Pharmacol 1996;119:330–334.

18   Hoyer D: Functional correlates of serotonin 5-HT1 recognition sites. J Rec Res 1988;8:59–81.

19   Hoyer D, Clarke DE, Fozard JR, Hartig PR, Martin GR, Mylecharane EJ, Saxena PR, Humphrey PP: International Union of Pharmacology classification of receptors for 5-hydroxytryptamine (Serotonin). Pharmacol Rev 1994;46:157–203.

20   Leysen JE, Gommeren W: In vitro receptor binding profile of drugs used in migraine; in Amery WK, Van Nueten JM, Wauquir A (eds): The Pharmacological Basis of Migraine Therapy. London, Pitman, 1984.

21   Leysen JE, Gommeren W, Heylen L, Luyten WH, Van de Weyer I, Vanhoenacker P, Haegeman G, Schotte A, Van Gompel P, Wouters R, Lesage AS: Alniditan, a new 5-hydroxytryptamine1D agonist and migraine-abortive agent: Ligand-binding properties of human 5-hydroxytryptamine1D alpha, human 5-hydroxytryptamine1D beta, and calf 5-hydroxytryptamine1D receptors investigated with [3H]5-hydroxytryptamine and [3H]alniditan. Mol Pharmacol 1996;50:1567–1580.

22   De Vries P, Villalon CM, Heiligers JP, Saxena PR: Characterization of 5-HT receptors mediating constriction of porcine carotid arteriovenous anastomoses: Involvement of 5-HT1B/1D and novel receptors. Br J Pharmacol 1998;123:1561–1570.

23   Müller-Schweinitzer E, Weidmann H: Basic pharmacological properties; in Berde B, Schild HO (eds): Handbook of Experimental Pharmacology: Ergot Alkaloids and Related Compounds. Berlin, Springer, 1978, pp 87–232.

24   Müller-Schweinitzer E: Ergot alkaloids in migraine: Is the effect via 5-HT receptors? in Olesen J, Saxena PR (eds): 5-Hydroxytryptamine Mechanisms in Primary Headaches. New York: Raven Press, 1992, pp 297–304.

25   Saxena PR, Cairo-Rawlins WI: Presynaptic inhibition by ergotamine of the responses to cardioaccelerator nerve stimulations in the cat. Eur J Pharmacol 1979;58:305–312.

26   Villalon CM, De Vries P, Rabelo G, Centurion D, Sánchez-López A, Saxena PR: Canine external carotid vasoconstriction to methysergide, ergotamine and dihydroergotamine: Role of 5-HT1B/1D receptors and α2-adrenoceptors. Br J Pharmacol 1999 (in press).

27   Johnston BM, Saxena PR: The effect of ergotamine on tissue blood flow and the arteriovenous shunting of radioactive microspheres in the head. Br J Pharmacol 1978;63:541–549.

28   Cortijo J, Marti-Cabrera M, Bernabeu E, Domenech T, Bou J, Fernandez AG, Beleta J, Palacios JM, Morcillo EJ: Characterization of 5-HT receptors on human pulmonary artery and vein: Functional and binding studies. Br J Pharmacol 1997;122:1455–1463.

29   Ostergaard JR, Mikkelsen E, Voldby B: Effects of 5-hydroxytryptamine and ergotamine on human superficial temporal artery. Cephalalgia 1981;1:223–228.

30   MaassenVanDenBrink A, Reekers M, Bax WA, Ferrari MD, Saxena PR: Coronary side-effect potential of current and prospective antimigraine drugs. Circulation 1998;98:25–30.

31   Andersen AR, Tfelt-Hansen P, Lassen NA: The effect of ergotamine and dihydroergotamine on cerebral blood flow in man. Stroke 1987;18:120–123.

32   Dixon RM, Meire HB, Evans DH, Watt H, On N, Posner J, Rolan PE: Peripheral vascular effects and pharmacokinetics of the antimigraine compound, zolmitriptan, in combination with oral ergotamine in healthy volunteers. Cephalalgia 1997;17:639–646.

33   Gnecchi-Ruscone T, Lorenzoni R, Anderson D, Legg N, Tousoulis D, Winter PD, Crisp A, Camici PG: Effects of ergotamine on myocardial blood flow in migraineurs without evidence of atherosclerotic coronary artery disease. Am J Cardiol 1998;81:1165–1168.

34 Bulow PM, Ibraheem JJ, Paalzow G, Tfelt-Hansen P: Comparison of pharmacodynamic effects and plasma levels of oral and rectal ergotamine. Cephalalgia 1986;6:107–111.

35 Buzzi MG, Moskowitz MA: Evidence for 5-HT1B/1D receptors mediating the antimigraine effect of sumatriptan and dihydroergotamine. Cephalalgia 1991;11:165–168.

36 Buzzi MG, Moskowitz MA, Peroutka SJ, Byun B: Further characterization of the putative 5-HT receptor which mediates blockade of neurogenic plasma extravasation in rat dura mater. Br J Pharmacol 1991;103:1421–1428.

37 Goadsby PJ, Edvinsson L: The trigeminovascular system and migraine: Studies characterizing cerebrovascular and neuropeptide changes seen in humans and cats. Ann Neurol 1993;33:48–56.

38 Hoskin KL, Kaube H, Goadsby PJ: Central activation of the trigeminovascular pathway in the cat is inhibited by dihydroergotamine. A c-fos and electrophysiological study. Brain 1996;119:249–256.

39 Ibraheem JJ, Paalzow L, Tfelt-Hansen P: Low bioavailability of ergotamine tartrate after oral and rectal administration in migraine sufferers. Br J Clin Pharmacol 1983;16:695–699.

40 Sanders SW, Haering N, Mosberg H, Jaeger H: Pharmacokinetics of ergotamine in healthy volunteers following oral and rectal dosing. Eur J Clin Pharmacol 1986;30:331–334.

41 Little PJ, Jennings GL, Skews H, Bobik A: Bioavailability of dihydroergotamine in man. Br J Clin Pharmacol 1982;13:785–790.

42 Winner P, Dalessio D, Mathew N, Sadowsky C, Turkewitz LJ, Sheftell F, Silberstein SD, Solomon S: Office-based treatment of acute migraine with dihydroergotamine mesylate. Headache 1993;33:471–475.

43 Humbert H, Cabiac MD, Dubray C, Lavene D. Human pharmacokinetics of dihydroergotamine administered by nasal spray. Clin Pharmacol Ther 1996;60:265–275.

44 Silberstein SD: The pharmacology of ergotamine and dihydroergotamine. Headache 1997;37(suppl 1):S15–S25.

45 Ghali R, De Lean J, Douville Y, Noel HP, Labbe R: Erythromycin-associated ergotamine intoxication: Arteriographic and electrophysiologic analysis of a rare cause of severe ischemia of the lower extremities and associated ischemic neuropathy. Ann Vasc Surg 1993;7:291–296.

46 Delaforge M, Riviere R, Sartori E, Doignon JL, Grognet JM: Metabolism of dihydroergotamine by a cytochrome P-450 similar to that involved in the metabolism of macrolide antibiotics. Xenobiotica 1989;19:1285–1295.

47 Francis H, Tyndall A, Webb J: Severe vascular spasm due to erythromycin-ergotamine interaction. Clin Rheumatol 1984;3:243–246.

48 Pessayre D: Effects of macrolide antibiotics on drug metabolism in rats and in humans. Int J Clin Pharmacol Res 1983;3:449–458.

49 Christians U, Schmidt G, Bader A, Lampen A, Schottmann R, Linck A, Sewing KF: Identification of drugs inhibiting the in vitro metabolism of tacrolimus by human liver microsomes. Br J Clin Pharmacol 1996;41:187–190.

50 Ostfeld AM: A study of migraine pharmacotherapy. Am J Med Sci 1961;241:192–198.

51 Ryan RE: Double-blind clinical evaluation of the efficacy and safety of ergostine-caffeine, ergotamine-caffeine, and placebo in migraine headache. Headache 1970;9:212–220.

52 Hakkarainen H, Vapaatalo H, Gothoni G, Parantainen J: Tolfenamic acid is as effective as ergotamine during migraine attacks. Lancet 1979;2:326–328.

53 Kinnunen E, Erkinjuntti T, Farkkila M, Palomaki H, Porras J, Teirmaa H, Freudenthal Y, Andersson P: Placebo-controlled double-blind trial of pirprofen and an ergotamine tartrate compound in migraine attacks. Cephalalgia 1988;8:175–179.

54 Sargent JD, Baumel B, Peters K, Diamond S, Saper JR, Eisner LS, Solbach P: Aborting a migraine attack: Naproxen sodium vs ergotamine plus caffeine. Headache 1988;28:263–266.

55 Friedman AP, Di Serio FJ, Hwang DS: Symptomatic relief of migraine: Multicenter comparison of Cafergot P-B, Cafergot, and placebo. Clin Ther 1989;11:170–182.

56 Reches A and the Eletriptan Steering Committee: Comparison of the efficacy, safety and tolerability of oral eletriptan and Cafergot® for the acute treatment of migraine. Cephalalgia 1999;19:355.

57 Waters WE: Controlled clinical trial of ergotamine tartrate. Br Med J 1970;1:325–327.

58 Cortelli P, Pierangeli G, Corsini R, Prologo G, Limido GL: Pain control in migraine attacks: Results from a double-blind, randomized, within-patient, placebo-controlled trial comparing diclofenac-K and ergotamine-caffeine. Cephalalgia 1996;16:359.

59 McNeely W, Goa KL: Diclofenac-potassium in migraine – A review. Drugs 1999;57:991–1003.
60 Hakkarainen H, Gustafsson B, Stockman O: A comparative trial of ergotamine tartrate, acetyl salicylic acid and a dextropropoxyphene compound in acute migraine attacks. Headache 1978;18: 35–39.
61 Hakkarainen H, Quiding H, Stockman O: Mild analgesics as an alternative to ergotamine in migraine. A comparative trial with acetylsalicylic acid, ergotamine tartrate, and a dextropropoxyphene compound. J Clin Pharmacol 1980;20:590–595.
62 Yuill GM, Swinburn WR, Liversedge LA: A double-blind crossover trial of isometheptene mucate compound and ergotamine in migraine. Br J Clin Pract 1972;26:76–79.
63 Adams M, Aikman P, Allardyce K: General practitioner clinical trials: Treatment of migraine. Practitioner 1971;206:551–554.
64 Le Jeunne C, Gomez JP, Pradalier A, Titus i Albareda F, Joffroy A, Liano H, Henry P, Lainez JM, Geraud G: Comparative efficacy and safety of calcium carbasalate plus metoclopramide versus ergotamine tartrate plus caffeine in the treatment of acute migraine attacks. Eur Neurol 1999;41: 37–43.
65 Titus F, Lainez JM, Leira R, Diez E, Monteiro P, Dexeus I: Double-blind, multicentric, comparative study of lysin acetylsalicylate (1,620 mg equivalent to 900 mg aspirin) + metoclopramide (10 mg) versus ergotamine (2 mg) + caffeine (200 mg) in the treatment of migraine. Cephalalgia 1999;19: 371.
66 The Multinational Oral Sumatriptan and Cafergot Comparative Study Group: A randomized, double-blind comparison of sumatriptan and Cafergot in the acute treatment of migraine. Eur Neurol 1991;31:314–322.
67 Crooks J, Stephen SA, Brass W: Clinical trial of inhaled ergotamine tartrate in migraine. Br Med J 1964;1:221–224.
68 Kangasniemi P, Kaaja R: Ketoprofen and ergotamine in acute migraine. J Intern Med 1992;231: 551–554.
69 The Swedish Medicines Agency: Sumatriptan versus cafergot suppositories. http://www.mpa.se/sve/mono/imig.shtml 1998.
70 Tulunay FC, Karan O, Aydin N, Culcuoglu A, Guvener A: Dihydroergotamine nasal spray during migraine attacks. A double-blind crossover study with placebo. Cephalalgia 1987;7:131–133.
71 Ziegler D, Ford R, Kriegler J, Gallagher RM, Peroutka S, Hammerstad J, Saper J, Hoffert M, Vogel B, Holtz N: Dihydroergotamine nasal spray for the acute treatment of migraine. Neurology 1994;44:447–453.
72 Dihydroergotamine Nasal Spray Multicenter Investigators: Efficacy, safety, and tolerability of dihydroergotamine nasal spray as monotherapy in the treatment of acute migraine. Headache 1995; 35:177–184.
73 Gallagher RM: Acute treatment of migraine with dihydroergotamine nasal spray. Dihydroergotamine Working Group. Arch Neurol 1996;53:1285–1291.
74 Glaxo Study No S2B-T60: Data on file with Glaxo Wellcome Research and Development.
75 Dahlöf C: Sumatriptan nasal spray in the acute treatment of migraine: A review of clinical studies. Cephalalgia 1999 (in press).
76 Touchon J, Bertin L, Pilgrim AJ, Ashford E, Bes A: A comparison of subcutaneous sumatriptan and dihydroergotamine nasal spray in the acute treatment of migraine. Neurology 1996;47:361–365.
77 Winner P, Ricalde O, Le Force B, Saper J, Margul B: A double-blind study of subcutaneous dihydroergotamine vs subcutaneous sumatriptan in the treatment of acute migraine. Arch Neurol 1996;53:180–184.
78 Carleton SC, Shesser RF, Pietrzak MP, Chudnofsky CR, Starkman S, Morris DL, Johnson G, Rhee KJ, Barton CW, Chelly JE, Rosenberg J, Van Valen MK: Double-blind, multicenter trial to compare the efficacy of intramuscular dihydroergotamine plus hydroxyzine versus intramuscular meperidine plus hydroxyzine for the emergency department treatment of acute migraine headache. Ann Emerg Med 1998;32:129–138.
79 Klapper JA, Stanton J: Current emergency treatment of severe migraine headaches. Headache 1993; 33:560–562.
80 Meyler WJ: Side effects of ergotamine. Cephalalgia 1996;16:5–10.

81   Lipton RB: Ergotamine tartrate and dihydroergotamine mesylate: Safety profiles. Headache 1997; 37(suppl 1):S33–S41.

82   Netzer P, Binek J, Hammer B: Diffuse abdominal pain, nausea and vomiting due to retroperitoneal fibrosis: A rare but often missed diagnosis. Eur J Gastroenterol Hepatol 1997;9:1005–1008.

83   Peroutka SJ: Drugs effective in the therapy of migraine; in Hardman JG, Limbird LE, Molinoff PB, Ruddon RW, Gilman AG (eds): Goodman & Gilman's The Pharmacological Basis of Therapeutics ed 9. New York, McGraw-Hill, 1996, pp 487–502.

84   Mathew NT: Dosing and administration of ergotamine tartrate and dihydroergotamine. Headache 1997;37(suppl 1):S26–S32.

85   Silberstein SD, Young WB: Safety and efficacy of ergotamine tartrate and dihydroergotamine in the treatment of migraine and status migrainosus. Working Panel of the Headache and Facial Pain Section of the American Academy of Neurology. Neurology 1995;45:577–584.

86   Nakasa H, Nakamura H, Ono S, Tsutsui M, Kiuchi M, Ohmori S, Kitada M: Prediction of drug-drug interactions of zonisamide metabolism in humans from in vitro data. Eur J Clin Pharmacol 1998;54:177–183.

87   Iribarne C, Berthou F, Baird S, Dreano Y, Picart D, Bail JP, Beaune P, Menez JF: Involvement of cytochrome P450 3A4 enzyme in the N-demethylation of methadone in human liver microsomes. Chem Res Toxicol 1996;9:365–373.

88   Elkind AH: Drug abuse and headache. Med Clin North Am 1991;75:717–732.

89   Gallagher RM: Ergotamine withdrawal causing 'rebound headache'. J Am Osteopath Assoc 1983; 82:677.

90   Mathew NT: Drug-induced headache. Neurol Clin 1990;8:903–912.

91   Iniguez C, Larrode P, Mauri JA, Morales F: Clinical features of daily chronic headache. Rev Neurol 1997;25:1034–1037.

92   Evers S, Schmidt F, Bauer B, Voss H, Grotemeyer KH, Husstedt IW: The impact of ergotamine-induced headache and ergotamine withdrawal on information processing. Psychopharmacology 1999;142:61–67.

93   Di Stefano R: Prophylactic treatment of vascular headaches. Prensa Med Argent 1965;52:1376–1379.

94   Beubler E: Migraine: Dihydroergotamine nasal spray – An alternative. Wien Med Wochenschr 1995; 145:326–331.

95   Silberstein SD, Schulman EA, Hopkins MM: Repetitive intravenous DHE in the treatment of refractory headache. Headache 1990;30:334–339.

Carl G.H. Dahlöf, MD, PhD, Associate Professor, Gothenburg Migraine Clinic,
Sociala Husset, Uppg. D, SE-411 17 Gothenburg (Sweden)
Tel. +46 31 774 1375, Fax +46 31 774 1086, E-Mail carl.dahlof@migraineclinic.se

Diener HC (ed): Drug Treatment of Migraine and Other Headaches.
Monogr Clin Neurosci. Basel, Karger, 2000, vol 17, pp 83–92

....

Sumatriptan – Pharmacology

Helen E. Connor

Glaxo Wellcome R&D Ltd, Stevenage, Herts, UK

Sumatriptan (Imigran[TM] or Imitrex[TM]), a $5\text{-}HT_{1B/1D}$ receptor agonist, is the first of a novel class of drug for the acute treatment of migraine. The efficacy of sumatriptan in alleviating both the headache, and the associated symptoms of a migraine attack, is now well established by data from many rigorously designed, placebo-controlled clinical trials [see 1, 2 for review and chapter 7.2 of this book]. Sumatriptan was first made widely available in Europe for the acute treatment of migraine and cluster headache in 1991. To date, sumatriptan has been used worldwide by more than 9 million patients in the treatment of more than 180 million attacks of migraine. This review will describe the pharmacology of sumatriptan, focusing particularly on the preclinical and clinical pharmacology that is most relevant to its use in the treatment of migraine.

The hypothesis behind the discovery of sumatriptan was based on the knowledge that vasoconstrictor agents, including 5-HT (5-hydroxytryptamine, serotonin), effectively alleviate a migraine attack and that several commonly used anti-migraine drugs (e.g. ergotamine and methysergide) interact with 5-HT receptors [3]. Early research revealed differences in the 5-HT receptor subtypes mediating vasoconstriction in the cranial compared to the peripheral vasculature. Hence it was hypothesized that a drug which selectively constricted the cranial vasculature without the undesirable effects of 5-HT (e.g. peripheral vasoconstriction, bronchoconstriction, effects in the gastro-intestinal system) would have benefit as a novel acute treatment for migraine [4].

Receptor-Binding Profile of Sumatriptan

Sumatriptan was designed as a selective agonist for the $5\text{-}HT_1$ receptor mediating vasoconstriction in the cranial vasculature [4]. Sumatriptan (fig. 1) is

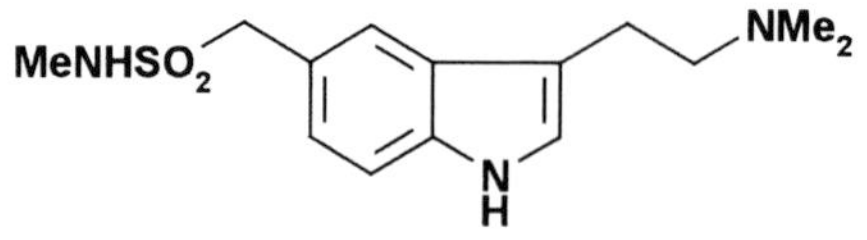

Sumatriptan (3-[2-dimethylamino]ethyl-N-methyl-1H indole-5-methane sulphonamide)

Fig. 1. Chemical structure of sumatriptan.

chemically related to the endogenous hormone, 5-HT and was first synthesized in the mid 1980s. Sumatriptan was discovered from a chemical programme, using 5-HT as a starting point, which aimed to identify novel com- pounds with activity at 5-HT$_1$ receptors but without activity at other 5-HT receptor subtypes, many of which mediate undesirable effects of 5-HT. Recent advances in the classification of 5-HT receptors, primarily driven by the molecular cloning of several new subtypes, have now identified 14 different 5-HT receptor subtypes, divided into seven different families (5-HT$_{1-7}$) [5]. The 5-HT$_1$ receptor group is now known to be heterogeneous, consisting of five different subtypes: 5-HT$_{1A}$, 5-HT$_{1B}$ (previously 5-HT$_{1D\beta}$), 5-HT$_{1D}$ (previously 5-HT$_{1D\alpha}$), 5-HT$_{1E}$ and 5-HT$_{1F}$.

Sumatriptan is a potent, selective 5-HT$_{1B/1D/1F}$ receptor agonist, having high affinity for human 5-HT$_{1B}$, and 5-HT$_{1D}$ receptors, slightly lower affinity at 5-HT$_{1F}$ receptors, and weak activity at 5-HT$_{1A}$ and 5-HT$_{1E}$ receptors (table 1) [6, 7]. At clinically relevant doses, concentrations of sumatriptan achieved doses (Cmax of 54–77 ng/ml, equivalent to 0.1–0.2 μM; [8]) are unlikely to be within the range required to activate 5-HT$_{1A}$ or 5-HT$_{1E}$ receptors. Sumatriptan has no significant activity at other 5-HT$_1$ receptor types (5-HT$_{2-7}$; table 1), or at a wide range of other non 5-HT receptors and ion channels (e.g. adrenergic, dopaminergic and histamine receptors) [6, 7 and Glaxo Wellcome unpublished data]. Recent research has focused on the relative importance of 5-HT$_{1B}$, 5-HT$_{1D}$ and 5-HT$_{1F}$ receptors in mediating the clinical efficacy of sumatriptan.

Sumatriptan Pharmacodynamics

Vasoconstrictor Effects of Sumatriptan
Cranial Vasoconstrictor Effects. There is now extensive preclinical data to show that sumatriptan contracts isolated intracranial arteries from a variety

---

Connor

Table 1. Affinity of sumatriptan at 5-HT and non-5-HT receptors

Receptor	Sumatriptan affinity (pK_i or pIC_{50})
5-HT$_{1A}$	6.0
5-HT$_{1B}$	7.9
5-HT$_{1D}$	7.9
5-HT$_{1E}$	5.6
5-HT$_{1F}$	7.6
5-HT$_{2A}$	<5
5-HT$_3$	<5
5-HT$_4$	<5
5-HT$_5$	<6.8
α1-adrenoceptors	<5
α2-adrenoceptors	<5
Dopamine D1	<5
Dopamine D2	<5
Muscarinic	<5

See [6] for more information and individual references for above data.

of species, including man [4, 6]. Hence sumatriptan contracts human isolated basilar artery (EC_{50} value of approx 0.3 μM) and causes vasoconstriction of the human isolated perfused dura mater via activation of 5-HT$_1$ receptors [6]. Use of antagonists and experiments to look at distribution of the various 5-HT$_1$ receptor subtypes have shown that this cranial vasoconstrictor effect of sumatriptan is mediated via activation of 5-HT$_{1B}$ receptors on the cranial vascular smooth muscle [6, 9]. Sumatriptan also constricts large pial arteries in anaesthetized cats following local application to the perivascular space. However, no vasoconstrictor effects on pial arteries were seen if sumatriptan was administered systemically in these studies [6]. In anaesthetized dogs, sumatriptan selectively constricts the carotid vasculature (increase in carotid vascular resistance; the dose of sumatriptan causing 50% maximum effect is 39 µg/kg i.v.; [4]).

The cranial vasoconstrictor effect of sumatriptan has now been confirmed in several clinical studies. For example using a transcranial Doppler technique, sumatriptan (6 mg s.c.) significantly increased blood flow velocity in the internal carotid and middle cerebral arteries of migraineurs, indicative of vasoconstriction [10, 11]. In a more recent study using angiography, evidence was obtained to show that sumatriptan (after s.c. or intra-arterial injection) had a vasoconstrictor effect on dural vessels in humans [12]. However importantly, both preclinical and clinical data show that sumatriptan does not reduce regional cerebral blood flow [11, 13]. The intracranial vasoconstrictor action of sumatriptan occurs at the level of the large conducting cerebral arteries and not at the level of the resistance arterioles in the cerebral circulation. Hence sumatriptan does not cause changes in cerebral nutrient blood flow.

Peripheral Vasoconstrictor Effects. Sumatriptan has little or no vasoconstrictor effect in a variety of peripheral blood vessels [4, 6]. This is because 5-HT_{2A} receptors, at which sumatriptan has no significant effect, predominantly mediate peripheral vasoconstriction. The selective carotid vasoconstrictor effect of sumatriptan in anaesthetized dogs, with little effect in other vascular beds (e.g. coronary) and little or no change in arterial blood pressure confirms the lack of generalized peripheral vasoconstriction with this compound [4, 6]. This is in marked contrast to the effects of ergotamine which, after i.v. administration, causes vasoconstriction in several vascular beds and marked increases in blood pressure, indicative of widespread vasoconstrictor effects [4, 6].

Sumatriptan, and other compounds of the 5-$HT_{1B/1D}$ class, cause small contractions of human epicardial coronary arteries [14, 15]. This reflects the presence of a small population of 5-HT_{1B} receptors in these vessels, although 5-HT_{2A} receptors, at which sumatriptan has no significant effect, predominantly mediate the contractile effects of 5-HT [14]. A recent study, using human epicardial isolated coronary arteries, compared the magnitude of contraction achieved with several 5-$HT_{1B/1D}$ receptor agonists, colloquially known as triptans, and showed that all these compounds produced a small, but similar maximum response at high concentrations [15]. However, at concentrations equivalent to therapeutic plasma levels achieved on clinical dosing, there was little or no contraction of coronary arteries [15]. Nevertheless, these data account for the labelling restriction where sumatriptan and other drugs of this class are contra-indicated in patients with coronary artery disease.

Cranial Vasoconstriction: Relevance to Mechanism of Action in Migraine. The selective intracranial vasoconstrictor action of sumatriptan has been proposed as the mechanism underlying its clinical efficacy in migraine [16]. This is explained on the basis of activation of the trigeminovascular system during a migraine headache where large intracranial arteries are distended, oedematous and pain-sensitive. Sumatriptan, via cranial vasoconstriction, is thought to normalize vessel tone and reduce afferent noxious firing in the trigeminal nerve, leading to relief of headache and other migraine symptoms (fig. 2). However, direct inhibition of trigeminal nerves either peripherally or centrally (see below) has also been proposed to account for the clinical efficacy of sumatriptan (fig. 2) [17]. To date, it is not clear which of these actions is most important for clinical efficacy [18], and indeed it may be that a combination

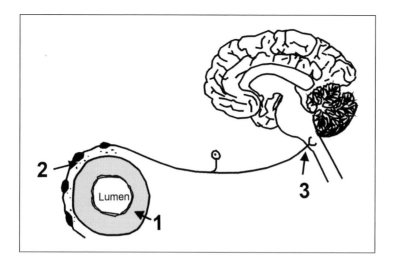

Fig. 2. Schematic diagram to illustrate the three possible mechanisms of action of sumatriptan in migraine. *1* Selective constriction of large intracranial arteries, *2* inhibition of neuropeptide release from peripheral trigeminal nerve terminals and *3* central inhibition of trigeminal nerve firing. See text for more details.

of effects (vasoconstriction and trigeminal inhibition) accounts for the effective relief of migraine with sumatriptan, and other compounds of this class.

Effects of Sumatriptan on Peripheral Trigeminal Nerves

Moskowitz et al. [19] developed a rodent model to try and mimic the peripheral consequences of trigeminal nerve activation in the cranial circulation during a migraine attack. This involved electrical stimulation of the trigeminal nerve to elicit neuropeptide release from peripheral trigeminal nerve terminals and the subsequent development of plasma protein extravasation in intracranial (dura) and extracranial tissues. Sumatriptan inhibits the development of plasma protein extravasation in the dura mater at doses that are similar to clinically effective doses [19]. This effect of sumatriptan is attributed to activation of prejunctional inhibitory receptors on trigeminal nerve terminals to cause inhibition of transmitter release and hence blockade of trigeminal nerve firing (fig. 2) [17, 19]. Recently the predictive value of this dural plasma protein extravasation model for clinical efficacy in migraine has been questioned [20] and to date cranial neurogenic inflammation has not been shown to occur in man during a migraine attack [e.g. 20]. However, there is preclinical data to show that sumatriptan can directly inhibit neuronal release of CGRP (calcitonin gene-related peptide) and substance P, for example in rat isolated spinal cord [21]. Furthermore, sumatriptan (6 mg s.c.) inhibits the increase in CGRP levels measured in plasma from the external jugular vein of patients during a migraine attack [22]. Hence despite concerns about the clinical validity of the dural plasma extravasation model, peripheral inhibition of neuropeptide release from peripheral trigeminal nerve terminals by sumatriptan may contribute to its clinical efficacy in migraine.

There has been a lot of interest in identifying which 5-HT receptor subtype mediates the neuronal inhibitory effect of sumatriptan. This would provide further understanding of sumatriptan's mechanism of action, and perhaps more importantly, could identify a molecular target for novel drugs that would inhibit the trigeminal nerve without having concomitant vasoconstrictor effects. Studies to date have suggested that 5-HT_{1D} [23] and 5-HT_{1F} receptors [24] may play a role in peripheral inhibition of the trigeminal nerve. However, a role for 5-HT_{1B} receptors has not yet been excluded. Clinical trials with selective 5-HT_{1D} and 5-HT_{1F} receptor agonists in migraine patients are currently ongoing and results will be key to understanding the importance of these receptors as targets for migraine treatment.

Central Effects of Sumatriptan

In anaesthetized cats, sumatriptan inhibits neuronal firing in the trigeminal nucleus caudalis after i.v. administration only when the blood-brain barrier is disrupted [25]. The trigeminal nucleus caudalis is the first central site of termination of trigeminal fibres arising from the cranial vasculature and synapse with second order fibres. Furthermore, direct iontophoretic application of sumatriptan to nerve cells in the trigeminal nucleus caudalis of anaesthetized cats markedly inhibits nerve firing [26]. Sumatriptan, a relatively hydrophilic drug, only very poorly penetrates the blood-brain barrier under normal circumstances [6, 25]. In contrast, some of the more recently identified $5\text{-HT}_{1B/1D}$ agonists (e.g. naratriptan, zolmitriptan) are slightly more lipophilic, and hence can more readily gain access to centrally inhibit trigeminal neuronal firing [27], possibly via an action at central 5-HT_{1D} or 5-HT_{1F} receptors. Whether this central site of action contributes to the clinical efficacy of $5\text{-HT}_{1B/1D}$ agonists is currently a subject of debate [27]. However, it has been suggested that there may be some breakdown of the blood-brain barrier during a migraine attack such that sumatriptan could then gain access to the trigeminal nucleus caudalis (fig. 2).

Effects of Sumatriptan in Animal Models of Pain

Whether sumatriptan has antinociceptive activity has been studied in a range of animal models, using various noxious (thermal, pressure, inflammatory) stimuli. However, even after very high doses administered peripherally

Table 2. Summary of sumatriptan pharmacokinetics

Route of administration (single dose)	Sub-cutaneous [32] 6 mg	Oral [32] 25 mg	Oral [29] 100 mg	Suppos [32] 25 mg	Intranasal [32] 20 mg
C_{max} (ng/ml)	69.5	16.5	54	22.9	12.9
t_{max} (h)	0.17	1.5	1.5	1.0	1.5
F relative to sub-cut (%)	–	14.3	14[a]	19.2	15.8
$t_{1/2}$ (h)	1.9	1.7	2	1.8	1.8
AUC (ng/ml h^{-1})	89.3	53.3	197	71.3	47.5

[a] Absolute bioavailability.

AUC = Area under the plasma concentration-time curve; C_{max} = peak plasma concentration; F = bioavailability; t_{max} = time to peak plasma concentration.

and directly into the CNS, sumatriptan had no generalized anti-nociceptive actions in rodent pain models [28]. Hence sumatriptan appears to be selective for migraine pain.

Sumatriptan Pharmacokinetics

The pharmacokinetic properties of sumatriptan following oral, subcutaneous, intranasal and rectal administration to healthy volunteers and patients have been presented and reviewed previously in detail [e.g. 1, 8, 29]. This review will highlight only the key points from the many pharmacokinetic clinical studies that have been performed to date. Pharmacokinetic parameters for the various formulations of sumatriptan are summarized in table 2.

Sumatriptan 50 and 100 mg tablets are available; 25 mg sumatriptan tablets are available in some markets. The oral bioavailability of sumatriptan is relatively low (14% mean absolute oral bioavailability) [8]. This primarily reflects extensive first pass metabolism [8]. Mean t_{max} values range from 1.0–2.3 h after oral dosing [2, 8, 29]; however 80% of C_{max} plasma levels are achieved within 45 min of oral administration of sumatriptan to healthy subjects [29]. Administration of oral sumatriptan with food did not significantly change absorption of the drug in healthy subjects [29]. Furthermore, oral absorption of sumatriptan was not significantly changed during (compared to outside), a migraine attack in patients [30], despite delayed gastric emptying being reported to occur in migraine.

After subcutaneous administration, sumatriptan (6 mg) is rapidly absorbed, with a t_{max} of 0.17–0.23 h and high bioavailability (mean value of 96%)

[2, 8, 29]. The subcutaneous formulation of sumatriptan provides very rapid relief of migraine headache [2]. Intranasal administration of sumatriptan produces faster absorption than oral administration, although maximum plasma levels (t_{max}) occur after 1.0–1.5 h and bioavailability is similar [31, 32]. The nasal spray sumatriptan formulation (20 mg dose) provides a quick onset, non-oral alternative for patients who, for example, are nauseous/vomiting during their migraine. Sumatriptan (25 mg) suppositories are available in some markets; C_{max}, t_{max}, $t_{0.5}$ and AUC values reported after rectal administration of sumatriptan are similar to values obtained after oral dosing [2, 32, 33].

Sumatriptan has a relatively large volume of distribution, indicating that the drug is extensively distributed in tissues [29]. Sumatriptan is mainly metabolized to the pharmacologically inactive indole acetic acid analogue, which is mainly excreted in the urine with a small amount excreted in the faeces. After oral administration, 3% of the sumatriptan dose is excreted unchanged in the urine, and 9% of unchanged drug is excreted in the faeces [8, 29]. The plasma half-life ($t_{0.5}$) of sumatriptan is about 2 h, irrespective of route of administration [2, 32]. In vitro plasma protein binding of sumatriptan is low over a wide range of drug concentrations [29].

Drug Interactions

Studies to date indicate that the pharmacokinetics of sumatriptan are not modified by concomitant administration of dihydroergotamine, propranolol, flunarizine, pizotifen, butorphanol, naratriptan and paroxetine, or by alcohol (ethanol) (reviewed in [2]). However, systemic sumatriptan exposure was increased in healthy subjects treated with the monoamine oxidase inhibitor, moclobemide [34].

Conclusions

Sumatriptan, the first of a novel class of drug, has provided a significant advance in the acute treatment of migraine. Sumatriptan is a selective 5-$HT_{1B/1D/1F}$ agonist and causes selective cranial vasoconstriction, via 5-HT_{1B} activation, and inhibition of the trigeminal nerve. The 5-HT_1 receptor subtype responsible for the neuronal inhibitory effect of sumatriptan still has not been definitively identified. The discovery of sumatriptan has stimulated a lot of research, both preclinical and clinical, into its mechanism of action in migraine. However, the debate as to whether cranial vasoconstriction or trigeminal neuronal inhibition is most important for clinical efficacy is still ongoing.

Future studies on the pathological mechanisms underlying migraine and clinical testing of 5-HT$_1$ receptor subtype selective agonists will provide valuable insight into this question.

Acknowledgement

The assistance of Dr. Eliane Fuseau, Clinical Pharmacology, Glaxo Wellcome, Greenford in the preparation of this manuscript is gratefully acknowledged.

References

1 Tfelt-Hansen P: Efficacy and adverse events of subcutaneous, oral, and intranasal sumatriptan used for migraine treatment: A systematic review based on number needed to treat. Cephalalgia 1998; 18:532–538.
2 Perry CM, Markham A: Sumatriptan. An updated review of its use in migraine. Drugs. 1998;55: 889–922.
3 Humphrey PPA: 5-Hydroxytryptamine and the pathophysiology of migraine. J Neurol 1991; 238(suppl 1):S38–S44.
4 Humphrey PPA, Feniuk W, Perren MJ, Connor HE, Oxford AW: The pharmacology of the novel 5-HT$_1$-like receptor agonist, GR43175. Cephalalgia 1989; 9(suppl 9):23–33.
5 Hoyer D, Martin GR: 5-HT receptor classification and nomenclature: Towards a harmonisation with the human genome. Neuropharmacol 1997;36:419–428.
6 Beattie DT, Connor HE, Feniuk W, Humphrey PPA: The pharmacology of sumatriptan. Rev Contemp Pharmacother 1994;5:285–294.
7 Connor HE, Beattie DT: 5-Hydroxytryptamine receptor subtypes: Relation to migraine; in Edvinsson L (ed): Migraine Pathophysiology. London, Martin Dunitz Ltd, 1999, pp 43–52.
8 Lacey LF, Hussey EK, Fowler PA: Single dose pharmacokinetics of sumatriptan in healthy volunteers. Eur J Clin Pharmacol 1995;47:543–548.
9 Longmore J, Shaw D, Smith D, Hopkins R, McAllister G, Pickard JD, Sirinathsinghji DJ, Butler AJ, Hill RG: Differential distribution of 5HT1D- and 5HT1B-immunoreactivity within the human trigemino-cerebrovascular system: Implications for the discovery of new antimigraine drugs. Cephalalgia 1997;17:833–842.
10 Caekebeke JF, Ferrari MD, Zwetsloot CP, Jansen J, Saxena PR: Antimigraine drug sumatriptan increases blood flow velocity in large cerebral arteries during migraine attacks. Neurology 1992;42: 1522–1526.
11 Friberg L, Olesen J, Iversen HK, Sperling B: Migraine pain associated with middle cerebral dilatation: Reversal by sumatriptan. Lancet 1991;338:13–17.
12 Henkes H, May A, Kühne D, Berg-Dammer E, Diener HC: Sumatriptan: Vasoactive effect on human dural vessels, demonstrated by subselective angiography. Cephalalgia 1996;16:224–230.
13 Perren MJ, Feniuk W, Humphrey PPA: The selective closure of feline carotid arteriovenous anastomoses (AVAs) by GR43175. Cephalalgia 1989;9(suppl 9):41–46.
14 Connor HE, Feniuk W, Humphrey PPA: 5-Hydroxtryptamine contracts human coronary arteries predominantly via 5-HT$_2$ receptor activation. Eur J Pharmacol 1989;161:91–94.
15 MaassenVanDenBrink A, Reekers M, Bax WA, Ferrari MD, Saxena PR: Coronary side-effect potential of current and prospective antimigraine drugs. Circulation 1998;98:25–30.
16 Humphrey PPA, Feniuk W: Mode of action of the anti-migraine drug sumatriptan. Trends Pharmacol Sci 1991;12:444–446.
17 Moskowitz MA: Neurogenic versus vascular mechanisms of sumatriptan and ergot alkaloids in migraine. Trends Pharmac Sci 1992;13:307–311.

18   Humphrey PPAH, Goadsby PJ: The mode of action of sumatriptan is vascular? A debate. Cephalalgia 1994;14:401–410.

19   Buzzi MG, Moskowitz MA: The anti-migraine drug sumatriptan (GR43175) selectively blocks neurogenic blocks plasma extravasation from blood vessels in dura mater. Br J Pharmacol 1990; 99:202–206.

20   May A, Shepheard SL, Knorr M, Effert R, Wessing A, Hargreaves RJ, Goadsby PJ, Diener HC: Retinal plasma extravasation in animals but not in humans: Implications for the pathophysiology of migraine. Brain 1998;121:1231–1237.

21   Arvieu L, Mauborgne A, Bourgoin S, Oliver C, Feltz P, Hamon P, Cesselin F: Sumatriptan inhibits the release of CGRP and substance P from the rat spinal cord. Neuroreport 1996;7:1973–1976.

22   Edvinsson L, Goadsby PJ: Neuropeptides in migraine and cluster headache. Cephalalgia 1994;14: 320–327.

23   MacLeod AM, Street LJ, Reeve AJ, Jelley RA, Sternfeld F, Beer MS, Stanton JA, Watt AP, Rathbone D, Matassa VG: Selective, orally active 5-HT$_{1D}$ receptor agonists as potential antimigraine agents. J Med Chem 1997;40:3501–3503.

24   Johnson KW, Schaus JM, Durkin MM, Audia JE, Kaldor SW, Flaugh ME, Adham N, Zgombick JM, Cohen ML, Branchek TA, Phebus LA: 5-HT$_{1F}$ receptor agonists inhibit neurogenic dural inflammation in guinea pigs. Neuroreport 1997;8:2237–2240.

25   Kaube H, Hoskin KL, Goadsby PJ: Inhibition by sumatriptan of central trigeminal neurones only after blood-brain barrier disruption. Brit J Pharmacol 1993;109:788–792.

26   Storer RJ, Goadsby PJ: Microiontophoretic application of serotonin (5HT)1B/1D agonists inhibits trigeminal cell firing in the cat. Brain 1997;120:2171–2177.

27   Hoskin KL, Goadsby PJ: Comparison of more and less lipophilic serotonin (5HT$_{1B/1D}$) agonists in a model of trigeminovascular nociception in cat. Exp Neurol 1998;150:45–51.

28   Skingle M, Birch PJ, Leighton GE, Humphrey PP: Lack of antinociceptive activity of sumatriptan in rodents. Cephalalgia 1990;10:207–212.

29   Fowler P, Lacey LF, Thomas M, Keene ON, Tanner RJ, Baber NS: The clinical pharmacology, pharmacokinetics and metabolism of sumatriptan. Eur Neurol 1991;31:291–294.

30   Sramek JJ, Hussey EK, Clements B, Cutler NR: Oral sumatriptan pharmacokinetics in the migraine state. Clin Drug Invest 1999;17:137–144.

31   Moore KHP, Hussey EK, Shaw S, Fuseau E, Duquesnoy C, Pakes GE: Safety, tolerability and pharmacokinetics of sumatriptan in healthy subjects following ascending single intranasal doses and multiple intranasal doses. Cephalalgia 1997;17:541–550.

32   Duquesnoy C, Mamet JP, Sumner D, Fuseau E: Comparative clinical pharmacokinetics of single doses of sumatriptan following subcutaneous, oral, rectal and intranasal administration. Eur J Pharm Sci 1998;6:99–104.

33   Kunka RL, Hussey EK, Shaw S, Warner P, Aubert B, Richard I, Fowler PA, Pakes GE: Safety, tolerability and pharmacokinetics of sumatriptan suppositories following single and multiple doses in healthy volunteers. Cephalalgia 1997;17:532–540.

34   Williams P, Fuseau E, Cosson V, Barrow A: Sumatriptan pharmacokinetics are significantly altered by monoamine oxidase inhibitor co-administration. Cephalalgia 1997;17:408.

Helen E. Connor, PhD, Glaxo Wellcome R&D Ltd, Stevenage, Herts, SG1 2NY (UK)
Tel. +44 1438 745 745, Fax +44 1438 763 363, E-Mail hec4466@glaxowellcome.co.uk

Diener HC (ed): Drug Treatment of Migraine and Other Headaches.
Monogr Clin Neurosci. Basel, Karger, 2000, vol 17, pp 93–109

··························

Sumatriptan – Therapy

H.C. Diener

Department of Neurology, University of Essen, Essen, Germany

Sumatriptan, the first selective $5HT_{1B/1D}$ agonist marketed for the treatment of migraine, was introduced in 1991 in injectable form. Sumatriptan is now available in tablet, nasal spray, injectable, and in some countries, suppository formulations. Through December 1998, more than 60,000 patients and healthy volunteers have used sumatriptan to treat more than 300,000 migraine attacks in clinical trials, and sumatriptan injection or tablets were used to treat an estimated 180 million migraine attacks in worldwide practice for more than 90 million patient exposures. This chapter reviews pivotal data on the efficacy and tolerability of sumatriptan.

Efficacy

In controlled studies, approximately 80% of patients treated with sumatriptan injection (6 mg) [1, 2] and 70% (range 65 to 78%) of patients treated with sumatriptan tablets (25 mg, 50 mg, 100 mg) [3] or sumatriptan nasal spray (20 mg) [4] experience pain relief 2 h after dosing. The effectiveness of sumatriptan in alleviating migraine-associated symptoms such as nausea, photophobia, and phonophobia is similarly high. The times to onset of action for pain relief with sumatriptan injection, nasal spray, and tablets are 10 min, 15 min and 30 min, respectively. This section considers pivotal efficacy data on sumatriptan injection, tablets and nasal spray in the acute treatment of migraine.

Sumatriptan Injection

The evaluation of an optimal dosage regimen for sumatriptan was conducted in an international, multicenter, double-blind, placebo-controlled trial [1] (n = 639) by 'The Subcutaneous Sumatriptan International Study Group'.

Headache relief was rapid: 50 and 56% of patients receiving 6 or 8 mg sumatriptan injection reported headache relief 30 min post-dose compared with 16% of placebo patients. Headache relief 1 h post-dose was reported by 72 and 79% of patients receiving 6 and 8 mg sumatriptan, respectively, compared with 25% of placebo patients. Sumatriptan injection was significantly more effective than placebo beginning 10 min post-dose. Sumatriptan was similarly effective at relieving nausea, photophobia, and phonophobia as well as migraine-associated clinical disability. Neither migraine type (migraine with vs. without aura) nor attack duration before treatment (up to or more than 4 h) affected efficacy of sumatriptan injection.

The efficacy of sumatriptan injection 6 mg was further evaluated in two identical multicenter, double-blind, randomized, placebo-controlled studies [2] conducted in the United States. Results of the two studies were combined. Headache relief was reported by significantly more patients using sumatriptan injection 6 mg than placebo beginning 10 min post-dose. Headache relief 1 h post-dose was reported by 70% of patients using sumatriptan injection 6 mg compared with 22% of patients on placebo.

In a retrospective analysis of these two trials [5], 157 women were identified as treating menstrual migraine (migraine beginning 1 to 4 days from the onset of menstrual flow). A total of 104 patients were treated with subcutaneous sumatriptan 6 mg and 53 with placebo. One hour after treatment, 80% of menstrual migraine patients who received sumatriptan reported headache relief compared with 19% who received placebo (p < 0.001). These results were similar to those from 512 female patients in the same trials with non-menstrual migraine (sumatriptan 70%; placebo 20%). Sumatriptan also treated nausea and photophobia more effective than did placebo.

These early trials demonstrated that a single dose of sumatriptan injection 6 mg was effective in the acute treatment of migraine. Headache relief was rapid, commencing within 10 min of treatment. Approximately 50% of patients reported a response after 30 min, 70% or more after 1 h with over 80% responding 2 h after one or two doses. The extent of headache improvement was independent of migraine type and attack duration before treatment. Over 60% of sumatriptan-treated patients were headache-free within 2 h; by 6 h over 75% had complete resolution of headache. There was no significant benefit from giving a second 6 mg dose at 1 h to non-responders. There was no additional benefit in efficacy from 8 mg sumatriptan compared with the 6 mg dose.

As migraine is an intermittent, recurring disorder, most patients require repeated courses of acute therapy, a pattern of use which may affect the efficacy and tolerability of a drug. Tolerance, a reduced responsiveness to a drug as a consequence of repeated use, may quickly develop, and repeated courses of therapy can affect the type and severity of drug-related side effects. A multicenter, randomized, double-blind, placebo-controlled, crossover study [6] (n = 170) was conducted to investigate the efficacy and tolerability of single-dose sumatriptan injection 6 mg administered for multiple migraine attacks and to assess the impact of migraine on patients' lives and their perceptions of sumatriptan relative to their usual acute therapies. Patients were treated for four moderate or severe migraine attacks in the clinic in one of four sequences (P = placebo; S = sumatriptan): PSSS, SPSS, SSPS, or SSSP. Each study treatment was separated by a headache-free interval of at least 24 h. Similar proportions of patients receiving sumatriptan injection 6 mg (86 to 90%) reported headache relief 90 min after treatment across the four attacks, and significantly more (p < 0.001) than following placebo (9 to 38%). A total of 73% of patients responded after 1 h to all three attacks they treated with sumatriptan; 89% responded at least two out of three times; and 96% responded at least one out of three times.

Headache recurrence, where initial relief is followed within 24 h of dosing by the reappearance of moderate or severe headache, was reported by about 30 to 45% of patients in short-term trials with sumatriptan injection 6 mg. A large multicenter, double-blind, placebo-controlled trial [7] (n = 881) was therefore conducted to further investigate the incidence of headache recurrence after a 6-mg dose and the efficacy and tolerability of a second 6-mg dose in the treatment of headache recurrence. Patients treated up to three migraine attacks during a 3-month period, initially with an open 6-mg dose of sumatriptan injection. Patients were randomized at study entry to receive an optional second injection of either sumatriptan 6 mg or placebo in the event of headache recurrence (defined as an initial severe or moderate headache which improved to mild or none, 1 h after the initial sumatriptan dose but which then worsened to severe or moderate within 1 to 24 h). Over the three attacks, headache relief 2 h post-dose was reported by 76 to 83% of patients after the initial dose of sumatriptan. A minority of patients (10 to 16%) reported recurrence over the three attacks. Significantly more patients taking sumatriptan as their second dose reported relief of headache recurrence over all three attacks compared with those taking placebo. Over 80% of patients taking sumatriptan reported headache relief 1 h after their initial second dose.

The long-term efficacy of sumatriptan injection has also been evaluated. In one study [8], patients who treated a single migraine attack with sumatriptan injection 6 mg or placebo could treat all attacks over 6 months with sumatriptan injection 6 mg plus a further 6 mg after 1 h if necessary. Eighty migraine patients treated 1,566 migraine attacks during the 6 months. Headache relief 1 h post-dose was reported in a mean 77% of attacks during the 6 months – 83% in the first 3 months and 76% in the second 3 months. There was no evidence of tachyphylaxis over the 6-month treated period. Patients with very frequent migraine attacks, however, were excluded. Patients consistently reported headache relief with sumatriptan: 63% of patients responded in more than 80% of their attacks, and 49% of patients responded in more than 90% of attacks. These data show that the efficacy of sumatriptan injection administered over the long-term is similar to that observed in short-term, placebo-controlled trials.

Tfelt-Hansen [9] performed a meta-analysis of 12 randomized controlled trials (RCT) with subcutaneous sumatriptan. The success rate of sumatriptan after 1 h was 69% (1337/1927) and of placebo 19% (226/1200) resulting in a number needed to treat (NNT) of 2.0 (95% confidence interval 1.9–2.1) and a number needed to harm (NNH) of 3.0 (2.7–3.4).

Sumatriptan Tablets

Although sumatriptan injection provides highly effective and rapid relief of migraine, oral administration is a more convenient route for many patients. An early study [10] with sumatriptan tablets showed that doses of 100-mg, 200 mg, and 300 mg provided similar, effective degrees of headache relief within 2 h of dosing. The 100-mg dose was better tolerated than the 200-mg or 300-mg doses. Subsequent trials evaluated doses up to and including 100 mg. In two randomized, double-blind, placebo-controlled studies [11, 12] conducted in the United States, sumatriptan tablets (25 mg, 50 mg, 100 mg) compared with placebo alleviated migraine pain and associated symptoms such as nausea and photophobia. In the first study, headache relief 2 h post-dose was reported by 52, 50, and 56% of patients using sumatriptan tablets 25 mg, 50 mg, and 100 mg, compared with 38% of placebo patients (p < 0.05 each dose vs. placebo). In the second study, headache relief 2 h post-dose was reported by 52, 54 and 57% of patients using sumatriptan tablets 25 mg, 50 mg and 100 mg, compared with 19% of placebo patients (p < 0.05 each dose vs. placebo).

These two studies of the 25-mg, 50-mg and 100-mg doses did not have sufficient statistical power to distinguish among the three doses or to provide definitive data for the clinical profiles of the 25-mg and 50-mg doses. Therefore a larger, multinational, randomized, double-blind, placebo-controlled, parallel-group trial [3] evaluating the efficacy and tolerability of 25-mg, 50-mg and 100-mg doses of oral sumatriptan was carried out by Pfaffenrath and colleagues. The trial, conducted at 93 clinical centers in seven countries, involved 1,003 patients who treated up to three migraine attacks, using the same dose for all three attacks. The patients who received sumatriptan as initial treatment were independently randomized to receive either the same dose of sumatriptan or placebo to treat headache recurrence (which was defined as the return of

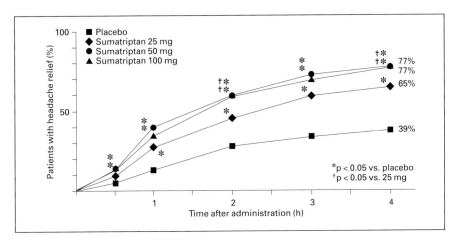

Fig. 1. Percentage of patients with headache relief as a function of time after dosing in a large study of sumatriptan tablets; adapted from Pfaffenrath et al. [3].

moderate or severe headache pain within 24 h of initial dosing in patients who had experienced headache relief during the first 4 h after dosing). The proportion of patients experiencing headache relief was significantly greater ($p < 0.05$) among sumatriptan-treated patients than among placebo-treated patients beginning as early as 30 min after dosing for the first attack, for patients taking the 50-mg and 100-mg doses (fig. 1). All of the doses of sumatriptan were significantly better than placebo at providing headache relief at 1, 2, 3 and 4 h after dosing for attack 1. In addition, the 50-mg and 100-mg doses were significantly better than the 25-mg dose at 2 and 4 h after dosing (this was also true for attack 3). By 4 h after dosing for attack 1, headache had been relieved in 65, 77 and 77% of patients in the 25-mg, 50-mg and 100-mg groups, respectively, and completely eliminated in 43, 55 and 58% of patients.

Across all attacks, sumatriptan 100 mg was significantly more effective than a 25-mg dose in providing headache relief beginning 30 min after dosing, when relief was experienced by 15, 12, 11 and 6% of patients in the 100-mg, 50-mg, 25-mg and placebo groups, respectively. Also, across all attacks the 50-mg dose was significantly better than the 25-mg dose beginning 2 h after dosing, when relief was experienced by 79, 78, 67 and 38% of patients in those respective groups.

Consistency of response was notably better for the 50-mg and 100-mg doses than for the 25-mg dose. For the 692 patients who treated three attacks and had all of the relevant data recorded, the proportions reporting headache relief 4 h after dosing in all three attacks, were 38%, 48% and 51% for the 25-mg, 50-mg and 100-mg doses, compared with 11% for placebo. Headache relief was experienced 2 h after dosing in at least two out of three attacks by 51, 61 and 64% of the patients treating three attacks in the 25-mg, 50-mg and 100-mg groups, respectively, compared with 26% in the placebo group; at 4 h after dosing, the corresponding figures were 67, 81 and 81%, compared with 40% in the placebo group.

The 50-mg and 100-mg doses of oral sumatriptan were also superior to the 25-mg dose in alleviating clinical disability (severe impairment of functioning or a need for bed rest) and photophobia or phonophobia.

Although the incidences of headache recurrence were similar across treatment groups, the time to recurrence increased with increasing dose-for attack 1, from 9.00 to 11.75 to 14.00 h for the 25-mg, 50-mg, and 100-mg doses, respectively, compared with 6.13 h for placebo; attacks 2 and 3 had times to recurrence that were similar to those for attack 1. All doses of sumatriptan provided better relief of recurrent headache than did placebo at 2 h after taking the optional second dose of study medication. Considered together, the efficacy data suggest that the 50 mg and 100 mg doses provide optimum efficacy.

Tfelt-Hansen [9] also reported a meta-anlysis of the twelve RCTs performed with 100 mg oral sumatriptan. The success rate was 58% (1067/1854) for sumatriptan compared to 25% (256/1036) for placebo resulting in an NNT of 3.0 (95% CI 2.8–3.4) and NNH of 8.3 (95% CI 6.3–12.2).

Sumatriptan Nasal Spray

Sumatriptan has been widely available around the world in both injectable and oral forms since the beginning of this decade. The recently introduced nasal formulation of sumatriptan complements the oral and injectable offerings and broadens the range of treatment options for migraine patients with nausea who do not want to swallow a tablet. The clinical efficacy of sumatriptan nasal spray was evaluated in five randomized, double-blind, placebo-controlled studies [13–16] employing the currently recommended dosing regimen with the marketed formulation, one active comparator with dihydroergotamine nasal spray [17], and one long-term open-label study [14]. Five randomized, double-blind, placebo-controlled, parallel-group studies were conducted to evaluate the efficacy and tolerability of sumatriptan nasal spray doses ranging from 2.5 mg to 20 mg (table 1). Across the five placebo-controlled studies, headache relief (moderate or severe pain reduced to mild or no pain) 2 h post-dose was reported in a significantly greater percentage of patients treated with sumatriptan nasal spray 20 mg (55 to 64%) compared with placebo-treated patients (25 to 36%; p < 0.05; fig. 2). Across studies, greater proportions of

Table 1. Summary of sumatriptan nasal spray clinical studies

Protocol number	Study design	Doses	No. of patients in intent-to-treat population
S2B-T47 Study 1 [13]	Randomized, double-blind, placebo-controlled, parallel-group, single-attack	Placebo Sumatriptan 2.5 mg Sumatriptan 5 mg Sumatriptan 10 mg Sumatriptan 20 mg	63 123 122 115 120
S2B-T50 Study 2 [14]	Randomized, double-blind, placebo-controlled, parallel-group, single-attack	Placebo Sumatriptan 10 mg Sumatriptan 20 mg	156 304 301
S2B-340 Study 3 [15]	Randomized, double-blind, placebo-controlled, parallel-group, single-attack	Placebo Sumatriptan 10 mg Sumatriptan 20 mg	100 106 202
S2B-341 Study 4 [15]	Randomized, double-blind, placebo-controlled, parallel-group, single-attack	Placebo Sumatriptan 10 mg Sumatriptan 20 mg	112 109 215
S2B-342 Study 5 [16] [33]	Randomized, double-blind, placebo-controlled, parallel-group, three-attack	Placebo Sumatriptan 5 mg Sumatriptan 10 mg Sumatriptan 20 mg	198 297 294 288
S2B-T60 [14]	Randomized, double-blind, two-attack crossover with dihydroergotamine comparator	Sumatriptan 20 mg Dihydroergotamine 1 mg	185 183
S2B-T51 [14]	Open-label, 12-month	Sumatriptan 20 mg	182

patients treated with sumatriptan nasal spray 20 mg compared with 10 mg or 5 mg, reported headache relief 2 h post-dose (fig. 2). Headache relief rates did not differ with gender, weight, or age of the patient; duration of migraine prior to treatment (<4 h or >4 h); presence or absence of aura; previous use of sumatriptan; or use of migraine prophylaxis. Onset of headache relief compared with placebo was observed as early as 15 min post-dose (the earliest time point measured) among patients treated with sumatriptan nasal spray 20 mg in three of the five placebo-controlled studies.

The efficacy of sumatriptan nasal spray administered for multiple attacks was examined in the S2B-342 study, in which the same dose of sumatriptan nasal spray or placebo was administered for up to three attacks occurring over a 6-month period. The results demonstrate that sumatriptan nasal spray

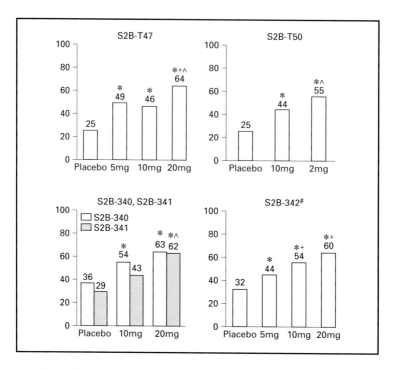

Fig. 2. Percentage of patients reporting headache relief 2 h post-dose in five placebo-controlled studies of sumatriptan nasal spray. Patient numbers per group ranged from 63 to 304. *$p < 0.05$ vs. placebo; ⁺$p < 0.05$ vs. 5 mg; ∧ $p < 0.05$ vs. 10 mg; # Data for all attacks combined. For details see table 1.

maintains its efficacy with repeated use for separate migraine attacks. Headache relief rates 60 and 120 min post-dose examined by individual attack were similar to relief rates for all attacks combined (fig. 3). Similar results were observed for the other efficacy endpoints (data not shown). Patients using sumatriptan nasal spray repeatedly for separate migraine attacks responded consistently to sumatriptan nasal spray. The percentages of patients treating three attacks and experiencing headache relief 2 h post-dose on at least two or three attacks in the sumatriptan 20 mg, 10 mg, 5 mg and placebo groups were 67, 59, 46 and 34%, respectively ($p < 0.05$ each sumatriptan group vs. placebo; sumatriptan 20 mg vs. 5 mg).

The efficacy and tolerability of sumatriptan nasal spray 20 mg (plus placebo optional dose after 30 min) and intranasal dihydroergotamine 1 mg plus 1 mg optional dose after 30 min) were compared in a 2-attack crossover study (S2B-T60). The optional second dose was taken by 81% of patients after initial treatment with dihydroergotamine and by 76% of patients after initial

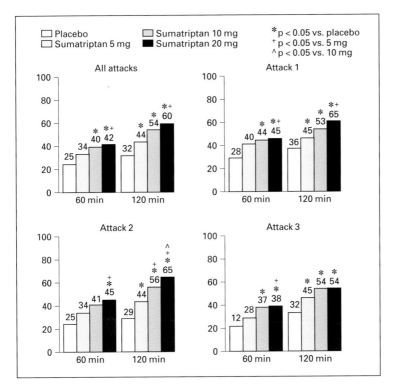

Fig. 3. Percentage of patients with headache relief 1 h and 2 h post-dose in a multiple-attack placebo-controlled study of sumatriptan nasal spray (number of patients see table 1). Adapted from [35].

treatment with sumatriptan nasal spray 20 mg. The results demonstrate that a significantly greater percentage of patients reported headache relief after treatment with sumatriptan nasal spray 20 mg compared with intranasal dihydroergotamine 1 mg beginning 45 min post-dose and continuing through 2 h post-dose (table 2). Although greater percentages of patients reported no associated symptoms (with the exception of vomiting) 2 h after dosing with sumatriptan nasal spray 20 mg compared with dihydroergotamine, these differences were not statistically significant (table 2). The results of this single study suggest that sumatriptan nasal spray is significantly more effective than intranasal dihydroergotamine in the acute treatment of migraine.

Long-term effectiveness of sumatriptan nasal spray 20 mg was examined in an open-label study of the acute treatment of migraine attacks in individual patients for up to 12 months (Study 7 in table 1). The patients enrolled in this continuation study had successfully completed participation in Study 1.

Table 2. Percentages of patients with headache and associated symptom relief in a study comparing the efficacy and tolerability of sumatriptan nasal spray with intranasal dihydroergotamine

	Sumatriptan 20 mg + placebo %	Dihydroergotamine 1 mg + 1 mg %
Headache relief		
15 min post-dose	13	9
30 min post-dose	26	22
45 min post-dose	38[a]	31
60 min post-dose	53[a]	41
90 min post-dose	60[a]	48
120 minutes post-dose	63[a]	51
Headache resolution 120 min post-dose	39	32
No or mild clinical disability 120 min post-dose	70	66
No nausea 120 min post-dose	64	60
No photophobia/phonophobia 120 min post-dose	63	59

[a] $p < 0.05$ vs. dihydroergotamine.

During the study, patients were requested to treat each moderate or severe migraine attack with a sumatriptan dose of 20 mg, with an option for a second 20-mg dose if the headache was not effectively treated or if it recurred within 2 to 24 h after the first dose. During the 12-month period of the study, 182 patients treated 6,382 moderate or severe migraine attacks (median, 33 attacks per patient). Headache relief was reported in 77% of attacks at 2 h after treatment, and in 58% of attacks at 1 h after treatment. The percentage of attacks in which headache relief was obtained within 2 h of dosing was about the same during the second 6 months of the study (75% of attacks) as during the first 6 months (78% of attacks) and about the same for patients with aura (75% of attacks) as for those without aura (77% of attacks).

Although data were available for relatively few patients, the study suggested that the incidence of headache relief for sumatriptan nasal spray 20 mg was not influenced by whether a patient had a high or low frequency of attacks during the study period. The mean percentage of attacks in which relief had been obtained 2 h after treatment was 67% among patients with fewer than 20 attacks over 12 months (n = 13) and 83% among patients with more than 60 attacks over 12 months (n = 36).

Tfelt-Hansen's meta-analysis [9] included 6 trials with intranasal sumatriptan. The success rate after 2 h was 61% (563/917) compared to placebo 30% (149/503) and an NNT of 3.1 (95% CI 2.7–3.8) was achieved.

Sumatriptan as Suppository

Sumatriptan as a suppository was tested in a double-blind placebo-controlled trial including 431 patients with dosages of 6, 12.5, 25, 50 and 100 mg. Dosages of 12.5 mg and upwards showed a significant improvement of headache within 2 h. However, there were no statistical differences between these dosages. Two hours following the drug administration 65, 72, 66 and 70% of the patients reported significant improvement of headache receiving 12.5, 25, 50 and 100 mg, respectively [17]. A randomized double-blind, parallel-group, placebo controlled trial in 184 patients compared 12.5 mg, 25 mg sumatriptan suppositories with placebo. Relief rates 2 h post-dose were 68% in the high dose group, 47% with 12.5 mg and 25% with placebo [18]. The approved dose of the sumatriptan suppository is 25 mg.

Sumatriptan in Pediatric Migraine

Both sumatriptan nasal spray [19] and sumatriptan tablets [20] have been studied in adolescent clinical trials. Two large, placebo-controlled studies (SUMA2002, SUMB2003) of sumatriptan tablets (25 mg, 50 mg, 100 mg) in adolescent migraine show that sumatriptan tablets were well tolerated among adolescents. The most common adverse events were nausea/vomiting and headache, which may have been symptoms of the migraine rather than effects of study medication. Although they were well tolerated, sumatriptan tablets were not consistently more effective than placebo at conferring headache relief through 4 h post-dose. Even when differences between sumatriptan and placebo were statistically significant, the magnitude of differences between active treatment and placebo was small compared with data from previous studies in the adult population. The incidences of headache relief after sumatriptan in these adolescent studies were consistent with those previously observed in adult patients, but there were unusually high placebo response rates (up to 65% of patients) in these adolescent studies relative to those reported with the adult population (approximately 30%).

One factor that may contribute to the high placebo effect observed in these studies compared with studies in adult migraineurs is the shorter attack duration, on average, among adolescent patients compared with adults. Many of the responders to placebo or to active treatment in these studies may have experienced spontaneous resolution of their headaches within a few hours of attack onset without any treatment or medical attention.

Based on these data, it was hypothesized that sumatriptan nasal spray, a more rapidly effective dosing form than triptan tablets, may be more markedly effective in the short-duration attacks characteristic of adolescent migraine. The efficacy and tolerability of sumatriptan nasal spray 5 mg, 10 mg and 20 mg in the acute treatment of migraine in adolescent patients (n = 510) were evaluated in a randomized, double-blind, placebo-controlled study [19]. IHS-diagnosed migraine patients 12 to 17 years of age were randomized to receive either suma-triptan nasal spray or placebo for the outpatient treatment of one moderate or severe migraine attack in a double-blind, parallel-group trial. Headache relief 1 h post-dose was reported by 47 to 56% of patients using sumatriptan nasal spray (any dose) compared with 41% of placebo patients. Headache relief 2 h post-dose (primary endpoint) was reported by significantly more patients using sumatriptan nasal spray 5 mg compared with placebo. Of the three nasal spray doses tested in this study, the 20-mg dose confers the best efficacy. Although the 20-mg dose of sumatriptan nasal spray was not statistically different from placebo on the primary endpoint of headache relief 2 h post-dose, the balance of the data suggest that the 20-mg dose is the most effective one, providing relief of headache as well as other symptoms such as photophobia and phonophobia. The 20-mg dose, but not the 5-mg dose, was more effective than placebo begin-ning 1 hour after dosing; and only the 20-mg dose was more effective than pla-cebo 2 h post-dose in conferring complete relief of pain. Sumatriptan nasal spray was well-tolerated at all three doses. When the adverse event 'bad taste' was not included in the calculation, the overall incidence of adverse events with sumatrip-tan nasal spray 20 mg was not different from that with placebo.

Sumatriptan nasal spray is the only $5HT_1$ agonist shown to be effective 2 h post-dose compared with placebo in the acute treatment of migraine in adolescent patients. The relatively quick onset of action of sumatriptan nasal spray (earliest onset 15 min post-dose in adult patients) compared with tablet triptans (earliest onset 30 min post-dose in adults) may contribute to superior ability of the nasal spray to alleviate the relatively short-duration migraine attacks typical of adolescent patients.

Tolerability

In all sumatriptan clinical trials, adverse events were collected using the prospective definition of any medical or clinical change (occurring or worsening post-dose) noted by the patient on diary cards or reported to or observed by the clinician during a clinical trial. Adverse events reported more frequently for sumatriptan than placebo and by ≥3% of patients in the active treatment group (highest dose administered) in short-term (usually single-attack), controlled clinical trials are listed in table 3. Most adverse events were not clinically serious, resolved spontaneously, and lasted fewer than 60 min. Sumatriptan injection and tablets have been used for migraine attacks for up to five years [20, 21] and sumatriptan nasal spray for up to one year [14] in four open-label studies. Two subcutaneous 6-mg doses (n = 412 patients in two studies), three 100 mg oral doses (n = 275 patients), or two 20-mg intranasal doses (n = 182 patients) could be used to treat each migraine attack experienced during the study periods. (Sumatriptan prescribing information indicates that the daily dose of sumatriptan tablets should not exceed 200 mg.) The results suggest that the type, incidence, and frequency of adverse events with each of the sumatriptan formulations in long-term studies are consistent with data from single-attack studies. The most frequently reported adverse events in three representative long-term trials with sumatriptan injection, tablets, and nasal spray are listed in table 4.

One indication of adverse event severity is whether the adverse event precipitates the patient's withdrawal from the study, either at the patient's own wish or by the investigator. Few patients (12% with injection, 7% with tablet, 4% with nasal spray) withdrew from the studies because of adverse events.

Safety

All triptans have vasoconstrictive action and are contraindicated in patients with vascular disease. Post-marketing surveillance studies and case reports indicate, that sumatriptan, albeit rarely, is associated with serious cardiovascular events including myocardial infarction [22–25], cardiac arrythmia [26], stroke [27–29] and ischemic colitis [30]. The frequency of serious adverse events is about 1:1 million treated attacks. Almost all serious adverse events occurred in patients with contraindications or other diseases than migraine. A positron emission tomography study in healthy volunteers showed, that 6-mg sumatriptan s.c. has no influence on myocardial perfusion [31]. Glaxo/Wellcome established a pregnancy register to obtain data from patients and newborns when sumatriptan was taken during pregnancy (although not recommended). Up to now the data from 96 pregnancies are available and indicate that there is no increased risk of major birth defects [32].

Summary and Practical Use of Sumatriptan

Migraine treatment was revolutionized early this decade with the introduction of sumatriptan. The availability of multiple sumatriptan formulations allows the clinician to tailor therapy to the needs of the individual patient. For the majority of patients, sumatriptan tablets, which offer consistent efficacy within 30 to 60 min of dosing in a convenient dosing form, may be an appropriate choice. Clinical trials found no difference in efficacy between groups of

Table 3. Adverse events[a] in sumatriptan injection, tablets, and nasal spray clinical trials

Adverse event	Sumatriptan injection	
	Placebo (n = 370) %	Sumatriptan 6 mg (n = 547) %
Injection site reaction	24	59
Tingling	3	14
Warm/hot sensation	4	11
Burning sensation	< 1	8
Feeling of heaviness	1	7
Pressure sensation	2	7
Flushing	2	7
Feeling of tightness (excluding chest)	< 1	5
Neck pain/stiffness	< 1	5
Weakness	< 1	5
Numbness	2	5
Dizziness	4	12
Tightness in chest	1	3
Throat discomfort	1	3

Sumatriptan tablets

Adverse event	Placebo (n = 309) %	Sumatriptan 25 mg (n = 417) %	Sumatriptan 50 mg (n = 771) %	Sumatriptan 100 mg (n = 437)
Paresthesia (all types)	2	3	5	3
Warm/cold sensation	2	3	2	3
Pain/tightness/pressure of neck/throat/jaw	2	1	1	3
Pressure/tightness/heaviness (excluding chest)	2	1	1	3
Malaise/fatigue	< 1	2	2	3

Sumatriptan nasal spray

Adverse event	Placebo (n = 704) %	Sumatriptan 5 mg (n = 496) %	Sumatriptan 10 mg (n = 1007) %	Sumatriptan 20 mg (n = 1212) %
Bad/unusual taste	2	14	19	25
Nausea/vomiting	11	12	11	14
Discomfort nasal cavity/sinus	2	3	3	4

[a] Events that occurred at least 1% more often in the active treatment group (highest dose administered) than the placebo group and that occurred in ≥ 3% of patients in the active treatment group (highest dose administered).

Table 4. Adverse events most frequently reported in long-term trials[a]

	Percentage of attacks with adverse events
Sumatriptan injection – 2-year study (13,277 attacks treated; n = 412)	
Dizziness/vertigo	3%
Paresthesia	2%
Malaise/fatigue	2%
Neck pain/stiffness	2%
Pressure sensation	2%
Feeling of heaviness	2%
Throat symptoms	2%
Weakness	2%
Sumatriptan tablets – 2-year study (11,501 attacks treated; n = 275)	
Malaise/fatigue	5%
Neck pain/stiffness	2%
Dizziness/vertigo	2%
Nausea and/or vomiting	2%
Feeling of heaviness	2%
Sumatriptan nasal spray – 1-year study (6,382 attacks treated; n = 182)	
Disturbance of taste	12%
Nausea and/or vomiting	2%

[a] Adverse events reported in ≥2% of attacks are listed.

patients taking the 50-mg and 100-mg dose of sumatriptan. Individual patients often display a clear preference for one dose over the other. Patients with good efficacy but moderate side effects may prefer the 25 mg dose of sumatriptan. For patients who desire particularly rapid relief that cannot be provided by a tablet form, sumatriptan injection or sumatriptan nasal spray with earliest onset of relief 10 min and 15–30 min post-dose, respectively, may be appropriate choices. Patients with very severe attacks and those with early vomiting benefit also from the injection. Patients with nausea who are afraid of injections may use the suppositories.

Clinical experience with sumatriptan showed some phenomena which were also observed with the other triptans. These observations are:

(1) Depending on the initial response headache recurrence is observed in between 20 and 40% of migraine attacks.

(2) Headache recurrence can be treated successfully with a second dose of sumatriptan.

(3) Headache recurrence can not be prevented by taking a second dose of sumatriptan in the headache-free period.

(4) Sumatriptan taken during the migraine aura does not influence the duration of migraine aura and does not prevent the occurrence of headache.

(5) Sumatriptan tablets are not effective in migraine attacks in children. Sumatriptan nasal spray, a more rapidly effective form than tablets, is effective in adolescents.

(6) Very frequent use of sumatriptan may lead in some patients to an increase in migraine frequency and finally to drug-induced headache (see chapter on drug-induced headache).

(7) Serious adverse events are rare and occur in most cases in patients with contraindications for 'triptans' (and ergots) or diagnoses other than migraine.

References

1   The Subcutaneous Sumatriptan International Study Group: Treatment of migraine attacks with sumatriptan. N Engl J Med 1991;325:316–321.
2   Cady RK, Wendt JK, Kirchner JF, Sargent JD, Rothrock JF, Skaggs H: Treatment of acute migraine with subcutaneous sumatriptan. JAMA 1991;265:2831–2835.
3   Pfaffenrath V, Cunin G, Sjonell G, Prendergast J: Efficacy and safety of sumatriptan tablets in the acute treatment of migraine: Defining the optimum doses of oral sumatriptan. Headache 1998;38: 184–190.
4   The Finnish Sumatriptan Group and The Cardiovascular Clinical Research Group: A placebo-controlled study of intranasal sumatriptan for the acute treatment of migraine. Eur Neurol 1991; 31:332–338.
5   Salonen R, Saiers J: Sumatriptan is effective in the treatment of menstrual migraine: A review of prospective studies and retrospective analyses. Cephalalgia 1999;19:16–19.
6   Cady RK, Dexter J, Sargent JD, Markley H, Osterhaus JT, Webster CJ: Efficacy of subcutaneous sumatriptan in repeated episodes of migraine. Neurology 1993;43:1363–1368.
7   Hulme A, Dalton DW: The efficacy of subcutaneous sumatriptan in the treatment of headache recurrence. Cephalalgia 1993;13(suppl 13):157.
8   O'Callaghan J, Cleal AL: Long-term efficacy of subcutaneous sumatriptan using a novel auto-injector. Cephalalgia 1993;13(suppl 13):161.
9   Tfelt-Hansen P: Efficacy and adverse events of subcutaneous, oral, and intranasal sumatriptan used for migraine treatment: A systematic review based on number needed to treat. Cephalalgia 1998; 18:532–538.
10 The Oral Sumatriptan Dose-Defining Study Group: Sumatriptan – An oral dose-defining study. Eur Neurol 1991;31:300–305.
11 Cutler N, Mushet GR, Davis R, Clements B, Whitcher L: Oral sumatriptan for the acute treatment of migraine: Evaluation of three dosage strengths. Neurology 1995;45(suppl 7):S5–S9.
12 Sargent J, Kirchner JR, Davis R, Kirkhart B: Oral sumatriptan is effective and well tolerated for the acute treatment of migraine: Results of a multicenter study. Neurology 1995;45(suppl 7):S10–S14.
13 Peikert A, Becker WJ, Ashford EA, Dahlöf C, Hassani H, Salonen R: Sumatriptan nasal spray: A dose-ranging study in the acute treatment of migraine. Eur J Neurol 1999;6:43–49.

14   Dahlöf C: Sumatriptan nasal spray: A review. Cephalalgia, in press.

15   Ryan R, Elkind A, Baker CC, Mullican W, DeBussey S, Asgharnejad M: Sumatriptan nasal spray for the acute treatment of migraine. Results of two clinical studies. Neurology 1997;49:1225–1230.

16   Diamond S, Elkind A, Jackson RT, Ryan R, DeBussey S, Asgharnejad M: Multiple-attack efficacy and tolerability of sumatriptan nasal spray in the treatment of migraine. Arch Fam Med 1998;7: 234–240.

17   Göbel H, on behalf of the Study Group: A placebo-controlled, dose defining study of sumatriptan suppositories in the acute treatment of migraine. Cephalalgia 1995;15(suppl 14):232.

18   Tepper SJ, Cochran A, Hobbs S, Woessner M, on behalf of the S2B351 Study Group: Sumatriptan suppositories for the acute treatment of migraine. Int J Clin Pract 1998;52:31–35.

19   Winner P: Sumatriptan nasal spray in the acute treatment of migraine in adolescent migraineurs. Headache 1999;39:386.

20   Glaxo Wellcome data on file.

21   Pilgrim AJ: Long-term tolerability and safety of sumatriptan during a 2-year period. Cephalalgia 1993;13:190.

22   O'Connor P, Gladstone P: Oral sumatriptan-associated transmural myocardial infarction. Neurology 1995;45:2274–2276.

23   Main ML, Ramaswamy K, Andrews TC: Cardiac arrest and myocardial infarction immediately after sumatriptan injection (letter). Ann Intern Med 1998;128:874.

24   Ottervanger JP, Paalman HJA, Boxma GL, Stricker BHC: Transmural myocardial infarction with sumatriptan. Lancet 1993;341:861–862.

25   Mueller L, Gallagher RM, Ciervo CA: Vasospasm-induced myocardial infarction with sumatriptan. Headache 1996;36:329–331.

26   Ottervanger JP, Stricker BHC: Cardiovascular adverse reactions to sumatriptan – Cause for concern? CNS Drugs 1995;3:90–98.

27   Cavazos JE, Carees JB, Chilukuri VR: Sumatriptan-induced stroke in sagittal sinus thrombosis. Lancet 1994;343:1105–1106.

28   Luman W, Gray RS: Adverse reactions associated with sumatriptan. Lancet 1993;341:1091–1092.

29   Jayamaha JEL, Street MK: Fatal cerebellar infarction in a migraine sufferer whilst receiving sumatriptan. Intensive Care Med 1995;21:82–83.

30   Knudsen JF, Friedman B, Chen M, Goldwasser JE: Ischemic colitis and sumatriptan use. Arch Intern Med 1998;158:1946–1948.

31   Lewis PJ, Barrington SF, Marsden PK, Maisey MN, Lewis LD: A study of the effects of sumatriptan on myocardial perfusion in healthy male migraineurs using 13NH3 positron emission tomography. Cephalalgia 1997;48:1542–1550.

32   Shuhaiber S, Pastuszak A, Schick B, Matsui D, Spivey G, Brochu J, Koren G: Pregnancy outcome following first trimester exposure to sumatriptan. Neurology 1998;51:581–583.

33   Ashford E, Salonen R, Saiers J, Woessner M: Consistency of response to sumatriptan nasal spray across patient subgroups and migraine types. Cephalalgia 1998;18:273–277.

34   Massiou H, on behalf of the Study G: A comparison of sumatriptan nasal spray 20 mg and intranasal dihydroergotamin in the acute treatment of migraine. Poster, 3rd European Headache Conference, Sardinia 1996:56–59.

35   Diamond S, Elkind A, Jackson RT, Ryan R, DeBussey S, Asgharnejad M: Multiple-attack efficacy and tolerability of sumatriptan nasal spray in the treatment of migraine. Arch Fam Med 1998;7: 234–240

Prof. Dr. H.C. Diener, Neurologische Universitäts-Klinik,
Hufelandstrasse 55, D–45122 Essen (Germany)
Tel. +49 201 723 2460, Fax +49 201 723 5901, E-Mail h.diener@uni-essen.de

Diener HC (ed): Drug Treatment of Migraine and Other Headaches.
Monogr Clin Neurosci. Basel, Karger, 2000, vol 17, pp 110–115

....

The Pharmacology of Zolmitriptan

Graeme R. Martin

Department of Molecular Pharmacology, Neurobiology Unit, Roche Bioscience,
Palo Alto, Calif., USA

Zolmitriptan (Zomig®: (*S*) 4-[3-[2-dimethylamino-ethyl]-1*H*-indol-5-yl]-methyl-2-oxazolidinone) was the first of the second generation 5-$HT_{1B/1D}$ receptor 'triptan' agonists to be developed after sumatriptan [1, 2]. The drug shares a clear chemical heritage with serotonin (fig. 1), but was designed by applying constraints imposed by a 5-$HT_{1B/1D}$ receptor pharmacophore and a theoretical model for oral bioavailability [1, 3] to produce a highly selective 5-$HT_{1B/1D}$ receptor partial agonist with a modest degree of CNS penetration, pharmacokinetic properties conducive to rapid, consistent oral bioavailability and a duration of action suitable for the acute treatment of migraine [4]. These attributes were expected to overcome a number of perceived shortcomings in sumatriptan, most notably low and erratic oral bioavailability (F = 14%), slow oral absorption (T_{max} = 2 h), a short plasma elimination half-life ($t_{1/2}$ = 2 h) possibly accounting for a headache recurrence rate of up to 40% [5, 6] and an inability to prevent migraine by early treatment [7, 8].

Receptor Specificity

Zolmitriptan is a potent, high affinity agonist at human recombinant 5-HT_{1B} (pKi = 8.3) and 5-HT_{1D} (pKi = 9.2) receptors. With the exception of modest affinity at 5-HT_{1A} (pKi = 6.5) and putative 5-ht_{1f} (pKi = 7.0) receptors, the drug displays at least 100-fold selectivity over a wide range of other G-protein coupled receptors and ion channels. In a variety of isolated vascular preparations known to contain vasoconstrictor 5-HT_{1B} receptors (saphenous vein, basilar artery, middle cerebral artery and coronary artery from various species, including man) zolmitriptan is one of the most potent triptans (pEC_{50} = 6.8–7.4), but behaves

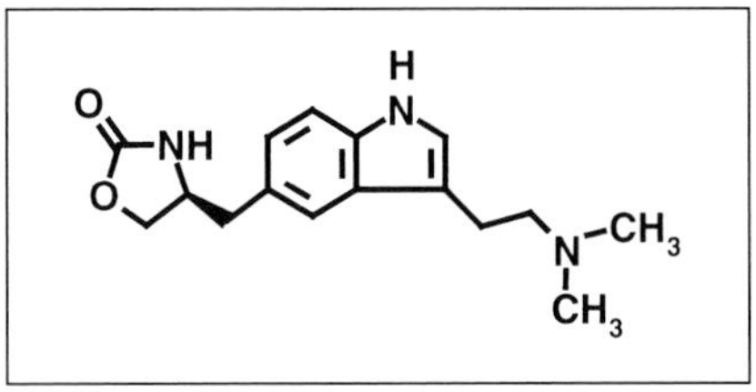

Fig. 1. Zolmitriptan.

in every case as a partial agonist with respect to 5-HT [9, 10]. Pharmacological efficacy is 60% of that for 5-HT, the same as for sumatriptan [9].

Effects on Cranial and Systemic Hemodynamics

Zolmitriptan potently and profoundly decreases carotid arterial conductance ($ED_{50} = 1$–3 $\mu g \cdot kg^{-1}$, i.v.) without affecting blood flow to the brain, myocardium, lungs or other vital organs [11]. These changes in carotid arterial conductance result from a selective constriction of cranial arterio-venous anastomoses, which normally carry more than 50% of the total carotid arterial blood supply. In anesthetized cats and dogs, A-V shunting is reduced by $\geq 90\%$, extra-cerebral blood flow is unaffected or modestly reduced (24% maximum reduction in cats) while cerebral microvascular blood flow remains unchanged [11]. Similar results have been described for other triptans as well as ergotamine [11–14] showing that although zolmitriptan is able to cross the blood-brain barrier, this property does not appear to adversely affect its actions on cranio-vascular dynamics.

In a wide variety of anesthetized and conscious animals (rats, rabbits, dogs and primates), zolmitriptan at doses 30–100 times higher than doses producing selective activation of $5\text{-HT}_{1B/1D}$ receptors in arterio-venous anastomoses, has little or no effect on either systemic blood pressure, heart rate or ECG [4]. In humans, zolmitriptan causes a modest increase in blood pressure (maximum mean change $= 4.3/11.5$ mmHg) but does not alter cardiac output, heart rate or stroke volume [4].

Effects on the Trigemino-Vascular System

The ability of zolmitriptan to modulate trigemino-vascular excitability has been examined using a number of experimental paradigms. When administered to anesthetized guinea-pigs prior to unilateral electrical stimulation of the trigeminal ganglion, the drug (3–30 µg · kg⁻¹, i.v.) produces dose-dependent inhibition of [¹²⁵I]-albumin extravasation within the ipsilateral dura mater and cranial vascular constriction as judged by decreases in ear arteriolar blood flow [3]. Interestingly, the vascular effects are transient, with complete recovery to the pre-drug state prior to stimulation of the trigeminal ganglion. Presuming that intracranial blood vessels respond to the drug in a similar manner, these results suggest that ongoing vessel constriction is not required for inhibition of plasma protein extravasation into the dura [see also 15].

In anesthetized cats, trigeminal ganglion stimulation produces frequency-dependent increases in cerebral blood flow concomitant with significant increases in CGRP and VIP concentrations in jugular venous blood (CGRP: 33 ± 3 to 68 ± 10 pmol · l⁻¹; VIP: 4 ± 1 to 20 ± 3 pmol · l⁻¹). Zolmitriptan (100 µg · kg⁻¹, i.v.) reverses both the increase in intracranial blood flow and the release of neuropeptides [16]. These results are consistent with the ability of zolmitriptan to inhibit CGRP release from perivascular terminals of the Vth (trigeminal) nerve by a pre-junctional, peripheral action, but they also imply that the drug must also act within the brainstem to block reflex activation of the VIIth cranial (facial) nerve, the source of VIP.

Confirmation of a central neuro-inhibitory effect of zolmitriptan has been provided by three types of experiments. Hence the drug, administered intravenously, has been shown to inhibit expression of c-fos immunoreactivity in lamina II of the trigeminal nucleus caudalis induced by electrical stimulation of the trigeminal ganglion [17]. In two additional types of experiment, the drug (30 and 100 µg · kg⁻¹, i.v., or applied iontophoretically onto brainstem neurons) decreases both the amplitude of trigeminal potentials and the probability of cell firing evoked by mild stimulation of the superior sagittal without affecting the latency to the fastest component [18, 19]. Except in the case of iontophoretic application, sumatriptan is unable to inhibit trigeminal excitability in these paradigms, consistent with its poor ability to penetrate the blood-brain barrier [17, 18].

Central Distribution of [³H]Zolmitriptan

In vitro autoradiography using [³H]zolmitriptan reveals a high density of specific binding in the nucleus tractus solitarius and outer laminae of the trigeminal nucleus caudalis in the brainstem, with lower density binding in the dorsal horns of the C1 and C2 cervical spinal cord. In the hindbrain, specific labeling of the subnucleus gelatinosus and area postrema was also observed. Very little binding was seen in the ventral grey matter or in the dorsal or ventral white matter [20–22]. Displacement studies exclude the possibility of binding to $5\text{-}HT_{1A}$ or $5\text{-}ht_{1f}$ recognition sites and confirm labeling of $5\text{-}HT_{1B}$ and/or $5\text{-}HT_{1D}$ receptors. However, the relative contributions of these two receptor subtypes to the total binding of [^{3}H]zolmitriptan remains unclear at this time [20, 21]. Interestingly, the same pattern of brainstem labeling is obtained ex vivo, confirming yet again that the drug accesses these structures following systemic administration [22].

Effects on Autonomic Function and Centrally Mediated Behaviors

In spite of its ability to modulate trigeminal sensory processing peripherally and centrally, zolmitriptan displays no generalized effects on the autonomic nervous system of animals or humans. However, local effects of $5\text{-}HT_{1B/1D}$ agonist drugs can be demonstrated in some vascular beds consistent, in some cases, with pre-junctional sympatho-inhibition and, in other cases, with inhibition of sympathetic ganglionic transmission [4]. Although the drug clearly crosses the blood-brain barrier, it produces no overt centrally mediated behaviors in mice, rats, rabbits or primates. Only beagle dogs exhibit transient, but specific behaviors after dosing with zolmitriptan. These appear to be typical for the triptan drug class, including sumatriptan, and include marked restlessness, agitation, frequent barking and a marked light-resistant mydriasis the mechanism for which remains unknown [4, 23].

Evidence for Central Effects of Zolmitriptan in Humans

Several studies have investigated the ability of zolmitriptan to modulate central serotonergic activity in humans [24–26]. In two studies using non-migraine volunteers, therapeutic doses of the drug have been shown to modify cortical potentials evoked by auditory stimulation without affecting global cortical processing [24, 25]. In a third study using transcranial magnetic stimulation, motor cortical excitability was shown to be [26]. In each case, the results suggest that even outside of a migraine attack, zolmitriptan can access central structures where it appears to modulate serotonergic neurotransmission resulting in changes in cortical excitability.

Discussion

Zolmitriptan (Zomig®), the first of the 'second generation' triptans to follow sumatriptan, was developed with the aim of building in a number of attributes considered to be desirable in a drug for the acute treatment of migraine. Potency and selectivity at the molecular target was achieved by reference to a pharmacophore model, which additionally provided the basis for designing a partial agonist drug. This combination of properties was expected to optimize the therapeutic window for this drug class, and appears to have achieved this objective since the drug has the lowest activity of any triptan at non-target vasculature [10]. Note was also taken of the molecular properties governing absorption across biological membranes to ensure that zolmitriptan is rapidly absorbed ($T_{max} = 2$ h) with good oral bioavailability (F = 40%) and penetrates the blood-brain barrier to access central components of the trigemino-vascular system. These attributes have now been shown to confer rapid, consistent relief from the symptoms of migraine, setting new standards for the acute management of this disabling condition.

References

1   Martin GR: 5-HT$_{1B/1D}$ agonists; in Leff P (ed): Receptor-based approaches to drug design. Drugs Pharm Sci, Dekker, 1998, vol 89, pp 173–194.
2   Martin GR: Pre-clinical pharmacology of zolmitriptan (Zomig®; formerly 311C90), a centrally and peripherally acting 5-HT$_{1B/1D}$ agonist for migraine. Cephalalgia 1997;17(suppl. 17):4–14.
3   Glen RC, Martin GR, Hill AP, Hyde RM, Woollard PM, Salmon JA, Buckingham J, Robertson AD: Computer-aided design and synthesis of 5-substituted tryptamines and their pharmacology at the 5-HT$_{1D}$ receptor: Discovery of compounds with potential anti-migraine properties. J Med Chem 1995;38:3566–3580.
4   Rolan PE, Martin GR: Zolmitriptan: A new acute treatment for migraine. Exp Op Invest Drugs 1998;7:633–652.
5   Hussey EK, Donn KH, Busch MA, Fox AW, Powell JR: Pharmacokinetics (PK) of oral sumatriptan in migraine patients during an attack and while pain free. Clin Pharmacol Ther 1991;49:134.
6   Fowler PA, Lacey LF, Thomas M, Keene ON, Tanner RJN, Baber NS: The clinical pharmacology, pharmacokinetics and metabolism of sumatriptan. Eur Neurol 1991;31:291–294.
7   Bates D, Ashford E, Dawson R, Ensink FB, Gilhus NE, Olesen J, Pilgrim AJ, Shevlin P: Subcutaneous sumatriptan during the migraine aura. Neurology 1994;44:1587–1592.
8   Monstad I, Krabbe A, Micieli G, Prusinski A, Cole J, Pilgrim A, Shevlin P: Preemptive oral treatment with sumatriptan during a cluster period. Headache 1995;35:607–613.
9   Martin GR, Robertson AD, MacLennan SJ, Prentice DJ, Barrett VJ, Buckingham J, Honey AC, Giles H, Moncada S: Receptor specificity and trigemino-vascular inhibitory actions of a novel 5-HT$_{1B/1D}$ receptor partial agonist, 311C90 (zolmitriptan). Br J Pharmacol 1997;121:157–164.
10 Maassen Van Den Brink A, Reekers M, Bax WA, Ferrari MD, Saxena PR: Coronary side-effect potential of current and prospective antimigraine drugs. Circulation 1998;98:25–30.
11 MacLennan SJ, Cambridge D, Whiting MV, Marston C, Martin GR: Cranial vascular effects of zolmitriptan, a centrally active 5-HT$_{1B/1D}$ receptor partial agonist for the acute treatment of migraine. Eur J Pharmacol 1998;361:191–197.
12 Villalon CM, De Vries P, Rabelo G, Centurion D, Sanchez-Lopez A, Saxena P: Canine external carotid vasoconstriction to methysergide, ergotamine and dihydroergotamine: Role of 5-HT$_{1B/1D}$ receptors and alpha$_2$-adrenoceptors. Br J Pharmacol 1999;126:585–594.
13 Willems E, De Vries P, Heiligers JP, Saxena PR: Porcine carotid vascular effects of eletriptan (UK-116,044): A new 5-HT$_{1B/1D}$ receptor agonist with anti-migraine activity. Naunyn-Schmiedeberg's Arch Pharmacol 1998;358:212–219.

14   den Boer MO, Villalon CM, Heiligers JP, Humphrey PP, Saxena PR: Role of 5-HT$_1$-like receptors in the reduction of porcine cranial arteriovenous anastomotic shunting by sumatriptan. Br J Pharmacol 1991;102:323–330.

15   Johnson KW, Schaus JM, Durkin MM, Audia JE, Kaldor SW, Flaugh ME, Adham N, Zgombick JM, Cohen ML, Branchek TA, Phebus LA: 5-HT$_{1F}$ receptor agonists inhibit neurogenic dural inflammation in guinea pigs. Neuroreport 1997;9–10:2237–2240.

16   Goadsby PJ, Edvinsson L: Peripheral and central trigeminovascular activation in cat is blocked by the serotonin (5HT)-1D receptor agonist 311C90. Headache 1994;34:394–399.

17   Hoskin KL, Goadsby PJ: Comparison of more and less lipophilic serotonin (5HT$_{1B/1D}$) agonists in a model of trigeminovascular nociception in cat. Exp Neurol 1998;150:45–51.

18   Goadsby PJ, Hoskin KL: Inhibition of trigeminal neurons by intravenous administration of the serotonin (5HT)$_{1B/1D}$ receptor agonist zolmitriptan (311C90): Are brain stem sites therapeutic target in migraine? Pain 1996;67:355–359.

19   Storer RJ, Goadsby PJ: Microiontophoretic application of serotonin (5HT)$_{1B/1D}$ agonists inhibits trigeminal cell firing in the cat. Brain 1997;120:2171–2177.

20   Mills A, Martin GR: Autoradiographic mapping of [^{3}H]sumatriptan binding in cat brain stem and spinal cord. Eur J Pharmacol 1995;280:175–178.

21   Martin GR, Rhodes P, Mills A: Autoradiographic mapping of receptors and recognition sites for established and putative antimigraine drugs; in Edvinsson L (ed): Migraine and Headache Pathophysiology. Dunitz, 1999, pp 63–79.

22   Goadsby PJ, Knight YE: Direct evidence for central sites of action of zolmitriptan (311C90): An autoradiographic study in cat. Cephalalgia 1997;17:153–158.

23   Humphrey PP, Feniuk W, Marriott AS, Tanner RJ, Jackson MR, Tucker ML: Preclinical studies on the anti-migraine drug, sumatriptan. Eur Neurol 1991;31:282–290.

24   Hughes AM, Dixon R, Dane A, Kemp J, Cummings L, Ytes RA: Effects of zolmitriptan (Zomig®) on central serotonergic transmission as assessed by active oddball auditory event-related potentials in volunteers without migraine. Cephalalgia 1999;19:100–106.

25   Proietti-Cecchini A, Afra J, Schoenen J: Intensity dependence of the cortical auditory evoked potentials as a surrogate marker of CNS serotonergic transmission in man: Demonstration of a central effect for the 5-HT$_{1B/1D}$ agonist zolmitriptan (311C90; Zomig®). Cephalalgia 1997;17:849–854.

26   Werhahn KJ, Förderreuther S, Straube A: Effects of the serotonin 1B/1D receptor agonist zolmitriptan on motor cortical excitability in humans. Neurology 1998;51:896–898.

Graeme R. Martin, PhD, Department of Molecular Pharmacology, Neurobiology Unit,
Roche Bioscience, Palo Alto, CA 94304 (USA)
Tel. +1 650 855 5360, Fax +1 650 852 3111, E-Mail Graeme.martin@roche.com

Diener HC (ed): Drug Treatment of Migraine and Other Headaches.
Monogr Clin Neurosci. Basel, Karger, 2000, vol 17, pp 116–123

....

Zolmitriptan – Therapy

John Edmeads

Sunnybrook Health Science Center, University of Toronto, Canada

The pharmacologic properties of zolmitriptan, described in the preceding chapter, suggest that it should be a useful agent for the treatment of acute attacks of migraine. The clinical utility of zolmitriptan has been determined by testing its efficacy and tolerability in dose-ranging studies and in phase II trials which compare it with placebo and, sometimes, other drugs.

Dose-Ranging Studies

In 1994, Schoenen et al. [1] reported an open study in which they gave zolmitriptan 25 mg by mouth to 18 inpatients as treatment for their acute attacks of migraine. Sixteen (82%) reported relief of headache at 2 h after taking the medication. 'Relief' was defined as a reduction in severity from severe (grade 3) or moderate (grade 2) to mild (grade 1) or no (grade 0) headache. Subsequently Visser et al. [2] reported a randomized, double-blind placebo-controlled parallel groups trial in which 84 outpatients were given either placebo or 1 mg, 5 mg or 25 mg of zolmitriptan for the treatment of one migraine attack, with an optional second dose for recurrent or persistent headache (no patient received more than 25 mg total). Fifteen percent had 2-h relief (defined above) from placebo, 27% from 1 mg zolmitriptan (not significantly better than placebo), 62% from 5 mg (p < 0.005 vs. placebo) and 81% from 25 mg (< 0.001 vs. placebo). Headache recurrence rates were 33% for placebo and 1 mg, 36% for 5 mg, and 7% for 25 mg. Adverse events were mild and infrequent. Dahlof et al. [3] performed a similar study in which 1,181 outpatients treated a single attack of migraine with either placebo, or 5, 10, 15 or 20 mg zolmitriptan; 19% of those who received placebo had a 2-h headache response, 66% with 5 mg, 72% with 10 mg, 69% with 15 mg, and 77% with 20 mg. Again, adverse effects were, in a roughly dose-dependent

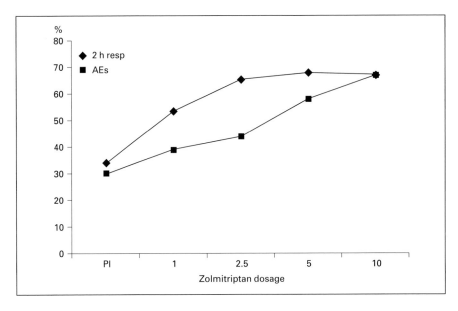

Fig. 1. Efficacy and tolerability.

fashion, 3–7% more frequent with zolmitriptan than with placebo, though none were severe. Rapoport et al. [4] studied the effects of placebo and of zolmitriptan in doses of 1, 2.5, 5 and 10 mg, in 999 evaluable outpatients who, in a randomized, double-blinded fashion, took one of these for an acute attack of migraine. Patients had the option of repeating the dose for persistent or recurrent headache. The headache response rates with zolmitriptan in doses of 2.5 mg or more were 44 to 51% at 1 h, 65 to 67% at 2 h and 75 to 78% at 4 h, all significantly better than placebo. The 1 mg dose of zolmitriptan was not better than placebo at 1 h, but was better at 2 and 4 h (53 and 57% for 1 mg vs. 34 and 32% for placebo. The adverse event rate was 30% with placebo, 39% with 1 mg, 44% with 2.5 mg, 58% with 5 mg and 67% with 10 mg. The authors concluded that the 2.5 mg dose was on the shoulder of the dose-response curve and at the point of widest separation between response rate and adverse event rate, and therefore recommended this as the optimal initial dose for the treatment of an acute attack of migraine (see figure 1).

Phase III Trials

Randomized controlled double-blinded studies have been done comparing zolmitriptan with placebo and, in some cases, with sumatriptan. Endpoints in the various studies were not only headache relief, but freedom from headache, and relief of associated symptoms such as nausea and phonophotophobia. Recurrence rates and adverse events were documented.

Solomon et al. [5] studied 327 outpatients who were randomized to receive either placebo or zolmitriptan 2.5 mg for a moderate or severe attack of migraine. Zolmitriptan was taken by 219 patients, and placebo by 108. The headache response at 2h was 62% for zolmitriptan and 36% for placebo; at 4h the headache response was 70% for zolmitriptan and 37% for placebo. Unlike the study of Rapoport et al. [4], zolmitriptan 2.5 mg produced no statistically significant benefit over placebo in terms of headache response at 1 h. 'Pain-free' rates were 6% for zolmitriptan and 2% for placebo (n.s.) at 1 h, 22% for zolmitriptan and 10% for placebo (p = 0.01) at 2 h, and 38% for zolmitriptan and 13% for placebo (p < 0.001) at 4 h. There were reductions in nausea, photophobia and phonophobia with zolmitriptan compared with placebo; wide confidence intervals were present. A subgroup analysis showed that among women with migraine associated with menses there was a 2-h headache response in 56% of those who took zolmitriptan compared with 41% of those who took placebo; among women in the reproductive age group whose migraine was not associated with menstruation, the 2-h response rate was 63% in those who took zolmitriptan and 33% in those who took placebo. Another subgroup analysis compared the 2-h headache response rates in those who awakened with migraine attack in progress and those who developed an attack while awake. In those who awakened in an attack, the response rate was 65% with zolmitriptan and 26% with placebo; in those who developed an attack while awake, the response rate was 59% with zolmitriptan and 46% with placebo. Recurrence rate was 22% for those who took zolmitriptan and 30% for placebo. The adverse event rate was 46% for zolmitriptan and 29% for placebo (see section on adverse events for details).

The long-term efficacy and tolerability of zolmitriptan was reported in 1998 [6]. In this open study, patients who had previously participated in placebo-controlled zolmitriptan studies were recruited to treat their migraine attacks, of any degree of intensity, with 5 mg tablets of zolmitriptan for up to a year. The initial dose was one tablet. For headache recurrences (headache improved but then came back within 2 to 24 h), a second 5 mg tablet could be taken, but for persistent headache (no improvement after 2 h from first dose) only escape medications could be taken. While this was primarily a study of long-term tolerability, data about efficacy were collected and analyzed. The 2,058 patients in this study treated 31,579 migraine attacks, an average of 15 attacks per patient.

Eighty-one percent of moderate or severe attacks treated showed a 2-h headache response from the first dose (89% of moderate attacks and 65%

of severe attacks). Complete clearing of headache from the first dose (pain-free in 2 h) occurred in 55% of attacks (35% of severe attacks, 57% of moderate, and 80% of mild). Overall, patients reported 'meaningful migraine relief' (a subjective global evaluation of response, incorporating all elements of the attack) in 73% of moderate or severe attacks in a mean time of one hour. Age, gender, association of migraine with menstruation, and the use of prophylactic medication appeared not to influence the efficacy of zolmitriptan. The consistency of zolmitriptan's efficacy over time was assessed by studying data from predetermined attack numbers (#1, #5, #15, #30 and #45). The authors reported that 'the rates of 2-h headache response and 2-h pain-free response suggested a trend for improved efficacy for zolmitriptan with increased number of attacks treated'. A likely explanation for this is that patients who were not getting satisfactory responses probably dropped out early from the study, so that those who stayed in and treated multiple attacks were self-selected for efficacy. It is noted that 11% of patients withdrew from this study because of 'inadequate response'. A subgroup analysis of patients who treated 30 or more attacks established that their 2-h response rates remained at 83–86% in attacks #1, 5, 15 and 30, their pain-free responses at 2 h remained at 52–54% across these attacks, and 'meaningful migraine relief' was recorded by 83–86% of these patients across the attacks. A clinically very relevant index is that 67% of patients reported zolmitriptan to be effective in at least four out of five treated attacks. Recurrence rate could not be accurately measured in this study since data concerning recurrent headaches were collected only for those taking a second dose (i.e. there might have been recurrences not treated with a second dose), but it was noted that patients chose to treat a recurrent headache in 32% of attacks; the second dose produced a 2-h headache response of 90% and a 2-h pain-free response of 65%. Data from this study on the tolerability of zolmitriptan are discussed below.

Quality of Life

The relationship between quality of life and response to zolmitriptan 5 mg was examined in two studies by Patrick and Hurst [7, 8] using the Migraine-Specific-Quality-of-Life (MSQoL) instrument. Approximately one-third of their 1,383 patients showed a 2-hour response in >90% of their attacks, and these patients had significant improvement in their MSQoL scores compared to the 5.6% of patients who had no response. In the 73% of patients who had 'meaningful migraine relief' in at least 60% of their attacks, there was also a statistically significant improvement in MSQoL scores.

Comparative Studies with Other Triptans

The single direct comparison study between zolmitriptan 5 mg and suma-triptan 100 mg and placebo showed no difference between the three groups in terms of the primary endpoint, 'complete response' (improvement in headache within 2 h, with no recurrence within the first 24 h). Probably this result occurred because the unusual randomization protocol (zolmitriptan:sumatriptan:pla-cebo = 8:8:1) produced a high placebo response rate for this endpoint (placebo 38% vs. sumatriptan 42% vs. zolmitriptan 41%) [9, 10].

Indirect comparison studies (i.e. comparison of results from different studies rather than of results from two agents in one study) are also unsatis-factory. One study [11] collected 10 patients whose headaches had not re-sponded to sumatriptan (or had had adverse effects or recurrences) and gave them 2.5 to 5.0 mg zolmitriptan; of the 17 attacks treated, 6 (35%) cleared completely in 2 h, with 2 (12%) recurrences. The authors concluded that unsuccessful treatment with one triptan did not preclude a response to others. Another study [12] compared data from a survey of one group of 207 patients (identified by their pharmacists) who were taking sumatriptan 25 or 50 mg for headaches, with data from an open phase III trial of zolmitriptan 2.5 and 5.0 mg used by 2,499 patients, and reported that the zolmitriptan patients used a smaller mean number of tablets per attack (sumatriptan 25 mg, 1.86 tablets; sumatriptan 50 mg, 1.94 tablets; zolmitriptan 2.5 mg, 1.5 tablets; zolmi-triptan 5.0 mg, 1.6 mg). Differences in all these comparisons are insignificant.

Recurrence

Recurrence rates with 2.5 and 5.0 mg zolmitriptan ranged from 22 to 36%, and with placebo from 30 to 44% [2, 5, 13]. In the open long-term study [6], 90% of moderate or severe recurrences responded to 5 mg of zolmitriptan within 2 h and 65% of these disappeared within 2 h.

Adverse Events

The adverse event rate of zolmitriptan in the various studies is dose-related; the overall rates are 46% with 2.5 mg, 58% with 5.0 mg, and 29% with placebo [14] (see fig. 1). The majority of adverse events occurred within 2 h of the dose; most were mild (59%) or moderate (35%) in intensity, and only 6% required action. In the placebo-controlled studies, 4% of patients on zolmi-triptan reported severe adverse effects, compared with 5% on placebo. The

Table 1. Adverse effects – percent of patients experiencing adverse effect*

Adverse effect	Placebo (%)	Zolmitriptan 2.5 mg (%)	Zolmitriptan 5.0 mg (%)	Sumatriptan 100 mg (%)
Paraesthesiae	1	6	8	7
Warmth/chills	2	4	5	6
Asthenia	3	3	10	11
Dizziness	4	8	8	7
Somnolence	3	6	8	6
Nausea	4	9	6	7
Chest symptoms	1.2	3.4	3.8	4.7

* From clinical studies [15] and package inserts.

spectrum of reported adverse events is shown in table 1. No significant changes in blood pressure and no cardiac events occurred, nor were there any significant ECG changes or alterations in cardiac enzymes. Despite the preclinical studies which demonstrated a dual central and peripheral action of zolmitriptan, there was no increased occurrence of central nervous system-related effects (such as drowsiness) compared with sumatriptan which has no central action; nor did zolmitriptan, even in high doses, produce any changes in psychometric scores.

Contradictions to Zolmitriptan

Like other triptans, zolmitriptan is contraindicated in patients with: ischemic cardiac, cerebrovascular or peripheral vascular syndromes; valvular heart disease; arrhythmias; uncontrolled or severe hypertension; hemiplegic, basilar and ophthalmoplegic migraine; within 24 h of treatment with another $5HT_{1B/1D}$ agonist; or a history of hypersensitivity (anaphylactoid) reaction to chemically related substances. Also like the other triptans, the lack of study of zolmitriptan in pregnancy militates against its use unless its potential benefit is deemed to outweigh its potential risk to the fetus. Like some of the other triptans, caution is advised in the following circumstances: with moderate or severe hepatic impairment use a loser dose; do not exceed a total dose of 5 mg zolmitriptan per day if also taking cimetidine or other CYP 1A2/P450 inhibitors; do not take zolmitriptan if taking an MAO inhibitor; if concomitant use of zolmitriptan and SSRIs is necessary, observe patient carefully. Like the other triptans, use in children is not recommended (because of inability to establish efficacy due to the high placebo response rate in children); and caution is urged when administering to nursing mothers (because of lack of knowledge reexcretion in breast milk).

Summary and Practical Advice

Zolmitriptan is a well-tolerated effective medication for treating the acute attack of migraine. Despite the pharmacologic evidence of a dual central and peripheral action, there is no increased incidence of 'central' side effects (such as drowsiness) compared with sumatriptan, which does not cross the intact blood-brain barrier. Nor, in the only published 'head-to-head' comparative trial, has there been any demonstrated difference between the efficacy of zolmitriptan and sumatriptan. Where and when should zolmitriptan be used? There are not enough data from well-designed direct comparative trials with the other triptans to give an evidence-based answer. The widespread impression of experienced clinicians, which will have to suffice until such studies can be completed and reported, is that zolmitriptan is as efficacious as any of the other presently available oral triptans, and has very acceptable tolerability and safety when used appropriately.

References

1   Schoenen J, Caekebeke P, Luis G, Monseu G, Phillips S, Pierre P: An open study to investigate the absorption and tolerability of oral 311C90 and to obtain a preliminary indication of efficacy in migraine patients; in Rose FC (ed): Proceedings of the 10th Migraine Trust Symposium, New Advances in Headache Research 4. London, Smith-Gordon, 1994:11–12.
2   Visser WH, Klein K, Cox RC, Jones D, Ferrari M: 311C90, a new central and peripherally acting 5HT$_{1D}$ receptor agonist in the treatment of migraine: A double-blind, placebo-controlled, dose-range finding study. Neurology 1996;46:552–556.
3   Dahlof C, Diener HC, Goadsby PJ, Massiou H, Olesen J, Schoenen J: A multicenter, double-blind, placebo-controlled, dose-range finding study to investigate the efficacy and safety of oral doses of 311C90 in the acute treatment of migraine. Headache 1995;35:292(abstract 19).
4   Rapoport A, Ramadan NM, Adelman JU, Mathew NT, Elkind AH, Kudrow DB, Earl NL: Optimizing the dose of zolmitriptan (Zomig, 311C90) for acute treatment of migraine. A multicenter, double-blind, placebo-controlled, dose range-finding study. Neurology 1997;49:1210–1218.
5   Solomon GD, Cady RK, Klapper JA, Early NL, Saper JR, Ramadan NM: Clinical efficacy and tolerability of 2.5 mg zolmitriptan for the acute treatment of migraine. Neurology 1997;49:1219–1225.
6   The International 311C90 Long-Term Study Group: The long-term tolerability and efficacy of oral zolmitriptan (Zomig, 311C90) in the acute treatment of migraine. An international study. Headache 1998;38:173–183.
7   Hurst BC, Patrick DL: Quality of life improvement in responders to long-term treatment with Zomig. Headache 1998;38:385–386.
8   Patrick DL, Hurst BC: Consistency of meaningful migraine relief and quality of life in patients treated with Zomig. Headache 1998;38:397.

9   Diener HC: Issues in migraine trial design: A case study. Proc European Headache Conference. Sardinia, June 5–8, 1996, pp 10–11.

10   Ferrari MD: 311C90: Increasing the options for therapy with effective antimigraine $5HT_{1B/1D}$ agonists. Neurology 1997;48(suppl 3):S21–S24.

11   Newman LC, Steiner DG, Berliner R, Kazmi MM: Zolmitriptan for the acute treatment of migraine in sumatriptan non-responders: An open label pilot study. Headache 1998;38:395.

12   Tepper S, Ward T, Maurer C: Patient-reported tablet utilization of zolmitriptan and sumatriptan. Headache 1998;38:408–409.

13   Schoenen J, Sawyer J: Zolmitriptan (Zomig, 311C90), a novel dual central and peripheral $5HT_{1B/1D}$ agonist: An overview of efficacy. Cephalalgia 1997;17(suppl 18):28–40.

14   Edmeads JG, Millson DS: Tolerability profile of zolmitriptan (Zomig, 311C90), a novel dual central and peripherally acting $5HT_{1B/1D}$ agonist. Cephalalgia 1997;17(suppl 18):41–52.

John Edmeads, MD, Sunnybrook Health Science Center, Room D 474,
2075 Bayview Avenue, Toronto, ON, M4N3M5 (Canada)
Tel. +1 416 480 4592, Fax +1 416 480 6191

Diener HC (ed): Drug Treatment of Migraine and Other Headaches.
Monogr Clin Neurosci. Basel, Karger, 2000, vol 17, pp 124–133

....

Naratriptan – Pharmacology

Helen E. Connor, David T. Beattie

Glaxo Wellcome R&D Ltd, Stevenage, Herts, UK

Naratriptan (Amerge™ or Naramig™) is a novel, highly selective
5-HT$_{1B/1D/1F}$ receptor agonist recently introduced for the acute treatment of
migraine. Naratriptan (see fig. 1 for chemical structure) was designed chemically to be resistant to metabolism [1] and to hence to have greater oral
bioavailability, compared to sumatriptan. Indeed, clinical data show naratriptan has high oral bioavailability (63–74%) and a long plasma half-life (6 h)
in man compared to sumatriptan (14% and 2 h, respectively) [2, 3]. Naratriptan
is highly effective when taken for the acute treatment of migraine and is well-
tolerated [4, 5]. This review summarizes the pharmacology of naratriptan,
focusing particularly on the pharmacology that is most relevant to its use in
migraine. More detailed information on much of the preclinical pharmacology
of naratriptan presented in this review is described by Connor et al. [1].

Preclinical Pharmacology of Naratriptan

Receptor Binding Profile

The in vitro binding affinity and functional potency of naratriptan at the
various 5-HT receptor subtypes (twelve different 5-HT receptor subtypes,
belonging to seven different families (5-HT$_{1-7}$), identified to date; [see 6])
and at a wide range of other, non-5-HT, receptors have been determined
[1]. Experiments have been conducted using recombinant human receptors
expressed in cells, or animal isolated tissues (table 1). These data show that
naratriptan is a highly selective agonist at several 5-HT$_1$ receptor subtypes,
having high affinity at human 5-HT$_{1B}$ (previously called 5-HT$_{1D\beta}$), 5-HT$_{1D}$
(previously called 5-HT$_{1D\alpha}$) and 5-HT$_{1F}$ receptors. Naratriptan has approximately 6-, 3- and 16-fold higher affinity than sumatriptan at the 5-HT$_{1B}$,

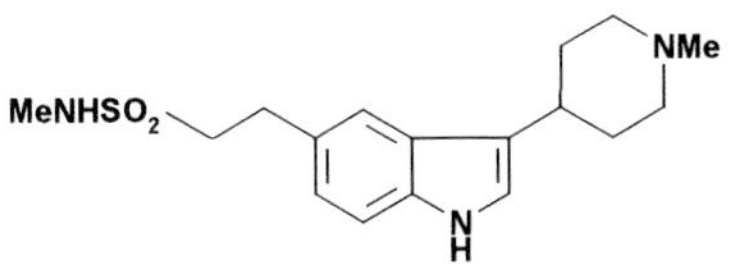

Naratriptan (GR85548; N-methyl-3-(1-methyl-4-piperidinyl)-1H-indole-5-ethane-sulphonamide)

Fig. 1. Chemical structure of naratriptan.

Table 1. Receptor binding profile of naratriptan at 5-HT receptor subtypes

5-HT receptor	Tissue	$pK_i/pIC_{50}/pEC_{50}$
5-HT$_{1A}$	Rat hippocampus	7.1
5-HT$_{1B}$	Human recombinant receptor	8.7
5-HT$_{1D}$	Human recombinant receptor	8.3
5-HT$_{1E}$	Human recombinant receptor	7.2
5-HT$_{1F}$	Human recombinant receptor	8.7
5-HT$_{2A}$	Rabbit aorta	<5
5-HT$_3$	Rat entorrhinal cortex	5.9
5-HT$_4$	Guinea-pig colon	<5
5-HT$_7$	Piglet vena cava	<4

$pIC_{50} \leq 5$ at adenosine A$_{1/2}$, adrenergic $\alpha_{1/2}$, $\beta_{1/2}$, bradykinin, CCK, dopamine D$_{1/2}$, GABA$_{A/B}$, muscarinic M$_{1/2}$, nicotinic, NK$_1$, neurotensin, NPY, opioid μ, σ and κ, NMDA, kainate, quisqualate, glycine and benzodiazepine receptors, and at a variety of uptake sites and ion channels. See [1] for more information.

5-HT$_{1D}$ and 5-HT$_{1F}$ receptor suptypes, respectively. Naratriptan has lower affinity at 5-HT$_{1A}$ and 5-HT$_{1E}$ receptors and such activity is thought to be of little physiological relevance at clinically effective plasma levels. Furthermore, even at high concentrations, naratriptan is devoid of functional activity at other 5-HT receptor types found in the cardiovascular system such as at 5-HT$_{2A}$ receptors mediating peripheral vasoconstriction, or at 5-HT$_7$ receptors mediating vascular relaxation and hypotension. In addition, naratriptan has little or no affinity (pK$_i$ values ≤ 6) at a wide variety of non-5-HT receptors and ion channels.

Vasoconstrictor Effects of Naratriptan

Like sumatriptan, naratriptan contracts large isolated cerebral arteries from dog (basilar and middle cerebral arteries; [1]), primate and man (Glaxo Wellcome unpubl. observ.). This effect is now known to be due to activation of 5-HT$_{1B}$ receptors on cranial vascular smooth muscle. Naratriptan is about 3-fold more potent than sumatriptan at contracting isolated cerebral arteries (EC$_{50}$ of around 0.1 μM for naratriptan in dog isolated cerebral arteries; [1]), in keeping with its higher affinity for 5-HT$_{1B}$ receptors. Naratriptan and sumatriptan cause similar maximum contractile effects in isolated cerebral arteries [1].

Like other 5-HT$_{1B/1D}$ agonists, naratriptan has little or no contractile effects in a number of peripheral blood vessels [1]. This reflects the differential distribution of 5-HT receptors where 5-HT$_{1B}$ receptors predominantly mediate vasoconstriction in the intracranial circulation and 5-HT$_{2A}$ receptors, at which naratriptan has no effect, predominantly mediate vasoconstriction in peripheral tissues. However, a small population of 5-HT$_{1B}$ receptors has been identified in some human peripheral vessels such as human epicardial coronary arteries [7]. This finding accounts for the ability of all 5-HT$_{1B/1D}$ agonists tested to date, including naratriptan, to cause small contractions of human isolated coronary arteries [1, 8]. The maximum contraction produced by naratriptan in these arteries is similar to that produced by sumatriptan, zolmitriptan and rizatriptan [1, 8]. Importantly, plasma concentrations of naratriptan achieved after clinical dosing (30 nM or less) cause little or no contractions of human coronary artery in vitro [1, 8]. However, this class of drug is contra-indicated in patients with coronary artery disease.

Preclinical data show that naratriptan has a selective vasoconstrictor effect in the cranial circulation. Naratriptan (1–300 μg/kg i.v.) produces dose-dependent, long lasting and selective vasoconstriction in the carotid vascular bed (increase in carotid vascular resistance and decrease in carotid artery blood flow) in anaesthetized dogs. The dose of naratriptan that caused 50% of the maximum carotid vasoconstriction is 19 μg/kg i.v. [1]. This value is about 2-fold lower than that for sumatriptan, in keeping with the slightly higher affinity of naratriptan, compared to sumatriptan, for the 5-HT$_{1B}$ receptor. The carotid vasoconstrictor effect is associated with little or no change in arterial blood pressure, demonstrating that the effect of naratriptan (like sumatriptan) is selective for the carotid vasculature and that naratriptan is not having a generalized vasoconstrictor effect [1]. This is in marked contrast to the effect of ergotamine where carotid vasoconstriction is accompanied by marked increases in systemic blood pressure [9].

The effects of naratriptan have been examined in other vascular beds in anaesthetized dogs. Like sumatriptan, naratriptan produces small vasocon-

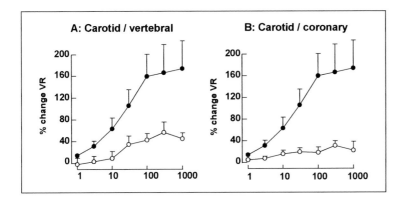

Fig. 2. Comparison of effects of naratriptan on carotid vascular resistance (●) with A: vertebral and B: coronary vascular resistance (○) in anaesthetized dogs. Values are means ± s.e. mean, n = 4.

strictor effects in the vertebral vascular bed but this effect is less than that produced in the carotid bed (fig. 2). Naratriptan produces only very small vasoconstrictor effects in the coronary circulation; these are markedly less than the carotid effects in the same animal (fig. 2).

Vasoconstriction of distended, pain-sensitive intracranial arteries to normalize vessel diameter and hence to reduce afferent firing of the trigeminal nerve may explain the clinical efficacy of 5-HT$_{1B/1D}$ agonists, colloquially known as 'triptans', in migraine. Alternatively, it is possible that the neuronal inhibitory effects of these compounds to reduce afferent trigeminovascular transmission may be important (see below). The debate as to which mechanism is most important is still ongoing, and indeed, it may be that a combination of effects underlies the clinical efficacy of these compounds in migraine.

Effects of Naratriptan on Neurogenic Inflammation

In the rodent model of cranial neurogenic inflammation, developed to mimic the peripheral consequences of trigeminal nerve activation in migraine [10], naratriptan, like other triptans, has an inhibitory effect on the development of neurogenic plasma protein extravasation in the dura mater following electrical stimulation of the trigeminal nerve. Naratriptan is equipotent with sumatriptan in this respect (ID$_{50}$ of 4 µg/kg i.v. [1]). The inhibitory effect appears to be specific for the dural circulation and is not seen in extracranial tissues [1]. This effect of the triptan compounds is thought to be attributable to activation of prejunctional inhibitory receptors (possibly 5-HT$_{1D}$ or 5-HT$_{1F}$ [11, 12] on peripheral trigeminal nerve terminals, leading to inhibition of peptide release, a reduction in oedema formation/neurogenic inflammation and an associated reduction in afferent trigeminal nerve firing.

The relevance of the rodent dural plasma protein extravasation to migraine pathogenesis has recently been questioned [13]. Several compounds that were effective in this model have subsequently been found to be ineffective clinically in the treatment of established migraine headache (e.g. NK_1 receptor antagonists [14] and an endothelin antagonist [15]). Hence the rodent cranial neurogenic inflammation model is probably not a good predictor of clinical efficacy. This may relate to species differences or, more likely, indicate that the antidromic method of gross electrical stimulation of the trigeminal nerve and the measurement of dural extravasation do not adequately reflect what happens during a migraine headache.

Central Effects of Naratriptan on Trigeminovascular Transmission

Naratriptan is slightly more lipophilic than sumatriptan (log D values at $pH_{7.4}$ of –0.3 and –1.3, respectively; 1), and so would be expected to cross the blood-brain barrier more easily. However, compared to typical CNS acting drugs (e.g. diazepam; Log D ($pH_{7.4}$) of around 3), naratriptan still has relatively low lipophilicity. Autoradiographic studies, using ^{14}C-labelled compound administered intravenously, to look at CNS penetration in rats have indicated that only low levels of naratriptan are found in brain following systemic administration (G. Somers, Glaxo Wellcome unpubl. data). However, at clinically relevant doses, naratriptan (30 and 100 µg/kg i.v.) inhibits firing of neurones within the trigeminal nucleus caudalis in the brain-stem of anaesthetized cats [16]. This is the first central site of termination for the primary afferent sensory nerve fibres arising from the cranial vasculature. The inhibitory effect of naratriptan is reversed by the selective $5\text{-HT}_{1B/1D}$ receptor antagonist, GR127935 (fig. 3; [16]). However, which 5-HT_1 receptor subtype is important for causing central inhibition of trigeminovascular transmission is at present unclear: 5-HT_{1D} and 5-HT_{1F} receptors may be involved [11, 17] although a role for 5-HT_{1B} receptors has not been excluded.

Whether this central inhibitory action of naratriptan in the trigeminal nucleus caudalis observed in preclinical experiments confers any clinical advantage is currently the subject of debate. Some of the other more recent triptans (e.g. zolmitripan and rizatriptan) also have this central pharmacological action within the trigeminal nucleus caudalis [18] whilst in contrast, sumatriptan only has inhibitory effects at this central site following disruption of the blood-brain barrier [19]. It has been suggested that the blood-brain barrier is disrupted during a migraine attack, allowing less lipophilic drugs such as sumatriptan to gain access across the cerebrovascular endothelium.

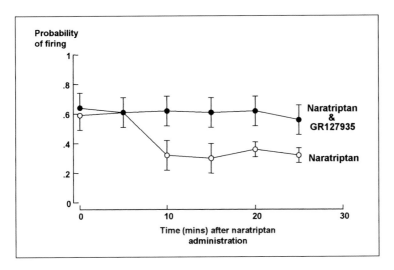

Fig. 3. Inhibitory effect of naratriptan (100 μg/kg i.v. (○)), and reversal by GR127935 (0.1 mg/kg i.v (●)), on cell firing in the trigeminal nucleus caudalis in response to electrical stimulation of the superior sagittal sinus in anaesthetized cats. From [16] with permission.

Action of Naratriptan in Animal Models of Pain

The anti-nociceptive effects of naratriptan (administered intravenously or intrathecally) have been examined in several animal models (mouse hot plate, mouse tail flick, guinea-pig paw pressure). However, even at relatively high doses and when administered directly into the CNS, naratriptan was without effect [1]. This demonstrates that naratriptan does not have generalized analgesic effects, and is specific for migraine pain.

Pharmacokinetics of Naratriptan

The pharmacokinetics of naratriptan in animals are shown in table 2 [5]. Naratriptan has high oral bioavailability in rat and dog and is excreted predominantly as unchanged drug in the urine.

The pharmacokinetics of oral naratriptan in female subjects are shown in table 3 [21]. Naratriptan has high oral bioavailability (74% in women and 63% in men) with an elimination half-life of 6–7 hours [1, 20]. The small gender differences in pharmacokinetics seen after tablet administration are not considered to be of clinical significance. Naratriptan pharmacokinetics are dose-proportional and plasma protein binding is low [2, 20]. A study of oral pharmacokinetics of naratriptan in migraine subjects during and outside

Table 2. Pharmacokinetic profile of naratriptan in rat and dog

Species	Dose	Bioavailability (%AUC p.o./i.v.)	Half-life (h)
Rat (n=3)	10 mg/kg i.v./p.o.	71	1.7
Dog (n=2)	0.5 mg/kg i.v./p.o.	95	1.7

Table 3. Derived naratriptan pharmacokinetic parameters after administration of a single dose of naratriptan 2.5 mg tablets in 15 female migraine patients outside an attack (see [21] for more information)

Parameter	Naratriptan dose, 2.5 mg tablet
AUC_∞ (ng/ml h^{-1}) (dose normalized)	86 (67–111)
C_{max} (ng/ml) (dose normalized)	8.7 (6.6–11.6)
t_{max} (h)	2.0 (0.5–4.0)
$T_{0.5}$ (h)	6.7 (6.3–7.2)
Cl/F (ml/min)	484 (433–541)

Values are geometric means and 95% confidence limits.

an attack, showed that there was no effect of the migraine attack on naratriptan exposure (C_{max}, AUC). However, the rate of absorption was decreased, as shown by an increased t_{max}, probably due to delayed gastric emptying [21].

After oral dosing, naratriptan is eliminated predominantly as an unchanged drug in the urine (50%) and faeces (20%) with 30% recovered as metabolites in the urine [2].

Drug Interaction Studies

In in vitro experiments, naratriptan is metabolized into inactive metabolites by a variety of cytochrome P450 (CYP450) isoenzymes and is not metabolized by monoamine oxidase. Naratriptan itself did not inhibit a wide range of P450 isoenzymes or monoamine oxidase A or B. Hence, induction or inhibition of a particular CYP450 isoenzyme by a co-administered drug would be unlikely to significantly affect naratriptan clearance, and naratriptan is unlikely to affect metabolism of other drugs. Furthermore, interactions between naratriptan and other drugs which interact with, or are metabolized by, monoamine oxidase are unlikely [2].

Clinical studies have been conducted to investigate the potential interaction of naratriptan 2.5 mg tablets with ergotamine (2 mg p.o.), dihydroergotamine (DHE; 1 mg i.m.) and sumatriptan (6 mg s.c) [see 22, 23 and 24, respectively]. Conclusions are:

1. Naratriptan and ergotamine co-administration was well-tolerated with no safety issues or clinically significant effects on the ECG or heart rate. Ergotamine co-administration did not affect the pharmacokinetics of naratriptan (AUC_∞, C_{max} or t_{max}); a small increase in the naratriptan half-life is unlikely to be of clinical significance. Ergotamine co-administration was not associated with an effect on diastolic blood pressure.
2. Co-administration of naratriptan and DHE was well-tolerated and was not associated with any safety issues or clinically significant effects on heart rate or the ECG. There was no significant interaction on blood pressure when naratriptan and DHE were co-administered, nor when DHE was administered 24 h after naratriptan. The naratriptan AUC_∞ and C_{max} were reduced by 15 and 20%, respectively, with DHE co-administration. This small effect is unlikely to be relevant in clinical use.
3. There was no evidence of an additive pressor response following co-administration of naratriptan and sumatriptan and the systemic exposure of each drug was not modifed. Co-administration of the two drugs was well-tolerated.

In addition, no pharmacokinetic interaction has been shown between naratriptan and β-blockers, selective serotonin re-uptake inhibitors (SSRIs) or tricyclic antidepressants in clinical studies [25].

Conclusions

Naratriptan is a potent, selective agonist at human $5\text{-}HT_{1B}$, $5\text{-}HT_{1D}$ and $5\text{-}HT_{1F}$ receptors. Preclinical data show that naratriptan causes selective cranial vasoconstriction, inhibits the development of peripheral neurogenic inflammation in the intracranial circulation and also acts centrally, within the trigeminal nucleus caudalis, to inhibit afferent trigeminal nerve firing. Each of these actions may contribute to the clinical efficacy of naratriptan in migraine. In addition, naratriptan has high oral bioavailability and a relatively long pharmacokinetic half-life (6 h) in man: this latter factor may contribute to lower headache recurrence rates reported with naratriptan in clinical studies [5].

References

1 Connor HE, Feniuk W, Beattie DT, North PC, Oxford AW, Saynor DA, Humphrey PPA: Naratriptan: Biological profile in animal models relevant to migraine. Cephalalgia 1997;17:145–152.

2 Fuseau E, Baille P, Kempsford R: A study to determine the absolute oral bioavailability of naratriptan. Cephalalgia 1997;17:417.

3 Lacey LF, Hussey EK, Fowler PA: Single dose pharmacokinetics of sumatriptan in healthy volunteers. Eur J Clin Pharmacol 1995;47:543–548.

4 Klassen A, Elkind A, Asgharnejad M, Webster C, Laurenza A: Naratriptan is effective and well tolerated in the acute treatment of migraine. Results of a double-blind, placebo-controlled, parallel-group study. Naratriptan S2WA3001 Study Group. Headache 1997;37:640–645.

5 Mathew NT, Asgharnejad M, Peykamian M, Laurenza A: Naratriptan is effective and well tolerated in the acute treatment of migraine. Results of a double-blind, placebo-controlled, crossover study. The Naratriptan S2WA3003 Study Group. Neurology 1997;49:1485–1490.

6 Hoyer D, Martin GR: 5-HT receptor classification and nomenclature: Towards a harmonisation with the human genome. Neuropharmacol 1997;36:419–428.

7 Connor HE, Feniuk W, Humphrey PPA: 5-Hydroxytryptamine contracts human coronary arteries predominantly via 5-HT2 receptor activation. Eur J Pharmacol 1989;161:91–94.

8 MaassenVanDenBrink A, Reekers M, Bax WA, Ferrari MD, Saxena PR: Coronary side-effect potential of current and prospective antimigraine drugs. Circulation 1998;98:25–30.

9 Feniuk W, Humphrey PPA, Perren MJ: The selective carotid arterial vasoconstrictor action of GR43175 in anaesthetised dogs. Br J Pharmacol 1989;96:83–90.

10 Buzzi MG, Moskowitz MA: The anti-migraine drug sumatriptan (GR43175) selectively blocks neurogenic blocks plasma extravasation from blood vessels in dura mater. Br J Pharmacol 1990; 99:202–206.

11 Longmore J, Shaw D, Smith D, Hopkins R, McAllister G, Pickard JD, Sirinathsinghji DJ, Butler AJ, Hill RG: Differential distribution of 5HT1D- and 5HT1B-immunoreactivity within the human trigemino-cerebrovascular system: Implications for the discovery of new antimigraine drugs. Cephalalgia 1997;17:833–842.

12 Johnson KW, Schaus JM, Durkin MM, Audia JE, Kaldor SW, Flaugh ME, Adham N, Zgombick JM, Cohen ML, Branchek TA, Phebus LA: 5-HT$_{1F}$ receptor agonists inhibit neurogenic dural inflammation in guinea pigs. Neuroreport 1997;8:2237–2240.

13 May A, Shepheard SL, Knorr M, Effert R, Wessing A, Hargreaves RJ, Goadsby PJ, Diener HC: Retinal plasma extravasation in animals but not in humans: Implications for the pathophysiology of migraine. Brain 1998;121:1231–1237.

14 Goldstein DJ, Wang O, Saper JR, Stoltz R, Silberstein SD, Mathew NT: Ineffectiveness of neurokinin-1 antagonist in acute migraine: A crossover study. Cephalalgia 1997;17:785–790.

15 May A, Gijsman HJ, Wallnofer A, Jones R, Diener HC, Ferrari MD: Endothelin antagonist bosentan blocks neurogenic inflammation, but is not effective in aborting migraine attacks. Pain 1996;67: 375–378.

16 Goadsby PJ, Knight Y: Inhibition of trigeminal neurones after intravenous administration of naratriptan through an action at 5-hydroxytryptamine (5-HT(1B/1D)) receptors. Br J Pharmacol 1997; 122:918–22.

17 Castro ME, Pascual J, Romon T, del Arco C, del Olmo E, Pazos A: Differential distribution of [^{3}H]sumatriptan binding sites (5-HT$_{1B}$, 5-HT$_{1D}$ and 5-HT$_{1F}$ receptors) in human brain: Focus on brainstem and spinal cord. Neuropharmacol 1997;36:535–542.

18   Hoskin KL, Goadsby PJ: Comparison of more and less lipophilic serotonin (5HT$_{1B/1D}$) agonists in a model of trigeminovascular nociception in cat. Exp Neurol 1998;150:45–51.

19   Kaube H, Hoskin KL, Goadsby PJ: Inhibition by sumatriptan of central trigeminal neurones only after blood-brain barrier disruption. Br J Pharmacol 1993;109:788–792.

20   Kempsford RD, Hoke JF, Huffman CS: The safety, tolerability and pharmacokinetics of oral naratriptan in healthy subjects. Cephalalgia 1997;17:416–417.

21   Fuseau E, Webster C, Asgharnejad M, Huffman C: Naratriptan oral pharmacokinetics in migraine subjects. J Neurological Sci 1997;150(suppl):S33.

22   Kempsford RJ, Nicholls B, Lam R, Wintermute S: A study to investigate the potential interaction of naratriptan and ergotamine. Cephalalgia 1997;17:416.

23   Kempsford RJ, Nicholls B, Lam R, Wintermute S: A study to investigate the potential interaction of naratriptan and dihydroergotamine. Cephalalgia 1997;17:416.

24   Williams P, Kempsford R, Fuseau E, Dow J, Smith J: Absence of significant pharmacodynamic or pharmacokinetic interaction with naratriptan and sumatriptan co-administration. Cephalalgia 1997; 17:417.

25   Fuseau E, Kempsford R, Winter P, Asgharnejad M, Sambol N, Liu CY: The integration of the population approach into drug development: A case study, naratriptan; in Aarons L (ed): European Co-operation in the Field of Scientific and Technical Research. The Population Approach: Measuring and Managing Variability in Response, Concentration and Dose. Brussels, European Commission, 1997, pp 203–214.

Helen E. Connor, PhD, Glaxo Wellcome R&D Ltd,
Stevenage, Herts, SG1 2NY (UK)
Tel. +44 1438 745 745, Fax +44 1438 763 363, E-Mail hec4466@glaxowellcome.co.uk

Diener HC (ed): Drug Treatment of Migraine and Other Headaches.
Monogr Clin Neurosci. Basel, Karger, 2000, vol 17, pp 134–140

Treatment of Acute Migraine Attacks with Naratriptan

Peter J. Goadsby

Institute of Neurology, National Hospital for Neurology and Neurosurgery, London, UK

This chapter will cover the clinical data available in naratriptan. Much of this is published in abstract form although several papers in peer reviewed journals are now available. Naratriptan was developed to have acceptable efficacy with excellent tolerability and the following will outline how that aim was achieved. The only therapeutic indication for naratriptan is in the treatment of acute attacks of migraine with and without aura. Naratriptan has no proven role in the preventative management of migraine although the author is aware of ongoing studies for indications such as menstrually-related migraine.

Clinical Studies

The clinical studies will be considered in order from the dose-ranging studies through the phase III studies, comparisons, side effect profile and contraindications. The methods used in the studies were rather similar and very consistent with what has been done in triptan development programmes in the last decade. They will be outlined before the studies are reviewed.

Study Methods

Naratriptan has been studied in an extensive clinical development programme that covered some 3,200 patients and a hundred fold in the oral dose range from 0.1 mg to 10 mg. At least one parenteral dose-ranging study was done [1] but this formulation has not been further developed. There have been five pivotal studies in phase II and III, some of which have been published [2, 3], and some important specific studies. The studies were conducted along what have become standard lines in the last decade. Patients usually between 18 and 65 years with up to six acute migraine attacks per month by International Headache Society Diagnostic Criteria [4] were recruited. The studies were placebo controlled and some had the active control of sumatriptan 100 mg. Patients were largely studied in the outpatient setting in parallel group placebo-controlled double-blinded design except where indicated and asked to treat a moderate or severe headache on a four-point pain scale of nil, mild, moderate and severe headache intensity. The effect on nausea, photophobia and phonophobia as well as functional responses was mirrored in the outcome for headache intensity which will be the main focus of this chapter. Although most studies in the Naratriptan development programme used the end-point of the number of patients who had moved from a severe or moderate headache to no or mild headache at 4 h in this chapter I will use the 2-h data which is the current recommendation of the International Headache Society Clinical Trials Committee [5]. The natural history of a migraine attack is to improve so that the 4-h data are more flattering but less realistic, as both the active and placebo arms get better with time [6], and we know from population-based studies that a short time to the onset of effect is highly valued by patients [7].

Dose-Finding Studies. The dose-response curve for Naratriptan was evaluated for both the parentral form and for the tablets. Doses evaluated by the subcutaneous route (s.c.) were from 0.5 mg to 10 mg with 2-h headache response rates from 65% to 91%, respectively (fig. 1). These can be compared with a placebo response of 41% and a contemporaneous sumatriptan 6 mg s.c. arm of 89% [1]. Oral naratriptan has been evaluated from 0.1 mg through 10 mg and there is a dose-dependent increase in headache response from a no-effect dose at 0.1 mg through the doses used (fig. 2). The subsequent development programme sought to exploit the low adverse event rate seen in the early studies by developing the now recommended 2.5 mg dose.

Phase III Studies. From a meta-analysis across the entire clinical programme the response of a reduction in headache intensity to nil or mild was 48% (95% CI, 45–51) with a corresponding therapeutic gain of 21% (17–25%) across the studies, obtained by subtraction of the placebo response [8]. For comparison the therapeutic gain for sumatriptan 100 mg in the studies done at the same time was 33% (27–39%). The latter data are broadly comparable with the published therapeutic gain for oral sumatriptan from a large meta-analysis [9]. The data are compared in figure 3. Naratriptan has good consistency within a patient with a large placebo controlled study involving 1,219 patients across the range of doses from 0.1–2.5 mg demonstrating a headache response in 2 of 3 attacks treated in 72% of patients for naratriptan 2.5 mg

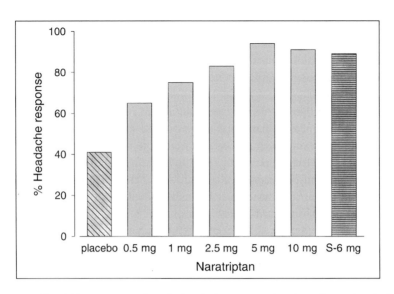

Fig. 1. Dose-response data for headache response (moderate/severe headache becoming nil or mild) at 2 h for subcutaneous naratriptan compared to placebo and sumatriptan 6 mg. There is a clear dose-dependence with a robust response at high doses comparable to sumatriptan [1].

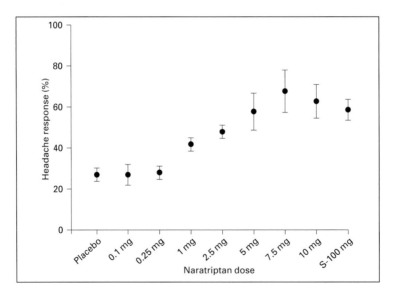

Fig. 2. Dose-response rates for the headache response (severe/moderate headache becoming nil/mild) at 2 h post-dose demonstrating the dose-dependent nature of the effect of naratriptan on headache intensity. The data are based on a meta-analysis of the phase II/III programme and cover 3,230 patients [16].

and 75% of patients for sumatriptan 100 mg compared with 22% for placebo. Unfortunately, only 4-h data are currently available, although as the study involved three attacks on each treatment in a parallel group design, it was a true test of individual consistency. A similar study demonstrated a headache response rate of 61% at 2 h for sumatriptan 50 mg in 2/3 attacks [10].

Associated Symptoms

In parallel with the data for headache relief patients experience reductions in nausea, photophobia and phonophobia. These were greater than what was seen in the placebo treated groups and were similarly prominent at the 4-h time point [2, 3]. Naratriptan is effective in treating the entire range of the usual symptoms of the acute attack of migraine.

Recurrence

The recurrence rate, the number of patients who have a headache response and then have the headache, return in a given period of usually 24 h, was observed to be relatively low in the large placebo controlled studies of naratriptan, and in comparison to sumatriptan still low after subcutaneous administration [11]. Historical comparisons of recurrence are plagued with the problems so that this important question was examined in a specific double-blind crossover study that enrolled patients with a high rate of headache recurrence ($>50\%$) compared to the more usual population rate of about 33% on sumatriptan 100 mg [12]. Headache recurrence was reduced from 57% to 45% ($p<0.005$) in the attack treated with naratriptan 2.5 mg but not significantly delayed [13]. This interesting outcome requires further consideration and study when naratriptan is used more widely.

Side Effects

To some extent the development brief for the naratriptan clinical trial programme focused on defining a dose with adequate efficacy and excellent tolerability. The adverse event profile of the 2.5 mg dose of naratriptan in the clinical studies was not different from placebo over the doses from 0.1 mg to 2.5 mg. At the recommended clinical dose the adverse event rate for the phase II/III studies after allowance for the placebo effect was 0.1% ($-4.0-+4.2\%$; fig. 3). Naratriptan has no significant interactions with preventative anti-migraine drugs, such as β-blockers and tricylic antidepressants, nor with selective serotonin reuptake inhibitors (SSRIs) and, although concurrent use with dihydroergotamine and sumatriptan is contraindicated, safety studies in fact demonstrated no significant interactions in volunteers [14].

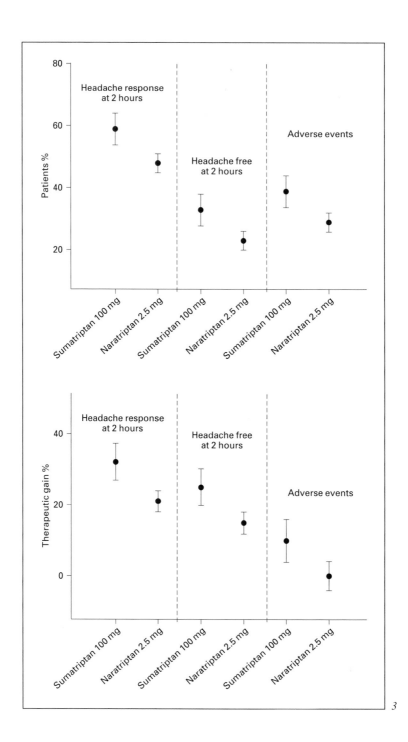

Contraindications

The contraindications for naratriptan are very similar to other triptans. It is important that while naratriptan is currently probably the best tolerated of the triptans, it is no safer in the cardiovascular sense than its cousins [15].

- Hypersensitivity to naratriptan or any component of the tablet;
- Ischemic heart disease;
- Previous myocardial infarction;
- Prinzmetal's angina or coronary vasospasm;
- Peripheral vascular disease;
- History of stroke or transient ischemic attacks;
- Uncontrolled hypertension;
- Severely impaired hepatic or renal function.

Practical Advice

In comparison with sumatriptan 100 mg, naratriptan 2.5 mg is slower in onset and probably has a lower response rate, however, it is better tolerated and has a lower recurrence rate. Given the clinical data naratriptan 2.5 mg is a good first step *triptan* in certain settings. Provided that speed of onset is not of overwhelming concern to an individual patient, then of those who respond to naratriptan they will do so consistently, be less likely to have a headache recurrence and certainly have a very well tolerated medicine. I use naratriptan when patients have been sensitive to other treatments, such as ergot derivatives or triptans, or those who report regular headache recurrence, particularly with sumatriptan.

Acknowledgments

The work of the author has been supported by the Wellcome Trust and the Migraine Trust. P.J.G. is a Wellcome Senior Research Fellow.

Fig. 3. Comparison of naratriptan 2.5 mg and sumatriptan 100 mg based on data from the naratriptan phase II/III clinical studies demonstrating the headache response (moderate/severe headache becoming nil or mild) and headache free data 2 h after treatment in placebo-controlled studies not corrected for the effect of placebo (see text). Also for comparison the adverse event rates across the studies are illustrated. All data are 95% confidence intervals [16]. In panel A the absolute raw data are presented and in panel B the therapeutic gain data are presented for comparison.

References

1 Dahlöf C, Hogenhuis L, Olesen J, Petit H, Ribbat J, Schoenen J, Boswell D, Fuseau E, Hassani H, Winter P: Early clinical experience with subcutaneous naratriptan in the acute treatment of migraine: A dose-ranging study. Eur J Neurol 1998;5:469–477.

2 Klassen A, Elkind A, Asgharnejad M, Webster C, Laurenza A: Naratriptan is effective and well tolerated in the acute treatment of migraine. Results of a double-blind, placebo-controlled, parallel group study. Headache 1997;37:640–645.

3 Mathew NT, Asgharnejad M, Peykamian M, Laurenza A: Naratriptan is effective and well tolerated in the acute treatment of migraine. Neurology 1997;49:1485–1490.

4 The Headache Classification Committee of The International Headache Society: Classification and diagnostic criteria for headache disorders, cranial neuralgias and facial pain. Cephalalgia 1988; 8(suppl 7):1–96.

5 The International Headache Society Committee on Clinical Trials in Migraine: Guidelines for controlled trials of drugs in migraine. Cephalalgia 1991;11:1–12.

6 Jhee SS, Salazar DE, Ford NF, Fulmor IE, Sramek JJ, Cutler NR: Monitoring of acute migraine attacks: Placebo response and safety data. Headache 1998;38:35–38.

7 Davies GM, Santanello NC, Kramer M, Matzura-Wolfe D, Lipton RB: Determinants of patient satisfaction with migraine treatment. Headache 1998;38:380.

8 Goadsby PJ: Naratriptan in the treatment of acute migraine attacks. Prescriber 1997;8:89–97.

9 Tfelt-Hansen P: Efficacy and adverse events of subcutaneous, oral, and intranasal sumatriptan used for migraine treatment: A systematic review based on number needed to treat. Cephalalgia 1998; 18:532–538.

10 Pfaffenrath V, Cunin G, Sjonell G, Prendergast S: Efficacy and safety of sumatriptan tablets (25 mg, 50 mg, and 100 mg) in the acute treatment of migraine: Defining the optimum doses of oral sumatriptan. Headache 1998;38:184–190.

11 Goadsby PJ, Winter P, Asgharnejad M: Twenty-four hour maintenance of headache relief after treatment of migraine with naratriptan tablets: A review of data from controlled clinical trials. Headache 1998;38:382.

12 Visser WH, Vriend RHMd, Jaspers NMWH, Ferrari MD: Sumatriptan in clinical practice. Neurology 1996;47:46–51.

13 Göbel H, Boswell D, Winter P, Crisp A: A comparison of the efficacy, safety and tolerability of naratriptan and sumatriptan. Cephalalgia 1997;17:426.

14 Kempsford R: Clinical pharmacology and pharmacokinetics of naratriptan. Cephalalgia 1997;17: 473.

15 MaassenVanDenBrink A, Reekers M, Bax WA, Ferrari MD, Saxena PR: Coronary side-effect potential of current and prospective antimigraine drugs. Circulation 1998;98:25–30.

16 Goadsby PJ: Place of naratriptan in clinical practice. Cephalalgia 1997;17:472–473.

Professor Peter J. Goadsby, Institute of Neurology,
Queen Square, London WC1N 3BG (UK)
Tel. +44 171 829 8749, Fax +44 171 813 0349, E-Mail peterg@brain.ion.ucl.ac.uk

Diener HC (ed): Drug Treatment of Migraine and Other Headaches.
Monogr Clin Neurosci. Basel, Karger, 2000, vol 17, pp 141–161

··························

The Pharmacology and Mechanisms of Action of Rizatriptan

R.J. Hargreaves, J. Longmore, M. Beer, S. Shepheard, M. Cumberbatch,
D. Williamson, J. Stanton, Z. Razzaque, B. Sohal, L. Street,
G. Seabrook, R. Hill

Merck Sharp & Dohme Research Laboratories, Harlow, Essex, UK

Migraine headache is a complex of symptoms that present clinically as discrete episodes of severe headache with associated features such as phonophobia, photophobia, nausea and emesis. Migraine can be broadly characterized as headache pain with associated disturbances in sensory sensitivity [1].

The specific cause of migraine headache is still unknown although a number of recently discovered genetic factors seem to be important in some patients [2–7]. These abnormalities involve neuronal ion channels that could regulate CNS excitability in response to migraine trigger factors [2, 8–11]. Considerably more is known about the mechanisms involved in the pathophysiology of migraine headache. Understanding of these mechanisms has resulted from increased knowledge of the anatomy and pharmacology of the trigeminal innervation of the intracranial circulation and from the introduction of receptor selective serotonin (5-HT) agonist drugs that are highly effective acute antimigraine agents.

The brain has a sparse sensory innervation and it is the superficial capsule structures comprising the meninges and dura mater that are the most significant pain-producing intracranial tissues [12–14]. Vasodilatation of intracranial, extracerebral blood vessels and consequent activation of perivascular trigeminal sensory nerves are likely to be one of the key factors underlying the generation of migraine headache pain [15–18]. The trigeminal sensory nerves arise from neurons in the trigeminal ganglia that have pseudo-unipolar morphology [19]. Nerve fibres arising from the trigeminal neurons innervate cranial blood vessels in the periphery [20, 21]. Trigeminal fibres relevant to nociception project centrally behind the blood brain barrier by way of the descending spinal trigeminal tract and terminate in the spinal trigeminal nucleus in the medulla. Due to somatotopic organization, sensory fibres which innervate the dura mater terminate within the most caudal region of the nucleus (i.e. trigeminal nucleus caudalis [22]). Thus, trigeminal sensory neurons provide a pathway to convey nociceptive information from distended blood vessels in the meninges into the central nervous system. This system is referred to as the trigeminovascular system.

When activated, perivascular sensory nerves release vasoactive neuropeptides (e.g. substance P, calcitonin gene related peptide, neurokinin A). In the periphery, these substances can cause perivascular inflammation and further increases in blood vessel diameter [23–27], thereby setting up a positive feedback system, a vicious cycle that amplifies the initial noxious dilator stimulus. In the CNS, neurons within the spinal trigeminal tract are uniquely concerned with perception of pain and thermal sensation [22]. Peptide release from these fibres can result in the transmission of nociceptive impulses to second-order sensory neurons in the trigeminal nucleus caudalis which then relay this information to higher CNS centres [15, 17, 19] where pain is experienced at the level of consciousness. Central pain transmission activates CNS autonomic nuclei in the brainstem and other ascending nervous pathways and this may, in turn, contribute to the production of the symptoms that are associated with migraine, namely nausea, emesis, phonophobia and photophobia [28, 29].

Serotonin Receptors

The serotonin receptor family is currently grouped into seven subfamilies ($5\text{-}HT_1$–$5\text{-}HT_7$) giving a total of 14 receptor subtypes that have different anatomical localization. $5\text{-}HT_1$ receptors have been characterized as $5\text{-}HT_{1A}$, $5\text{-}HT_{1B}$, $5\text{-}HT_{1D}$, $5\text{-}HT_{1E}$ and $5\text{-}HT_{1F}$ and all are G-protein coupled receptors that are negatively linked to adenylate cyclase [30[1]]. The ergot alkaloids were one of the first specific treatments for migraine and were shown to have high affinity for many monoaminergic (serotonergic, adrenergic, and dopaminergic) receptor subtypes [31, 32]. The receptor-binding profiles of ergotamine and dihydroergotamine at serotonergic, adrenergic and dopaminergic receptors is given in table 1 and shows the broad pharmacological activity of these agents.

[1] Receptor nomenclature can be confusing. Molecular cloning showed that two $5\text{-}HT_{1D}$ receptor subtypes exist intially called $5\text{-}HT_{1D\alpha}$- and $5\text{-}HT_{1D\beta}$, now reclassified as $5\text{-}HT_{1D}$ and $5\text{-}HT_{1B}$, respectively. The previous $5\text{-}HT_{1D\beta}$ receptor and the rat $5\text{-}HT_{1B}$ receptor are species homologues. Historically rizatriptan was termed a '$5\text{-}HT_{1D}$' receptor agonist and now should be reclassified as a $5\text{-}HT_{1B/1D}$-receptor agonist in line with the change in receptor nomenclature.

Table 1. Pharmacological activity of dihydroergotamine, ergotamine and rizatriptan at human monoaminergic receptors except where specified

	1A	1B	1D	1E	1F	2A	2C	3	gp 4
DHE	0.4	0.7	0.5	1,100	180	9.0	1.3	>3,700r	60
Ergot	0.3	1.0	0.8	840	170	n.d.	n.d.	>3,700r	65
Rizatriptan	300	7.2	2.3	87	138	7,200	7,300	4,100	n.d.

	α1a	α1b	α2a	α2b	α2c	β1	β2	β3	D2	D3	D4
DHE	6.6	8.3	1.9	3.3	1.4	3,100	2,700	271	1.2	6.4	8.7
Ergot	15	12	n.d.	n.d.	n.d.	n.d.	n.d.	n.d.	4	3.2	12
Rizatriptan	>10,000	>10,000	2,300	6,000	700	>10,000	>10,000	>10,000	>10,000	n.d.	>10,000

Top rows are 5-HT receptors, r is rat 5-HT$_3$ receptors and gp 4 is guinea pig 5-HT$_4$ receptors. Second row are alpha α (α1 rat liver, α2 human prostate) and cloned beta β adrenergic receptors and cloned dopamine D receptors. Data for rizatriptan at cloned 5-HT$_1$ receptor subtypes were modified from [42]. All values are affinity K$_i$ nM, n.d. = not determined.

It is noteworthy that alpha adrenergic activity in the ergots can be agonist or antagonist in nature, raising the interesting possibility that the low recurrence rates that have been reported with these agents may be due to modulation of the adrenoceptors on noradrenergic nuclei in the brainstem (locus coeruleus) that have been hypothesized to be involved in the initiation of a migraine attack [33].

The beneficial effects of the ergots as acute anti-migraine agents are likely to result from the activation of 5-HT$_{1B}$ and 5-HT$_{1D}$ receptors. This finding led to the design and development of sumatriptan, a selective 5-HT$_{1B/1D}$ agonist that lacked effects at the other ergot sensitive monoamine receptors that can mediate unwanted nausea, dysphoria, asthenia and vascular effects [1, 34, 35]. Although sumatriptan was a breakthrough drug designed specifically for the treatment of migraine it had some potential shortcomings in its pharmaco-kinetic profile. After oral dosing its bioavailability was low (14%) and the time taken to reach plasma concentrations was relatively slow (approx. 2–2.5 hours). The rizatriptan research program was designed to identify a 5-HT$_{1B/1D}$ receptor selective molecule with physicochemical characteristics that would lead to an improved oral bioavailability and faster absorption in the expectation that this could lead to faster and more consistent headache relief.

Anti-Migraine 5-HT$_{1B}$ and 5-HT$_{1D}$ Receptors in the Trigeminovascular System

Molecular biology investigations have shown that there is high expression of vasoconstrictor 5-HT$_{1B}$ receptors in the smooth muscle of meningeal blood vessels making activation of these receptors a good target to reverse the abnormal vasodilatation occurring during migraine [for review see 31]. These 5-HT$_{1B}$ receptors have also been found in coronary arteries and other peripheral blood vessels making it important to establish the relative contribution of this subtype to the contractile responses in coronary and other arteries as well as the target blood vessels [36]. Investigation of the receptor subtypes present in human trigeminal nerves has shown evidence for 5-HT$_{1D}$ receptors on their peripheral (ophthalmic branch that innervates pain-producing intracranial structures) and central terminals (descending trigeminal tract/nucleus caudalis) where they can regulate neurotransmitter release [37–40]. Activation of pre-junctional 5-HT receptors and the modulation of sensory neurotransmitter release could provide an additional break in the vicious cycle of trigeminal activation that, if left unchecked, would amplify the noxious vasodilator stimuli in the periphery and also centrally reduces neurotransmission within trigeminal pain relay nuclei. It is also noteworthy that 5-HT$_{1D}$ receptors were localized within the solitary tract and its nucleus that receives trigeminal inputs. This structure could be involved in the nausea and vomiting (clinically important aspects of migraine) associated with central pain transmission [37, 41]. The distribution 5-HT$_{1D}$ receptors prejunctionally in the trigeminal nervous system makes them an attractive target mechanism for the treatment of migraine and its associated symptoms of nausea and vomiting.

This article describes preclinical in vitro and in vivo receptor selectivity and functional pharmacology studies with the 5-HT$_{1B/1D}$ agonist rizatriptan that were conducted to assess its potential usefulness for and mode of action in the acute treatment of migraine. The experimental assays were designed to mimic some of the pathophysiological processes in the trigeminovascular systems that are hypothesized to occur in the generation of migraine headache pain.

5-HT$_{1B/1D}$ Receptor Activity of Rizatriptan

Radioligand binding and functional studies in vitro showed that rizatriptan was a potent, efficacious and selective ligand at human (h) cloned 5-HT$_{1B}$ and 5-HT$_{1D}$ receptors. Representative data from a single independent laboratory is given in tables 2 and 3 for the affinity and activity of rizatriptan at 5-HT$_1$ receptors [42]. This data has been compared with the activity of the reference compounds

Table 2. Serotonin receptor affinities of rizatriptan compared to 5-HT, DHE and other clinically used 5-HT$_{1B/1D}$ agonist anti-migraine agents

| | Binding affinities at recombinant human serotonin receptors (K$_i$ nM) | | | | |
	h5-HT$_{1A}$	h5-HT$_{1B}$	h5-HT$_{1D}$	h5-HT$_{1E}$	h5-HT$_{1F}$
5-HT	2.5	1.0	2.1	32	9
DHE	1.2	0.8	0.5	72	355
L-694,247	1.3	0.1	0.2	> 10,000	n.d.
Sumatriptan	45	3.2	2.1	646	12
Zolmitriptan	118	0.8	0.2	11	29
Naratriptan	51	0.5	0.7	11	4.0
Rizatriptan	302	7.2	2.3	87	138

Receptor binding affinities were measured as described in [42] and data presented was adapted from the same source.

Table 3. Functional activity of rizatriptan compared to 5-HT, DHE and other clinically used 5-HT$_{1B/1D}$ agonist anti-migraine agents

| | [^{35}S] GTPγS binding to membrane preparations containing recombinant receptors: | | | | Inhibition of forskolin (100 μM) stimulated cAMP formation in intact cells expressing: | |
| | h5-HT$_{1B}$ | | h5-HT$_{1D}$ | | h5-HT$_{1B}$ | h5-HT$_{1D}$ |
	EC$_{50}$ (nM)	E$_{max}$ (%)	EC$_{50}$ (nM)	E$_{max}$ (%)	EC$_{50}$ (nM)	EC$_{50}$ (nM)
5-HT	91.2	100	14.4	100	15.5	1.7
DHE	2.0	47.1	0.7	73.6	2.7	1.2
L-694,247	1.2	101.6	1.5	96.2	1.5	3.0
Sumatriptan	234.4	96.4	17.8	85.6	69.0	2.0
Zolmitriptan	60	98.8	1.6	85.5	30.9	0.3
Naratriptan	22.9	79.8	4.4	67.4	17.4	0.9
Rizatriptan	234.4	74.5	16.2	82.8	114.8	3.1

Data were generated as described in [42] and data presented have been adapted from the same source.

5-HT, the highly potent prototypic 5-HT$_{1B/1D}$ agonist L-694,247, dihydroergotamine and the other newer selective anti-migraine agents of the 5-HT$_{1B/1D}$ agonist class. It is very important to compare data from within one laboratory since there is considerable variation in the receptor reserve and responsivity of different h5-HT$_{1B}$ and h5-HT$_{1D}$ clonal cell lines to serotonin agonists. This can lead to erroneous conclusions when comparing the relative activity of the various agents if the experiments are not performed head to head in the same cell line.

Data in table 2 shows that all the clinically used triptan agents are selective for 5-HT$_{1B/1D}$ receptors but that they have somewhat different residual activity at 5-HT$_{1A}$ receptors (see below for implications). The affinity of rizatriptan at 5-HT$_{1B}$, and 5-HT$_{1D}$ receptors was at least 30-fold higher than 5-HT$_{1A}$ receptors (IC$_{50}$ = 7.2 nM, 2.3 nM, and 302 nM respectively). This profile differs from 5-HT, L-684,247 and DHE that retain marked 5-HT$_{1A}$ activity. Cross-screening at human serotonin receptor subtypes showed that rizatriptan also had some activity at human cloned 5-HT$_{1E}$ and 5-HT$_{1F}$ receptors where its affinities were 87 nM and 138 nM, respectively. Other notable activities were zolmitriptan and naratriptan at 5-HT$_{1E}$ sites and zolmitriptan, sumatriptan and naratriptan at 5-HT$_{1F}$ receptors.

Functional Pharmacology in h5-HT$_{1B}$ and h5-HT$_{1D}$ Clonal Cell Lines

In the functional assays L-694,247 was the only agonist that achieved the same maximal responses as 5-HT in the h5-HT$_{1B}$ and h5-HT$_{1D}$ receptor membrane preparations. At h5-HT$_{1D}$ receptors, rizatriptan, like sumatriptan and zolmitriptan, was slightly less efficacious than 5-HT (E$_{max}$ 83% of 5-HT) whereas efficacy of naratriptan was significantly less. At h5-HT$_{1B}$ receptors the maximal response to rizatriptan, and naratriptan were significantly less than 5-HT (E$_{max}$ 74.5 and 79.8%, respectively). It is noteworthy that of the clinically used 5-HT$_{1B/1D}$ agonists it was only rizatriptan that had similar balanced efficacy at h5-HT$_{1B}$ and h5-HT$_{1D}$ receptors. Sumatriptan, zolmitriptan and naratriptan appeared more efficacious at the h5-HT$_{1B}$ site with the maximum responses of sumatriptan and zolmitriptan being equal to that of 5-HT. The in vivo significance of differences in efficacy between the agonists is difficult to judge and may only manifest when receptor reserve (receptor coupling and receptor number) is low. The potency of the agonists to inhibit forskolin-stimulated cAMP formation in intact C6-glial cells expressing h5-HT$_{1D}$ receptors was 6–10 times higher than their potency to stimulate binding to membrane preparations from the same cells. In contrast, potencies at h5-HT$_{1B}$ receptors in the cAMP and [^{35}S] GTPγS assays were similar suggesting that the h5-HT$_{1B}$ receptor coupling be better preserved than the h5-HT$_{1D}$ receptor coupling in the membrane preparations. These findings underline the absolute need to compare the functional activity of compounds within any given clonal receptor cell line since differences often occur between cell lines in receptor expression and efficiency of coupling that can make efficacy and potency comparisons across laboratories and clonal expression systems completely meaningless.

Activity at Other Serotonin Receptors

At native mixed $5\text{-HT}_{1B/1D}$ receptors obtained from human cerebral cortex the binding affinity of rizatriptan (IC_{50}) was 12 nM. In human native tissues, as in the clonal cell lines, rizatriptan had 40-fold weaker affinity at cortical 5-HT_{1A} (IC_{50} 450 nM, [43]) compared to cortical $5\text{-HT}_{1B/1D}$ sites. This difference may be important since activation of central 5-HT_{1A} receptors can cause nausea and unwanted cardiovascular and behavioural effects [44, 45]. Further assessment in vitro of the nature of the functional 5-HT_{1A} receptor activity of rizatriptan showed it to be only a weak agonist in biochemical (inhibition of forskolin-stimulated adenylate cyclase activity in guinea pig hippocampus [43]) and electrophysiological (hyperpolarization of rat hippocampal CA1 neurons) assays. These findings indicate that in vitro, relative to the endogenous agonist 5-HT, rizatriptan has low efficacy at central 5-HT_{1A} receptors. Thus, rizatriptan is functionally as well as binding selective for its target anti-migraine receptors. The consequence of this selectivity is that it should be possible to select doses of rizatriptan that balance activation of central 5-HT_{1D} receptors without producing significant activation of the 5-HT_{1A} receptors that could mediate adverse effects such as nausea. At higher dose levels, unwanted central effects can be observed [46, 47] as concentrations adequate to activate 5-HT_{1A} receptors are reached.

Rizatriptan, like the other $5\text{-HT}_{1B/1D}$ selective agonists, had little affinity ($IC_{50} > 5,000$ nM) for human 5-HT_{2A} receptors that are thought to mediate many of the unwanted vasoconstrictor effects of unselective serotonin agonists [48, 49]. A practical clinical demonstration of the importance of removing 5-HT_{2A} agonist activity from the triptan molecules was reported by Siedelin [50] who compared the peripheral vasoconstrictor effects of rizatriptan (10 mg oral) to those of ergotamine (0.25 mg i.v.) by measuring changes in toe–arm blood pressure gradients. The studies showed that the response to rizatriptan was near to that of placebo, whereas ergotamine produced a pronounced vasoconstriction. As expected, since rizatriptan has no clinically relevant 5-HT_{2A} receptor activity, its co-administration with ergotamine did not cause any greater constriction than that to ergotamine alone.

Activity of Rizatriptan at Animal 5-HT_{1B} and 5-HT_{1D} Receptors

The activity of rizatriptan was assessed at rat and dog 5-HT_{1B} and 5-HT_{1D} receptors to support pharmacological and toxicological safety evaluations of rizatriptan. Overall affinities and maximum responses at animal 5-HT_{1D} receptors were similar to those at human receptors (see table 4). At rat 5-HT_{1B}

Table 4. Rizatriptan binding profile in pre-clinical species

	5-HT$_{1B}$	5-HT$_{1D}$
Rat	260 nM	12 nM
Rat ([^{35}S] GTPγS)	1700 nM/105%	12 nM/101%
Dog	17 nM	19 nM

Figures are affinity IC$_{50}$ nM. In the [^{35}S] GTPγS functional assay, potency is given as EC$_{50}$ nM and maximum responses expressed as a percentage of the response to 10 μM 5-HT (E$_{max}$ %). The assays used rat (r) or dog (d) cloned receptors: r5-HT$_{1D}$ in CHO, r5-HT$_{1B}$ in HeLa, d5-HT$_{1D}$ and d5-HT$_{1B}$ in CHO cell lines.

receptors, known to have a different pharmacology from h5-HT$_{1B}$ receptors due to a single amino acid difference in the binding domain [51, 52], rizatriptan had less affinity but gave a similar maximum response. At dog 5-HT$_{1B}$ receptors the activity of rizatriptan was similar to h5-HT$_{1B}$ receptors.

Plasma Protein Binding

Rizatriptan was poorly bound to human (14%) and animal (12–27%) plasma proteins and the binding was independent of concentration in the range 50–5,000 ng/ml. As a result, drug–drug interactions arising from displacement of rizatriptan from plasma proteins by co-administered drugs were not anticipated to be clinically significant.

Rizatriptan Metabolism

Rizatriptan is metabolized predominantly by the monoamine oxidase A (MAO-A) enzyme [53, 54]. The MAO-A route of metabolism has given rise to a contraindication on the co-administration of MAO inhibitors with rizatriptan (as with the other clinically used 5-HT$_{1B/1D}$ agonists: sumatriptan, zolmitriptan and naratriptan) as co-administration of the MAO inhibitor moclobemide can significantly increase exposure to both rizatriptan and its metabolites. A further recommendation arising from the MAO route of metabolism is that patients receiving propranolol should be given the lower 5 mg dose of rizatriptan as there is competition for the MAO-A enzyme between rizatriptan and the primary propranolol metabolite that is generated by CYP450 in the liver [55]. This competition results in an increased exposure to rizatriptan. If the 5 mg dose is used, then any increase in exposure (approx. 70%) when dosing with propranolol, would usually be expected to be within the exposure achieved with the 10 mg dosage form. There were no interactions with the other β-blockers nadolol or metoprolol that are commonly used for migraine prophylaxis, nor with oral contraceptive agents or serotonin reuptake inhibitors [55].

Radioligand Binding Studies on Metabolites

Radioligand binding studies on the human urinary metabolites of rizatriptan at animal and human 5-HT receptor sites showed that the major human metabolite, a carboxylic (indole acetic) acid was devoid of activity (IC_{50} > 10,000 nM) at all 5-HT sites tested. There was no evidence for metabolites with markedly different affinity profiles from the parent compound. Only a minor mono-desmethyl rizatriptan metabolite retained activity but its receptor affinity profile was similar to that of rizatriptan (5-HT$_{1B}$ IC_{50} 19 nM: 5-HT$_{1D}$ IC_{50} 9 nM [53]). Thus, the pharmacological activity of rizatriptan in vivo is predominantly due to the parent compound. It is also noteworthy that the plasma half-life of desmethyl rizatriptan is similar to that of the parent compound and this contributes to the simple predictable pharmacodynamics of rizatriptan in humans.

Oral Pharmacokinetics

The oral pharmacokinetics of rizatriptan were compared to those of sumatriptan [56–58]. The pre-clinical data are summarized in table 5. The studies showed that rizatriptan was rapidly and extensively absorbed after oral dosing suggesting an ability to provide rapid and consistent effects against migraine headache [57, 58]. Sumatriptan typically had a biphasic oral absorption profile and was more slowly and less extensively absorbed than rizatriptan [57]. It is noteworthy that the pharmacokinetic profile and oral bioavailability in the rhesus monkey was predictive of the profile later seen in humans. An important clinical pharmacokinetic study with rizatriptan also showed that its absorption during an attack was similar to its absorption between attacks [59] suggesting that, in contrast to some other serotonin receptor agonists [60, 61], its absorption and hence its performance as an anti-migraine drug, was unlikely to be affected by the gastrointestinal stasis that often accompanies migraine. This profile could contribute to the consistency of therapeutic effect that has been observed with rizatriptan.

Table 5. Pharmacokinetics of rizatriptan and sumatriptan in head to head studies in pre-clinical species

	Oral bioavailability (F%)		C_{max} (ng/ml)		T_{max} (h)	
	Rizatriptan	Sumatriptan	Rizatriptan	Sumatriptan	Rizatriptan	Sumatriptan
Rat	76	44	271	70	0.75	1.5 & 4
Dog	61	47	190	183	1.0	0.5 & 2
Rhesus	37	10	69	28	1.5	1.5 & 3

Oral pharmacokinetic studies were conducted head to head between rizatriptan and sumatriptan. C_{max} is the maximum plasma concentration reached after oral dosing and T_{max} is the time at which the maximum concentrations occurred after oral dosing. Sumatriptan typically produced a biphasic profile with two absorption peaks after oral dosing in all species.

Intracranial Extracerebral Vasoconstriction

Functional studies have shown conclusively that rizatriptan constricts intracranial extracerebral blood vessels and so has the potential to reverse the swelling of these vessels that is thought to activate trigeminal sensory nerves during a migraine attack [15, 17, 36].

The vasoconstrictor activity of rizatriptan was assessed in vitro using ring segments of human isolated middle meningeal arteries in comparison with 5-HT. These vessels are thought to be one of the targets for its anti-migraine effects. In the middle meningeal arteries the potency of rizatriptan (EC_{50} 90 nM) and the size of the maximal contractions evoked by 5-HT and rizatriptan were similar (see fig. 1 [36]). This indicates that the predominant contractile receptor in these intracranial blood vessels is of the 5-HT$_{1B}$ receptor subtype since this is the only serotonin receptor at which rizatriptan exerts significant vasoconstrictor activity (see table 1). Indeed immuno-histochemical studies have shown selective expression of 5-HT$_{1B}$ receptor immunoreactivity (but 5-HT$_{1D}$ receptor immunoreactivity) in these arteries [36, 37].

The haemodynamic effects of rizatriptan were assessed in vivo on carotid arteriovenous anastomoses and coronary blood flow. In this assay rizatriptan caused a highly selective vasoconstriction within the carotid artery vascular bed (ED_{50} 54 µg/kg giving an effective plasma concentration EC_{50} of 16 ng/ml) compared to the pulmonary and coronary artery vasculature [62]. This selectivity of vascular action occurred at relevant anti-migraine plasma concentrations since clinical studies showed that the anti-migraine plasma levels of

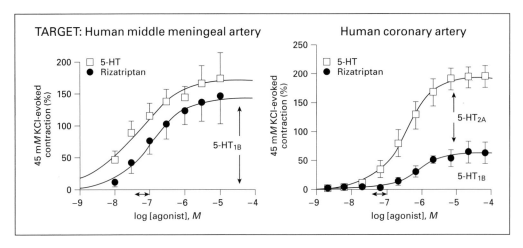

Fig. 1. The left-hand panel shows the contractile effects of serotonin and rizatriptan on isolated ring segments of human middle meningeal artery expressed relative to the reference response to 45 mM KCl. It can be seen that their maximum responses are similar. This indicates that the majority of the serotonergic contractile response in these vessels is mediated by the 5-HT$_{1B}$ receptor since this is the only contractile 5-HT receptor at which rizatriptan is active. The pharmacological data fits with the high density of 5-HT$_{1B}$ receptors that have been shown in these vessels using immunohistochemistry. The right hand panel shows the contractile responses to serotonin and rizatriptan in endothelium denuded ring segments of human coronary arteries relative to the response to 45 mM KCl. In this preparation, rizatriptan is a weak partial agonist relative to serotonin. The maximum response to rizatriptan is substantially lower than that to serotonin because rizatriptan is inactive at 5-HT$_{2A}$ receptors that mediate most of the contractile response to serotonin in this blood vessel and additionally the density of 5-HT$_{1B}$ receptors is lower than in the meningeal artery. These factors confer craniovascular selectivity. The arrows on the abscissa of both plots show the clinically relevant concentrations of rizatriptan. (Data is from references [36, 67, 68].)

rizatriptan achieved after dosing at 5 mg and 10 mg orally were 10–20 ng/ml (40–80 nM, [57, 59]).

The vasoconstrictor action of 5-HT$_{1B/1D}$ agonists is thought to be relatively specific to the intracranial extracerebral arteries. However, in the early stages of development of this class of drugs there was a potential concern that these agents could cause cerebral ischemia. This possibility was investigated with SPECT using [133]Xn-inhalation and showed, in a two-period two-treatment crossover study, that regional cerebral blood flow after dosing rizatriptan at 40 mg orally (compared to the 10 mg recommended therapeutic dose [55]) was not significantly different from placebo making it unlikely that rizatriptan has clinically relevant effects on cerebral blood flow [63].

Class Effect: All 5-HT$_{1B/1D}$ Agonists are Partial Agonists on Human Coronary Arteries in vitro

The demonstration that 5-HT$_{1B}$ receptors are present in the coronary arteries raised concerns over cardiac adverse event potential with the ergots and all the 5-HT$_{1B/1D}$ receptor selective agonists [36, 48, 64]. Clinical experience with sumatriptan over a number of years has however shown that adverse cardiac events are, however, rare with the 5-HT$_{1B/1D}$ agonist drugs. Drugs of this class are contraindicated for use in patients with known cardiovascular risk factors [55].

In order to address the potential coronary effects of rizatriptan, its vaso-constrictor activity was assessed in two independent academic studies using endothelium denuded ring segments of human isolated coronary arteries obtained from diseased hearts at the time of cardiac transplantation [66–68]. In both these studies the E$_{max}$ for 5-HT was 90.7 and 102% and for rizatriptan it was significantly less being 28.9 and 22.2%, respectively (fig. 1). It is noteworthy that in the in vitro experiment, drug concentrations causing contraction of the middle meningeal artery cover the clinically active range of plasma concentrations [36, 57, 59] and have no contractile effect on the coronary artery segments [57, 68]. The lower maximal contraction and the weak potency of rizatriptan compared to 5-HT in the coronary artery studies probably reflects an additional action of 5-HT at contractile 5-HT$_{2A}$ receptors. Studies using a polyclonal antibody specific for the 5-HT$_{1B}$ receptor clearly show that the density of 5-HT$_{1B}$ receptors is very much higher in the middle meningeal than in the coronary arteries [36]. This differential anatomical distribution, together with the absence of activity at contractile 5-HT$_{2A}$ receptors that are also present in coronary blood vessels [42, 49, 65], are the key factors which confer the craniovascular selectivity and cardiovascular safety for the class. At therapeutic concentrations there appear to be no marked differences between any of the triptan agents in their contractile effects on human coronary arteries in vitro [64, 69]. Any small differences reflect their relative therapeutic potency and occur at high concentrations that are supramaximal clinically and therefore probably irrelevant to their therapeutic use against migraine. It is noteworthy that all the triptan 5-HT$_{1B/1D}$ receptor selective agonists appear to be partial agonists in human coronary blood vessels in vitro [64, 68]. It should be noted chest symptoms/sensations that have sometimes been reported after dosing [70] may not be predominantly cardiac in origin but may be related to changes in pulmonary pressure or esophageal motility [71, 72].

Peripheral Trigeminal Nerve Inhibition

It has been hypothesized that excessive dilation of intracranial blood vessels could activate perivascular trigeminal nerves and thereby evoke the release of vasoactive neuropeptides (e.g. substance P, neurokinin A and calcitonin gene-related peptide (CGRP)) that can cause neurogenic inflammation within meningeal tissues such as the dura mater [15–17, 73, 74]. Substance P and neurokinin A cause increased blood vessel permeability and vasodilatation through endothelial receptors and nitric oxide release [15, 17, 75]. CGRP has no effects on vessel permeability but is one of the most potent endogenous vasodilator substances through its direct action on vascular smooth muscle and also through nitric oxide coupled mechanisms [76]. Experimental studies that showed effective acute anti-migraine agents to inhibit these processes led to the suggestion that they were important in the pathogenesis of migraine headache pain and gave rise to the neurogenic hypothesis of migraine [15–17, 73].

The effects of rizatriptan against these meningeal neurogenic processes were assessed in anaesthetized rats by (1) inducing neurogenic plasma protein extravasation (predominantly substance P-mediated [75, 78, 79]) in the dura mater by electrical stimulation of the trigeminal ganglion, and (2) by inducing neurogenic vasodilatation (proven to be CGRP-mediated [80–83]) in the middle meningeal artery through electrical stimulation of the dura mater. Rizatriptan caused a dose-dependent inhibition of extravasation and vasodilatation in the dura mater (fig. 2 [84]). Importantly, in the dural vasodilatation studies the responses to exogenously administered substance P and CGRP were unaffected by rizatriptan, at doses that inhibited neurogenic dilation, proving that this effect was through specific prejunctional inhibition of neuropeptide release [84]. The experimental findings on meningeal vasodilatation has clear parallels with the clinical observation that CGRP levels are raised in cranial venous effluent blood during migraine or cluster headache attacks and normalized by successful therapy with the 5-HT$_{1B/1D}$ agonist sumatriptan [74]. Indeed elevated levels of CGRP in cranial venous effluent blood have been one of the most reliable biochemical markers of trigeminal activation during migraine. In contrast, the relevance of plasma protein inhibition to migraine pathogenesis is not clear [85] as several compounds that were active against dural plasma protein extravasation (most notably substance P receptor antagonists and CP122, 288) are clinically ineffective in the acute treatment of migraine [78, 86–89]. Furthermore, the extravasation phenomenon has not been observed using in the meninges, gadolinium-enhanced MRI [90] or in the retina using a fluorescence technique during migraine headache attacks [91]. The key prejunctional inhibitory action of rizatriptan in the peripheral meningeal tissues

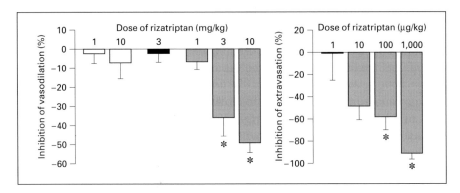

Fig. 2. Panel A shows data from intravital microscope studies on the inhibitory effects of rizatriptan on perivascular sensory nerves. Rizatriptan prevented CGRP-mediated vasodilatation of dural blood vessels evoked by electrical stimulation of the dura mater through a closed cranial window (hatched bars) but was inactive against exogenously administered substance P (open bars) and CGRP (filled bar). This profile indicates that rizatriptan acts as a vasoactive peptide release inhibitor (in this assay CGRP) through prejunctional 5-HT receptors and not as a peptide antagonist at postjunctional receptors. Panel B shows the inhibitory effects of rizatriptan on substance P mediated dural plasma extravasation evoked by electrical stimulation of the trigeminal ganglion. This effect is also mediated through an action at prejunctional 5-HT receptors. (Data are from reference [84].)

could thus be to break the dilator cycle that is driven by release of the vasoactive neuropeptide CGRP. This effect will promote normalization of meningeal blood vessel calibre and consequently decrease trigeminal sensory nerve activation thereby contributing to relief from headache pain [92].

Inhibition of Central Pain Processing and Trigeminal Sensitization

Trigeminal neurons are pseudo-unipolar in that as well as innervating intracranial blood vessels in the periphery they also have central projections that terminate behind the blood-brain barrier within the medulla [19]. It is therefore highly likely that the receptors that are expressed on peripheral trigeminal nerve fibres are also expressed on the central trigeminal terminals since both arise from the same neuronal cell body within the trigeminal ganglion. Electrophysiological studies in anaesthetized rats in vivo found that rizatriptan produced a dose-dependent inhibition of responses of single trigeminal neurons to noxious stimulation of the dura mater in the vicinity of the middle meningeal artery (fig. 3 [93]). This agreed with studies that have shown that other brain penetrant serotonin agonists inhibit the responses of neurons

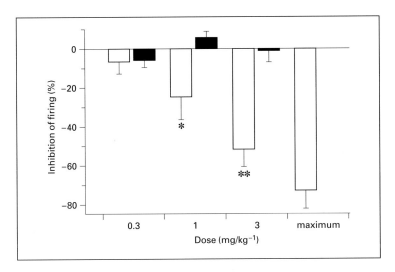

Fig. 3. The data shows evidence for central antinociceptive activity of rizatriptan in reducing the firing of single second order sensory neurons in the brainstem trigeminal nucleus caudalis caused by electrical stimulation of the dura mater. It is likely that this results from inhibition of neurotransmitter release from the central terminals of the trigeminal sensory fibers. Data are expressed relative to the pre-drug response and are taken from reference [93].

in the trigeminal nucleus caudalis to noxious stimulation of meningeal tissues or blood vessels [38–40, 94–96]. As in the periphery, it is likely that these inhibitory effects are due to prejunctional inhibition of neurotransmitter (peptide or glutamate) release that results in decreased activation of central sensory neurons. These findings indicate that rizatriptan is likely to have central anti-migraine effects by interrupting pain transmission within the medullary trigeminal nucleus caudalis.

Recent studies have also shown that sustained dural blood vessel dilation caused a sensitization of trigeminal neurons and a facilitation of facial sensory processing that could be blocked by a 5-HT$_{1B/1D}$ receptor agonist [97]. This data suggests that inhibition of central 'wind-up' in the medullary dorsal horn may also be an important feature of the action of the 5-HT$_{1B/1D}$ agonist anti-migraine agents in preventing the progression of headache pain intensity and the appearance of extracranial sensory disturbances during a migraine attack.

It is important to remember that although 5-HT$_{1B/1D}$ receptor agonists effectively block pain associated with migraine, they are not general analgesics. Naratriptan inhibits firing of nucleus caudalis cells after dural stimulation but it has no effect on nociceptive cell firing in the lumbar dorsal horn [40]. This selectivity is likely due to the highly specific trigeminal distribution of the 5-HT$_{1D}$ receptors within the CNS, and may explain the clinical observations that the 5-HT$_{1B/1D}$ agonists are specific craniovascular anti-nociceptive compounds rather than general analgesic drugs.

Conclusions

Preclinical studies have demonstrated that rizatriptan is a potent and selective 5-HT$_{1B/1D}$ receptor agonist that has good craniovascular over coronary selectivity in human isolated blood vessels and in vivo in pre-clinical assays. Pharmacological activity of rizatriptan has been shown to be due predominantly to the parent compound. The major human metabolite of rizatriptan (indole acetic acid) is devoid of activity at 5-HT receptors. Rizatriptan has three clear potential anti-migraine mechanisms of action. First, selective constriction of pain producing intracranial blood vessels that will reduce trigeminal sensory nerve activation. Second, inhibition of perivascular trigeminal sensory nerves that reduce neuropeptide release promoting normalization of vessel diameter. Third, central interruptions of nociceptive transmission within the brainstem trigeminal nucleus caudalis. The relative importance of each of these mechanisms to migraine headache relief can be debated, but it is very likely that they act simultaneously in a complimentary manner to reduce the intense trigeminal sensory input that occurs during a migraine headache attack. All three mechanisms are likely to be involved in providing rapid relief of headache pain and associated symptoms such as nausea.

References

1   Ferrari MD: Migraine. Lancet 1998;351:1043–1051.
2   Ophoff RA, Terwindt GM, Vergouwe MN, van Eijk R, Oefner PJ, Hoffman SMG, Lamerdin JE, Mohrenweiser HW, Bulman DE, Ferrari M, Haan J, Lindhout D, van Ommen G-JB, Hofker MH, Ferrari MD, Frants RR: Familial hemiplegic migraine and episodic ataxia type-2 are caused by mutations in the Ca^{2+}channel gene CACNL1A4. Cell 1996;87:543–552.
3   Valentino ML, Mochi M, Cevoli S, Montagna P: The genetics of migraine: A review. Confin Cephalalgia 1997;6:177–183.
4   Ogilvie AD, Russell MB, Dhall P, Battersby S, Ulrich V, Dale Smith CA, Goodwin GM, Harmar AJ: Altered allelic distributions of the serotonin transporter gene in migraine without aura and migraine with aura. Cephalalgia 1998;18:23–26.
5   Del Zompo M, Cherchi A, Palmas MA, Ponti M, Bocchetta A, Gessa GL, Piccardi MP: Association between dopamine receptor genes and migraine without aura in a Sardinian sample. Neurology 1998;51:781–786.
6   Gardner K: The genetic basis of migraine: How much do we know? Can J Neurological Sci 1999; 26(suppl 3):537–543.
7   Peroutka SJ: Genetic basis of migraine. Clin Neurosci 1998;5:34–37.

8   Nyholt DR, Lea RA, Goadsby PJ, Brimage PJ, Griffiths LR: Familial typical migraine. Linkage to chromosome 19p13 and evidence for genetic heterogeneity. Neurology 1998;50:1428–1432.

9   Spranger M, Spranger S, Schwab S, Benninger C, Dichgans M: Familial hemiplegic migraine with cerebellar ataxia and paroxysmal psychosis. Eur Neurol 1999;41:150–152.

10 Terwindt GM, Ophoff RA, Haan J, Sandkuijl LA, Frants RR, Ferrari MD: Migraine, ataxia and epilepsy: A challenging spectrum of genetically determined calcium channelopathies. Eur J Hum Genetics 1998;6:297–307.

11 Gardner K, Hoffman EP. Current status of genetic discoveries in migraine: Familial hemiplegic migraine and beyond. Curr Opin Neurol 1998;11:211–216.

12 Blau JN, Dexter SL: The site of pain origin during migraine attacks. Cephalalgia 1981;1:143–147.

13 Ray BS, Wolff HG: Experimental studies on headache. Pain sensitive structures of the head and their significance in headache. Arch Surgery 1940;41:813–856.

14 Wolff HG: Headache and Other Head Pain. 1963. New York, Oxford University Press, 1963.

15 Humphrey PPA, Feniuk W: Mode of action of the anti-migraine drug sumatriptan. Trends Pharmacol Sci 1991;12:444–446.

16 Friberg L, Olesen J, Iversen HK, Sperling B: Migraine pain associated with middle cerebral artery dilation: Reversal by sumatriptan. Lancet 1991;338:13–17.

17 Moskowitz MA: Neurogenic versus vascular mechanisms of sumatriptan and ergot alkaloids in migraine. Trends Pharmacol Sci 1992;13:307–312.

18 Lance JW: Migraine pain orginates from blood vessels; in Olesen J, Edvinsson L (eds): Headache Pathogenesis. Monoamines, Neuropeptides, Purines and Nitric Oxide. Frontiers in Headache Research, vol 7. New York, Lippincott-Raven, 1997, pp 3–9.

19 Hill RG: Current perspectives in pain. Sci Prog (Oxford) 1986;70:95–107.

20 Arrab MAR, Delgado T, Wiklund L, Svengaard NA: Brain stem terminations of the trigeminal and upper spinal innervation of the cerebrovascular system. J Cereb Blood Flow Metab 1988;8: 54–63.

21 Mayberg MR, Zervas NT, Moskowitz MA: Trigeminal projections to supratentorial pial and dural blood vessels in cats demonstrated by horseradish peroxidase histochemistry. J Comp Neurol 1984; 223:46–56.

22 Carpenter MB, Sutin J: The Autonomic Nervous System; in Human Neuroanatomy. Baltimore, Waverly Press, 1984, pp 209–231.

23 Jansen I, Uddman R, Ekman R, Olesen J, Ottoson A, Edvinsson L: Distribution and effects of neuropeptide Y, vasoactive intestinal polypeptide, substance P and calcitonin gene-related peptide in human middle meningeal arteries: Comparison with cerebral and temporal arteries. Peptides 1992;13:527–536.

24 Salt TE, Hill RG: Neurotransmitter candidates of somatosensory primary afferent fibres. Neurosci 1983;10:1083–1103.

25 Weihe E: Neuropeptides in primary afferent neurones; in Zenker W, Neuhuber W (eds): The Primary Afferent Neurone. New York, Plenum, 1990, pp 127–159.

26 Maggi CA, Patacchini R, Rovero P, Giachetti A: Tachykinin receptors and tachykinin receptor antagonists. Auto Pharmacol 1993;13:23–93.

27 Shepheard SL, Williamson DJ, Williams J, Hill RG, Hargreaves RJ: Comparison of the effects of sumatriptan and the NK_1 antagonist CP-99,994 on plasma protein extravasation in dura mater and c-fos mRNA expression in trigeminal nucleus caudalis of rats. Neuropharmacol 1995;34:255–261.

28 Goadsby PJ, Zagami AS, Lambert GA: Neural processing of craniovascular pain: A synthesis of the central structures involved in migraine. Headache 1991;31:365–371.

29 Goadsby PJ, Olesen J: Diagnosis and management of migraine. Br Med J 1996;312:1279–1283.

30 Hoyer D, Clarke DE, Fozard JR, Hartig PR, Martin GR, Mylecharane EJ, Saxena PR, Humphrey PPA: International union of pharmacology classification of receptors for 5-hydroxytryptamine (serotonin). Pharmacol Rev 1994;46:157–203.

31 Longmore J, Dowson AJ, Hill RG: Advances in migraine therapy – 5-HT receptor subtype specific agonists. Curr Opin Investigational Drugs 1999;1:39–53.

32 Silberstein S: The pharmacology of ergotamine and dihydroergotamine. Headache 1997;37:(suppl 1): S15–S25.

---

33 Weiller C, May A, Limmroth V, Jüptner M, Kaube H, Schayck RV, Coenen HH, Diener HC: Brain stem activation in spontaneous human migraine attacks. Nature Medicine 1995;1:658–660.

34 Connor HE, Beattie DT: Migraine: More advanced experimental models for drug development; in Olesen J, Moskowitz MA (eds): Frontiers in Headache Research, Experimental Headache Models. Philadelphia, Lippincott-Raven Press, 1996, vol 5, pp 19–26.

35 Moskowitz MA, Cutrer FM: Attacking migraine headache from beginning to end. Neurology 1997; 49:1193–1195.

36 Longmore J, Razzaque Z, Shaw D, Davenport AP, Maguire J, Pickard JD, Schofield WN, Hill RG: Comparison of the vasoconstrictor effects of rizatriptan and sumatriptan in using human isolated cranial arteries: Immunohistological demonstration of the involvement of 5-HT_{1B}-receptors. Br J Clin Pharmacol 1998;46:577–582.

37 Longmore J, Shaw D, Smith D, Hopkins R, McAllister G, Pickard JD, Sirinathsinghji DJS, Butler AJ, Hill RG: Differential distribution of 5-HT_{1D}- and 5-HT_{1B}-immunoreactivity within the human trigemino-cerebrovascular system: Implications for the discovery of new antimigraine drugs. Cephalalgia 1997;17:835–842.

38 Hoskin KL, Kaube H, Goadsby PJ: Central activation of the trigeminovascular pathway in the cat is inhibited by dihydroergotamine. A c-Fos and electrophysiological study. Brain 1996;119:249–256.

39 Goadsby PJ, Hoskin KL: Inhibition of trigeminal neurons by intravenous administration of the serotonin (5HT)-1D receptor agonist zolmitriptan (311C90): Are brain stem sites a therapeutic target in migraine. Pain 1996;67:355–359.

40 Cumberbatch MJ, Hill RG, Hargreaves RJ: Differential effects of the $5\text{-HT}_{1B/1D}$ receptor agonist naratriptan on trigeminal versus spinal nociceptive responses. Cephalalgia 1998;18:659–663.

41 Dahlof CGH, Hargreaves RJ: Pathophysiology and pharmacology of migraine. Is there a place for anti-emetics in future treatment strategies? Cephalalgia 1998;18:593–604.

42 Pauwels PJ, Tardif S, Palmier C, Wurch T, Colpaert FC: How efficacious are $5\text{-HT}_{1B/D}$ receptors ligands: An answer from GTP's binding studies with stably transfected C6-glial cell lines. Neuropharmacol 1997;36:499–512.

43 Beer M, Middlemiss D, Stanton J, Longmore J, Hargreaves RJ, Noble AJ, Scholey KS, Bevan Y, Hill RG, Baker R, Street LJ, Matassa VG, Iversen LL: In vitro pharmacological profile of the novel 5-HT_{1D} receptor agonist MK-462. Cephalalgia 1995;15(suppl):203P.

44 Grof P, Joffe R, Kennedy S, Persad E, Syrotiuk J, Bradford D: An open study of oral flesinoxan, a 5-HT_{1A} receptor agonist in treatment resistant depression. Int Clin Psychopharmacol 1993;8: 167–172.

45 De Voogd JM, Prager G: Early clinical experience with flesinoxan, a new selective 5-HT1A receptor agonist; in Saxena PR, Wallis DI, Wouters W, Bevan P (eds): Cardiovascular Pharmacology of 5-Hydroxytryptamine. Kluwer Academic Publishers, 1990, pp 355–359.

46 Visser WH, Terwindt GM, Reines SA, Jiang K, Lines CR, Ferrari MD: Rizatriptan vs sumatriptan in the acute treatment of migraine. Arch Neurol 1996;53:1132–1137.

47 Gijsman H, Kramer MS, Sargent J, Tuchmann M, Matzura-Wolfe D, Polis A, Teall J, Block G, Ferrari MD: Double-blind, placebo-controlled, dose-finding study of rizatriptan (MK-462) in the acute treatment of migraine. Cephalalgia 1997;17:647–651.

48 Kaumann AJ, Frenken M, Posival H, Brown AM: Variable participation of 5-HT_1-like receptors and 5-HT_2 receptors in serotonin-induced contraction of human isolated coronary arteries. Circulation 1994;90:1141–1153.

49 Connor HE, Feniuk W, Humphrey PPA: 5-Hydroxytryptamine contracts human coronary artery predominantly via 5-HT_2 receptor activation. Eur J Pharmacol 1992;161:91–94.

50 Siedelin KN, Tfelt-Hansen P, Mendel CN, Stepanavage M: Peripheral hemodynamic study of MK-462, ergotamine and their combination in humans. Presented at the International Headache Congress, Toronto, 1995.

51 Parker EM, Grisel DA, Iben LG, Shapiro RA: A single amino acid difference accounts for the pharmacological distinction between rat and human $5\text{-hydroxytryptamine}_{1B}$ receptors. J Neurochem 1993;60:380–383.

52   Adham N, Romanienko P, Hartig P, Weinshank R, Branchek T: The rat 5-hydroxytryptamine$_{1B}$ receptor is the species homologue of the human 5-hydroxtryptamine$_{1D\beta}$ receptor. Mol Pharmacol 1992;41:1–7.

53   Rodgers JD, Lee Y, Goldberg MR, Olah TV, Musson DG, Birk KM, McLoughlin DA, Beer M, Slaughter D, Halpin RA, Vyas KP: Human pharmacokinetics of rizatriptan, a 5-HT$_{1B/1D}$ receptor agonist. Functional Neurol 1998;13:179.

54   Liu L, Cheng H, Chavez C, Matuszewski B, Guiblin A, Polrino W, Chen T, Rogers J: Identification of urinary metabolites of N,N-dimethyl-2-[5-(1,2,4-triazol-1-ylmethyl)-1H-indol-3-yl] ethylamine benzoate (MK-462) in humans. Pharm Res 1994;11(suppl):S409.

55   Merck A Co., Inc. MAXALT ® (Rizatriptan Benzoake) tablets. MAXALT ® – MLT (Rizatriptan Benzoate) orally disintegrating tablets. Physicians Desk Reference. Medical Economics Company. Montrale NJ, Edition 53, 1999, pp 1822–1827.

56   Street LJ, Baker R, Davey WB, Guiblin AR, Jelley RA, Reeve AJ, Routledge H, Sternfeld F, Watt AP, Beer MS, Middlemiss DN, Noble AJ, Stanton JA, Scholey K, Hargreaves RJ, Sohal B, Graham M, Matassa V: Synthesis and serotonergic activity of N,N-dimethyl-2-[5-(1,2,4-triazol-1-ylmethyl)-1H-indol-3-yl]ethamine and analogues: Potent agonists for 5-HT$_{1D}$ receptors. J Med Chem 1995;38: 1700–1810.

57   Scriberras DG, Polvino, WJ, Gertz BJ, Cheng H, Stepanavage M, Wittreich J, Olah T, Edwards M, Mank T: Initial human experience with MK-462 (rizatriptan): A novel 5-HT$_{1D}$ agonist. Br J Clin Pharmacol 1997;43:49–54.

58   Lee Y, Conroy JA, Stepanavage ME, Mendel CM, Somers G, McLoughlin DA, Olah TV, De Smet M, Keymeulen B, Rogers JD: Pharmacokinetics and tolerability of oral rizatriptan in healthy male and female volunteers. Br J Clin Pharmacol 1999;47:373–378.

59   Cutler NR, Jhee SS, Majumdar AK, McLoughlin D, Bruker MJ, Carides AD, Kramer MS, Matzura-Wolfe D, Reines SA, Goldberg MR: Pharmacokinetics or rizatriptan tablets during and between migraine attacks. Headache 1999;39:264–269.

60   Palmer KJ, Spencer CM: Zolmitriptan. CNS Drugs 1997;7:468–478.

61   Johnson BF, Shah A, Law G: The absorption kinetics of eletriptan. Cephalalgia 1997;17:415.

62   Shepheard S, Williamson D, Cook D, Baker R, Street L, Matassa V, Beer M, Middlemiss D, Iversen L, Hill R, Hargreaves R: In vivo pharmacology of the novel 5-HT$_{1D}$ receptor agonist MK-462. Cephalagia 1995;15(suppl):205P.

63   Sperling B, Tfelt-Hansen P, Lines C: Lack of effect of MK-462 on cerebral blood flow in humans. Cephalagia 1995;15(suppl):206P.

64   MaassenVanDenBrink A, Reekers M, Bax WA, Ferrari MD, Saxena PR: Coronary side-effect potential of current and prospective antimigraine drugs. Circulation 1998;98:25–30.

65   Martin GR, Rhodes P, Mills A: Autoradiographic mapping of receptors and recognition sites for established and putative antimigraine drugs; in Edvinsson L (ed): Migraine and Headache Pathophysiology, chap 7. Martin Dunitz, 1999, pp 63–79.

66   Ferro A, Longmore J, Hill RG, Brown MJ: A comparison of the contractile effects of 5-hydroxy-tryptamine, sumatriptan and MK-462 on human coronary artery in vitro. Br J Clin Pharmacol 1995;40:245–251.

67   Longmore J, Boulanger CM, Desta B, Hill RG, Schofield WN, Taylor AA: 5-HT$_{1D}$ receptor agonists and human coronary artery reactivity in vitro: Crossover comparisons of 5-HT and sumatriptan with MK-462 and L-741,519. Br J Clin Pharmacol 1996;42:431–441.

68   Longmore J, Hargreaves RJ, Boulanger CM, Brown MJ, Desta B, Ferro A, Schofield WN, Taylor AA, Hill RG: Comparison of the vasoconstrictor properties of the 5-HT$_{1D}$-receptor agonists rizatriptan (MK-462) and sumatriptan in human isolated coronary artery: Outcome of two independent studies using different experimental protocols. Functional Neurol 1997;12:3–9.

69   Longmore J, Maguire JJ, MacLeod A, Street L, Schofield WN, Hill RG: Comparison of the vaso-constrictor effects of the selective 5-HT$_{1D}$-receptor agonist L-775,606 with the mixed 5-HT$_{1B/1D}$-receptor agonist sumatriptan and 5-HT in human isolated coronary artery. Br J Clin Pharmacol 1999; in press.

70   Visser WH: 5-HT$_1$ receptor agonists in the acute treatment of migraine. Clinical epidemiological and pharmacological aspects. 1996, PhD Thesis, Delft: Eburon-Delft.

71   Houghton LA, Foster JM, Whorwell PJ, Morris J, Fowler P: Is chest pain after sumatriptan oesophageal in origin. Lancet 1994;344:985–986.

72   MacIntyre PD, Bhagrave B, Hogg KJ, Gemmill JD, Hillis WS: Effect of subcutaneous sumatriptan, a selective 5-HT-1 agonist, on the systemic, pulmonary and coronary circulation. Circulation 1993; 87:401–405.

73   Goadsby PJ, Edvinsson L, Ekman R: Vasoactive neuropeptide release in the extracerebral circulation of humans during migraine headache. Ann Neurol 1990;28:183–187.

74   Goadsby PJ, Edvinsson L: The trigeminovascular system and migraine: Studies characterizing cerebrovascular and neuropeptide changes seen in humans and cats. Ann Neurol 1993;33:48–56.

75   Moskowitz MA, Buzzi MG: Neuroeffector functions of sensory fibres: Implications for headache mechanisms and drug action. J Neurol 1991;238:S18–S22.

76   Van Rossum D, Hanisch U-K, Quirion R: Neuroanatomical localization, pharmacological characterization and functions of CGRP, related peptides and their receptors. Neurosci Behav Rev 1997;21: 649–678.

77   Lassen LH, Ashina M, Christiansen I, Ulrich V, Olesen J: Nitric oxide synthase inhibition in migraine. Lancet 1997;349:401–402.

78   Shepheard SL, Williamson DJ, Hill RG, Hargreaves RJ: The non-peptide neurokinin-1 receptor antagonist, RP 67580, blocks neurogenic plasma extravasation in the dura mater of rats. Br J Pharmacol 1993;108:11–12.

79   O'Shaughnessy CT, Connor HE: Investigation of the role of tachykinin NK1, NK2 receptors and CGRP receptors in neurogenic plasma protein extravasation in dura mater. Eur J Pharmacol 1994; 263:193–198.

80   Kurosawa M, Messlinger K, Pawlak M, Schmidt RF: Increase in meningeal blood flow after electrical stimulation of rat dura mater encephali: Mediation by calcitonin gene-related peptide. Br J Pharmacol 1995;114:1397–1402.

81   Williamson DJ, Hargreaves RJ, Hill RG, Shepheard SL: Intravital microscope studies on the effects of neurokinin agonists and calcitonin gene-related peptide on dural vessel diameter in the anaesthetized rat. Cephalalgia 1997;17:518–524.

82   Goadsby PJ: Inhibition of calcitonin gene-related peptide by h-CGRP(8-37) antagonises the cerebral dilator response from nasocilary nerve stimulation in the cat. Neurosci Lett 1993;151:13–16.

83   Escott KJ, Beattie DT, Connor HE, Brain SD: Trigeminal ganglion stimulation increases facial skin blood flow in the rat: A major role for calcitonin gene-related peptide. Brain Res 1995;669: 93–99.

84   Williamson DJ, Shepheard SL, Hill RG, Hargreaves RJ: The novel anti-migraine agent rizatriptan inhibits neurogenic dural vasodilation and extravasation. Eur J Pharmacol 1997;328:61–64.

85   Hargreaves RJ, Williamson DJ Shepheard SL: Neurogenic inflammation: Relation to novel antimigraine drugs; in Edvinsson L (ed): Migraine and Headache Pathophysiology, chap 7. Martin Dunitz, 1999, pp 93–101.

86   Goldstein DJ, Wang O, Saper JS, Stolz R, Silberstein SD, Mathew NT: Ineffectiveness of neurokinin-1 antagonist in acute migraine. Cephalalgia 1997;17:785–790.

87   Connor HE, Bertin L, Gillies S, Beattie DT, Ward P and the GR205171 Clinical Study Group: Clinical evaluation of a novel, potent, CNS penetrating NK_1 receptor antagonist in the acute treatment of migraine. Cephalalgia 1998;18:392.

88   Beattie DT, Connor HE: The pre- and postjunctional activity of CP-122,288, a conformationally restricted analogue of sumatriptan. Eur J Pharmacol 1995;276:271–276.

89   Roon K, Diener HC, Ellis P: CP 122,288 blocks neurogenic inflammation but is not effective in aborting migraine attacks: Results of two controlled clinical trials. Cephalalgia 1997;17:24.

90   Nissila M, Parkkola R, Sonninen P, Saloene R: Intracerebral arteries and gadolinium enhanced MRI in migraine without aura. Cephalalgia 1996;16(suppl):362.

91   May A, Shepheard SL, Knorr M, Effert R, Wessing A, Hargreaves RJ, Goadsby PJ, Diener HC: Retinal plasma extravasation in animals but not in humans: Implications for the pathophysiology of migraine. Brain 1998;121:1231–1237.

92   Moskowitz MA: Interpreting vessel diameter changes in vascular headache. Cephalalgia 1992;12: 5–7.

93   Cumberbatch MJ, Hill RG, Hargreaves RJ: Rizatriptan has central antinociceptive effects against durally evoked responses. Eur J Pharmacol 1997;328:37–40.

94   Martin GR: Pre-clinical pharmacology of zolmitriptan (Zomig; formerly 311C90), a centrally and peripherally acting 5-HT$_{1B/1D}$ agonist for migraine. Cephalalgia 1997;18(suppl):4–14.

95   Cumberbatch MJ, Hill RG, Hargreaves RJ: The effects of 5-HT$_{1A}$, 5-HT$_{1B}$ and 5-HT$_{1D}$ receptor agonists on trigeminal nociceptive neurotransmission in anaesthetised rats. Eur J Pharmacol 1998; 362:43–46.

96   Goadsby PJ, Hoskin KL: Serotonin inhibits trigeminal nucleus activity evoked by craniovascular stimulation through a 5-HT$_{1B/1D}$ receptor: A central action in migraine. Ann Neurol 1998;43:711–718.

97   Cumberbatch MJ, Williamson DJ, Mason GS, Hill RG, Hargreaves RJ: Dural vasodilation causes a sensitization of rat caudal trigeminal neurones in vivo that is blocked by a 5-HT$_{1B/1D}$ agonist. Br J Pharmacol 1999;126:1478–1486.

Dr. R. Hargreaves, Merck & Co Inc,
PO Box 4, 770, Sumneytown Pike, West Point, PA 19486 (USA)
Tel. +1 215 652 4314, Fax +1 215 652 6913, E-Mail richard_hargreaves@merck.com

Diener HC (ed): Drug Treatment of Migraine and Other Headaches.
Monogr Clin Neurosci. Basel, Karger, 2000, vol 17, pp 162–172

....

Rizatriptan – Therapy

Carl Dahlöf[a], *Christopher Lines*[b]

[a] Gothenburg Migraine Clinic, Sociala Huset, Gothenburg, Sweden
[b] Clinical Research, Merck and Co., Inc., West Point, PA, USA

Rizatriptan is a novel 5-HT$_{1B/1D}$ receptor agonist for the acute treatment of migraine, which received approval for marketing in the United States, Europe, and other countries worldwide in 1998. The drug is available in two oral dosage strengths of 10 mg and 5 mg, with 10 mg being the recommended primary dose in most countries. As well as conventional tablets, rizatriptan is available in a rapidly-dissolving wafer formulation which can be taken without water. The wafer provides convenience of administration, and may be of utility in patients who have difficulty swallowing a tablet due to migraine-associated nausea.

In humans, rizatriptan is 40 to 45% bioavailable, has a T_{max} of approximately 1 h, and a $t_{1/2}$ of approximately 2 h [1, 2]. This pharmacokinetic profile is superior to sumatriptan, which has a T_{max} of 2.5 h and oral bioavailability of approximately 14% [1]. The dose-response profile of rizatriptan was established in two phase II studies, which covered a range of doses from 2.5 to 40 mg [3, 4]. Rizatriptan 10 mg and 5 mg had the most favorable benefit/risk profiles and were selected for subsequent development. The phase III trials confirmed that the 10-mg dose was more effective than 5 mg. This chapter discusses the efficacy and safety of rizatriptan 10 mg and 5 mg, in comparison to both placebo and sumatriptan, as investigated in phase III studies [5–10].

Clinical Trial Procedures

The trial methodology for the evaluation of rizatriptan as an acute symptomatic treatment for migraine was based on the procedures established for the development of sumatriptan, and followed guidelines from the International Headache Society [11, 12] (see table 1). Over 5,000 patients participated in the

Table 1. Design and methodology of phase III clinical trials with rizatriptan

Patient selection	Outpatients, age 18 years or older IHS diagnostic criteria for migraine with or without aura [12] 1–8 migraine attacks per month Otherwise healthy
Trial design	Short-term studies [5–9]: Single attack (4 attacks in 1 study [6]) Double-blind Placebo-controlled Randomized Parallel groups or crossover Active comparator = sumatriptan (various doses) [7–9] Long-term extensions [10]: Intermittent attacks over periods of up to 12 months Single-blind or open-label Randomized Parallel groups Active comparator = standard care (patient's usual migraine medication(s))
Symptom evaluation	Patient-reported symptoms at 0, 0.5, 1, 1.5, 2, 3 and 4 hours: Headache severity (4-grade scale) Functional disability (4-grade scale) Associated symptoms (presence or absence)
Primary endpoints	For comparisons to placebo: pain relief at 2 h (reduction from moderate or severe pain at baseline to mild or no pain) For comparisons to sumatriptan: time-to-pain-relief within 2 h

short-term, placebo-controlled, double-blind, studies (table 1). Approximately 1,800 of these patients continued in the long-term extensions (table 1), and treated over 46,000 migraine attacks. In all studies, patients were instructed to take test medication when they experienced a moderate or severe migraine headache. Escape medications, consisting of standard analgesics or anti-emetics, were allowed from 2 h post-dose and this compromises interpretation of efficacy results beyond the 2-h time-point.

Efficacy and Safety Evaluation

Efficacy data were gathered using patient-completed diary cards. The primary assessment of efficacy was based on patients' self-rating of headache severity on the standard 4-grade scale (0 = no headache, 1 = mild pain, 2 = moderate pain, 3 = severe pain) at time points up to 4 h (table 1). Additional outcome parameters (table 1) included functional disability (4-grade scale: 0 = normal, 1 = daily activities mildly impaired, 2 = daily activities severely impaired, 3 = unable to carry out daily activities, requires bedrest), and presence or absence of associated symptoms of photophobia, phonophobia, nausea, and vomiting.

The pre-determined primary or co-primary hypothesis in each study involved a comparison of rizatriptan to placebo for the percentage of patients with 'pain relief' at the 2-h time-point (defined as a reduction of headache severity from moderate or severe pain at baseline, to no headache or mild pain at 2 h). The 2-h time-point was the last occasion before escape medication was allowed, and efficacy results at this time-point therefore allow the clearest uncontaminated perspective on drug effects. However, response rates at later time-points are also important because they give an indication of the response rates that can be expected in 'real life' clinical practice when rizatriptan is administered according to the labeling instructions, which do not prohibit the use of escape medications. For studies involving sumatriptan, an additional pre-specified co-primary analysis was 'time-to-pain-relief' within 2 h (see 'Efficacy of Rizatriptan vs. Sumatriptan' below).

Safety was assessed by patient reports of clinical adverse events.

Efficacy of Rizatriptan versus Placebo in Short-Term Studies

Headache Pain

Treatment of a Single Migraine Attack. Rizatriptan 10 and 5 mg are clearly effective in the acute treatment of a moderate or severe migraine headache, both with regard to the percentage of patients experiencing pain relief and on the more stringent measure of the percentage of patients who became pain-free. Onset of relief was apparent from 30 min after dosing (the earliest time-point assessed) and was maintained over the 4-h evaluation period [8]. The greatest differences from placebo were observed at 2 h. On the pain relief measure at this time-point, across all studies, the difference from placebo was 34 percentage points for rizatriptan 10 mg, and 30 percentage points for rizatriptan 5 mg; on the pain-free measure, the difference from placebo was 33 percentage points for 10 mg, and 23 percentage points for 5 mg. At 4 h (the last evaluation time-point), after escape medication had been allowed, up to 84% of patients on rizatriptan 10 mg [7] and 79% of patients on rizatriptan 5 mg [8] had pain relief, while up to 65% (10 mg) [7] and 48% (5 mg) [8] of patients were pain-free.

Treatment of up to 4 Migraine Attacks. In a placebo-controlled short-term study of the efficacy of rizatriptan 10 mg when used to treat up to 4 attacks (with an additional interspersed placebo-treated attack in most patients), over 90% of patients responded to treatment during their first or second attack [6]. Of those who did not respond to the first attack within 2 h, most (70%) did respond during the second attack. This indicates that non-response during an initial attack does not predict non-response during a subsequent attack and it is therefore worthwhile for patients to treat with rizatriptan over several attacks, even if they do not initially respond.

The consistency of response following treatment with rizatriptan 10 mg was also good in this short-term study. Of the 252 patients who treated 3 attacks with rizatriptan (with an additional interspersed placebo-treated attack in most patients), 96, 86 and 60% reported pain relief at 2 h in 1 out of 3, 2 out of 3, and 3 out of 3 attacks, respectively. This appears to be more favorable than the consistency of response obtained in previous studies with sumatriptan 100 mg or 50 mg, in which about 30 to 40% of patients who treated 3 attacks had pain relief at 2 h in all attacks [13], and about 60% had pain relief at 2 h in 2 out of 3 attacks [14].

Treatment of Headache Recurrence. The main efficacy drawback of acute migraine therapies, including 5-$HT_{1B/1D}$ agonists, is that headache recurs within 24 h in approximately 30 to 40% of patients who initially experience pain relief after dosing [8, 15, 16]. (Note, the definition of recurrence is not standardized within the field of migraine research. For instance, a study of naratriptan used a definition corresponding to the return of headache in patients who experienced relief at 4 h [17], rather than at 2 h as used in the rizatriptan studies. The appropriate evaluation of recurrence rates requires direct comparison studies.) In a placebo-controlled, randomized investigation of the treatment of headache recurrence, rizatriptan was effective in treating headache recurrence, with the 10-mg dose appearing more effective than 5 mg (e.g. differences from placebo for percentage of patients pain-free at 2 h after randomized treatment of recurrence = 34 percentage points for 10 mg, and 21 percentage points for 5 mg) [5]. Thus, patients taking rizatriptan may experience headache recurrence, but if they do there is a high likelihood that a second dose of rizatriptan will be effective in treating it.

Associated Symptoms

The associated symptoms that accompany a migraine headache can be as bothersome to the patient as the headache itself, and can occur in up to 80% of untreated patients [18]. Rizatriptan 10 mg and 5 mg were consistently effective in reducing the incidence of associated symptoms of nausea, photophobia, and phonophobia at 2 h after dosing (e.g. differences from placebo for 10 mg/5 mg of 21/15 percentage points (nausea), 27/20 percentage points (photophobia), and 21/16 percentage points (phonophobia), respectively [5]). In some studies, the incidence of vomiting was also reduced, although, as this only occurred in a small minority of patients, it was not always possible to undertake formal statistical testing. The time course of rizatriptan's effects on associated symptoms generally paralleled that for headache relief with differences from placebo being apparent from 30 min after dosing in some instances and being maintained over the 4-h evaluation period [8]. Again, the greatest differences from placebo tended to be observed at 2 h.

Functional Disability

Migraine is not a life-threatening condition, but the cost of loss of productivity associated with an attack is high and has been estimated at over 700 million pounds per year in the United Kingdom [19]. Rizatriptan 10 mg and 5 mg were effective in enabling more patients to have normal functional ability than patients on placebo (e.g. difference from placebo at 2 h = 28 percentage points for 10 mg, and 20 percentage points for 5 mg [5]). The difference was apparent from as early as 30 min after dosing and persisted up to the last 4-h evaluation time point.

Efficacy of Rizatriptan 10 mg vs. 5 mg in Short-Term Studies

The comparative efficacy of rizatriptan 10 mg vs. rizatriptan 5 mg was investigated in two phase III studies [5, 7]. While both doses of rizatriptan were clearly effective in comparison to placebo, the 10-mg dose of rizatriptan was superior to the 5-mg dose on most efficacy measures, including the percentage of patients with pain relief, who were pain-free, or who were without associated symptoms. The superiority was sufficiently consistent across the two phase III studies which included the comparison (and also in the long-term extensions; see below) to indicate that 10 mg is more effective than 5 mg [5, 7]. For example, the 10-mg dose was superior to 5 mg on the percentage of patients who were pain-free at 2 h in both studies: 42% vs. 33% [5], and 40% vs. 25% [7].

Efficacy of Rizatriptan vs. Sumatriptan in Short-Term Studies

As oral sumatriptan was the standard prescription drug specifically targeted for the acute treatment of migraine, during its development rizatriptan was compared to oral sumatriptan in three studies [7–9]. These studies encompassed the range of recommended oral sumatriptan doses (100 mg, 50 mg, and 25 mg) and included the following comparisons: rizatriptan 10 mg and 5 mg vs. sumatriptan 100 mg in parallel treatment groups [7]; rizatriptan 5 mg vs. sumatriptan 50 mg in parallel treatment groups [8]; crossover comparison of rizatriptan 10 mg vs. sumatriptan 50 mg, and of rizatriptan 5 mg vs. sumatriptan 25 mg [9].

The primary pre-specified analysis for the comparison of rizatriptan to oral sumatriptan was 'time-to-pain-relief' over the 2 h after dosing. This is a time-to-event analysis based on the variable of 'time to first report of pain relief'. The analysis defined the likelihood of pain relief over the 2 h period following treatment, and quantified the difference between treatments in terms of a hazard ratio. A hazard ratio >1 for treatment X vs. treatment Y indicates an advantage in terms of speed of action for treatment X. For instance, a hazard ratio of 1.21 for treatment X vs. treatment Y indicates that, for a patient who has no pain relief up to a particular time point, the probability of pain relief in the near future is 21% higher with drug X than drug Y.

On this measure, rizatriptan 10 mg was significantly better than oral sumatriptan 100 mg (hazard ratio of 1.21) [7]) and oral sumatriptan 50 mg (hazard ratio of 1.14 [8]), while rizatriptan 5 mg was significantly better than oral sumatriptan 25 mg (hazard ratio of 1.16 [8]). The differences between rizatriptan 5 mg and sumatriptan 100 mg or 50 mg were not statistically significant (hazard ratios of 0.97 [7] and 0.94 [9], respectively). The faster onset of action demonstrated by these findings for rizatriptan 10 mg vs. oral sumatriptan 100 mg and 50 mg, and for rizatriptan 5 mg vs. oral sumatriptan 25 mg, is likely to be of considerable importance to patients [20].

In addition to faster onset of action over 2 h, the highest 10-mg dose of rizatriptan was more effective than the highest 100-mg dose of oral sumatriptan, on a number of efficacy parameters at individual time-points within 2 h (table 2) [7, 21]. These findings generally support the early onset of action of rizatriptan vs. oral sumatriptan. For example, at 1 h, significantly more patients experienced pain relief following rizatriptan 10 mg compared with sumatriptan 100 mg (37 vs. 28%), were without nausea (59 vs. 47%), or had normal functional ability (14 vs. 9%) [7]. At 2 h, significantly more patients on rizatriptan 10 mg were pain-free compared with sumatriptan 100 mg (40 vs. 33%), were without nausea (75 vs. 67%), and had normal functional ability (42 vs. 33%). By contrast, there was no measure at any time-point on which the highest 100-mg dose of oral sumatriptan was significantly better than the highest 10-mg dose of rizatriptan [7].

Rizatriptan 5 mg was more effective than oral sumatriptan 25 mg on a number of efficacy parameters at individual time-points within 2 h, including measures of headache severity, associated symptoms, and functional disability

Table 2. Measures on which rizatriptan 10 mg was more effective than sumatriptan 100 mg (p < 0.05) [7, 21]

	0.5 hour	1 hour	1.5 hours	2 hours
Time-to-pain-relief		$\longrightarrow$		
Pain relief		X		
Pain-free			X	X
Improvement in functional disability		X	X	X
Elimination of nausea	X	X	X	X
Elimination of photophobia		X	X	
Elimination of phonophobia		X	X	

Note: At no time point was sumatriptan 100 mg more effective than rizatriptan 10 mg.

[8]. Rizatriptan 5 mg generally showed equivalent efficacy to the 50- and 100-mg oral doses of sumatriptan through 2 h post-dose, but was more effective in reducing the associated symptom of nausea (e.g. percentage of patients without nausea at 2 h = 77% for rizatriptan 5 mg vs. 67% for sumatriptan 100 mg [7], and 70% for rizatriptan 5 mg vs. 63% for sumatriptan 50 mg [9]). The advantage for rizatriptan over oral sumatriptan with regard to nausea relief is potentially important, since nausea occurs in more than 80% of untreated patients and is the symptom that most bothers patients, after headache [22]. The reason for the difference between rizatriptan and oral sumatriptan is unknown, but may conceivably be suggestive of greater central exposure with rizatriptan.

Over the three sumatriptan comparison studies, the only instance of a measure on which any dose of oral sumatriptan was significantly better than rizatriptan 10 mg was in relation to the small incidence of vomiting at 4 h (1% for sumatriptan 50 mg vs. 3% for rizatriptan 10 mg), after escape medication was allowed [7]. Additionally, although not a consistent finding, sumatriptan 100 mg and 50 mg were significantly better than the lower 5-mg dose of rizatriptan on several other measures at 3 and 4 h after dosing in some studies (e.g. percentage of patients with pain relief, who were pain-free, or who were without phonophobia at 4 h = 84 vs. 73%, 58 vs. 45%, and 80 vs. 70% for sumatriptan 100 mg versus rizatriptan 5 mg, respectively [7]. Interpretation of this data is confounded by the use of escape medication at 2 h, but it is possible that the findings may be related to the later T_{max} of sumatriptan. There was also a small advantage for oral sumatriptan 25 mg over rizatriptan 5 mg in the percentage of patients who were pain-free at 30 min after dosing in one study (1.6 vs. 0.4%) [8]. However, this advantage was not maintained at subsequent time-points. In fact, as noted above, over the 2-h evaluation period rizatriptan 5 mg showed overall faster time-to-pain-relief [8].

Similar recurrence rates (approximately a third of patients) and mean time to recurrence (approximately 11 h) were noted for both rizatriptan and oral sumatriptan [7–9].

Long-Term Efficacy of Rizatriptan

During the long-term extension trials rizatriptan was compared to patients' usual standard care treatment(s) over periods of up to 12 months (table 1) [10]. Standard care mainly consisted of sumatriptan (76% of patients; approximately two thirds of the sumatriptan taken was in the oral tablet form, with the remaining third consisting of a subcutaneous injection) or NSAIDs (50% of patients).

Rizatriptan 10 mg was superior to standard care and rizatriptan 5 mg on pain relief and pain-free measures at 2 h. The median patient on rizatriptan 10 mg at 2 h post-dose had headache relief 90% of the time and was pain-free 50% of the time, vs. 70 and 29%, respectively, for standard care. After rizatriptan 5 mg, the median patient achieved pain relief in 80% of attacks and became pain-free by 2 h 35% of the time. The response to rizatriptan during long-term treatment was consistent. Overall, 73% of patients on rizatriptan 10 mg reported pain relief in more than three fourths of their treated attacks, while this was true for 56% of patients on rizatriptan 5 mg and only 43% of those on standard care. Thus, the superior efficacy of the 10-mg dose of rizatriptan apparent in short-term treatment was confirmed in long-term use. The distinction between the two rizatriptan doses was further supported by the finding that during the extensions only 4% of patients on rizatriptan 10 mg withdrew due to lack of efficacy, whereas 12% of those on rizatriptan 5 mg did. As in the short-term studies, headache recurrence was noted in approximately one third of treated attacks.

Safety and Tolerability of Rizatriptan

Both doses of rizatriptan were generally well-tolerated, as is illustrated by the combined safety data from four of the short-term treatment studies [5–7, 9]. During these studies, one or more clinical adverse events occurred in 42% of patients on rizatriptan 10 mg, 33% of patients on rizatriptan 5 mg, and 25% of patients on placebo treatment. There was a slightly higher incidence of clinical adverse events following rizatriptan 10 mg compared to 5 mg, but otherwise the character, severity and duration of clinical adverse events were comparable after the two doses. The most common clinical adverse events reported after rizatriptan were related to the central nervous system or digestive system and included dizziness, somnolence, asthenia/fatigue, and nausea. These occurred in less than 10% of patients. Clinical adverse events were typically of mild or moderate intensity and were short-lasting. The clinical adverse event profile of rizatriptan was generally comparable to that observed for oral sumatriptan, although rizatriptan 10 mg and 5 mg were associated with significantly fewer drug-related clinical adverse events than oral sumatriptan 100 mg in a study where a direct comparison was undertaken (33, 27 and 41%, respectively) [7]. Rizatriptan was safe and well-tolerated when used over periods of up to 12 months for the treatment of intermittent migraine attacks [10]. The safety profile was similar to that observed in the short-term studies.

Rapidly-Dissolving Wafer Formulation

In addition to conventional tablets, rizatriptan is available in a rapidly-dissolving wafer formulation which can be taken without water. As well as providing convenience of administration, the wafer formulation may be of utility in patients who have difficulty swallowing a tablet due to migraine-associated nausea. In a phase III study, the wafer formulation had a comparable clinical profile to the tablet formulation, and was effective from 30 min onwards [23].

Conclusions

Rizatriptan is an effective and well-tolerated acute treatment for migraine which acts rapidly, from as early as 30 min after dosing, and offers consistency of response over multiple attacks. Rizatriptan 10 mg is more effective than rizatriptan 5 mg, whereas rizatriptan 5 mg is associated with a lower incidence of adverse events than rizatriptan 10 mg, even though both doses are generally well-tolerated. Overall, rizatriptan 10 mg appears to have the most favorable therapeutic ratio. As with other 5-HT$_{1B/1D}$ receptor agonists, migraine recurs in a third of patients who initially report pain relief following rizatriptan, but rizatriptan is effective in treating the recurrence.

Rizatriptan 10 mg provides faster pain relief, and is generally more effective in the 2 h after dosing, than oral sumatriptan 100 mg and 50 mg; the same is true for rizatriptan 5 mg vs. oral sumatriptan 25 mg. Rizatriptan 5 mg and sumatriptan 50 mg show comparable overall efficacy, except for an advantage of rizatriptan 5 mg in terms of nausea relief. The superior efficacy of rizatriptan 10 mg over oral sumatriptan 100 mg and 50 mg, and of rizatriptan 5 mg over oral sumatriptan 25 mg, is not compromised by an increase in adverse events. Indeed, rizatriptan 10 mg resulted in fewer drug-related adverse events than sumatriptan 100 mg in a direct comparative trial.

In conclusion, oral rizatriptan is a rapidly and consistently effective, well-tolerated, new treatment for the acute therapy of intermittent migraine attacks, which may offer clinical benefits over oral sumatriptan, particularly with regard to speed of pain relief and relief of nausea.

References

1   Sciberras DG, Polvino WJ, Gertz BJ, Cheng H, Stepanavage M, Wittreich J, Olah T, Edwards M, Mant T: Initial human experience with MK-462 (rizatriptan): A novel 5-HT$_{1D}$ agonist. Br J Clin Pharmacol 1997;43:49–54.
2   Cheng H, Polvino WJ, Sciberras D, Yogendran L, Cerchio KA, Christie K, Olah TV, McLoughlin D, James I, Rogers JD: Pharmacokinetics and food interaction of MK-462 in healthy males. Biopharm Drug Disp 1996;17:17–24.
3   Visser WH, Terwindt GM, Reines SA, Jiang K, Lines CR, Ferrari MD: Rizatriptan vs sumatriptan in the acute treatment of migraine. Arch Neurol 1996;53:1132–1137.
4   Gijsman H, Kramer MS, Sargent J, Tuchman M, Matzura-Wolfe D, Polis A, Teall J, Block G, Ferrari MD: Double-blind, placebo-controlled, dose-finding study of rizatriptan (MK-462) in the acute treatment of migraine. Cephalalgia 1997;17:647–651.
5   Teall J, Tuchman M, Cutler N, Gross M, Willoughby E, Smith B, Jiang K, Reines S, Block G: Rizatriptan (MAXALT) for the acute treatment of migraine and migraine recurrence. A placebo-controlled, outpatient study. Headache 1998;38:281–287.
6   Kramer MS, Matzura-Wolfe D, Polis A, Getson A, Amaraneni PG, Solbach MP, McHugh W, Feighner J, Silberstein S, Reines SA: A placebo-controlled crossover study of rizatriptan in the treatment of multiple migraine attacks. Neurology 1998;51:773–781.
7   Tfelt-Hansen P, Teall J, Rodriguez F, Giacovazzo M, Paz J, Malbecq W, Block GA, Reines SA, Visser WH: Oral rizatriptan versus oral sumatriptan: A direct comparative study in the acute treatment of migraine. Headache 1998;38:748–755.
8   Goldstein J, Ryan R, Jiang K, Getson A, Norman B, Block GA, Lines C: Crossover comparison of rizatriptan 5 mg and 10 mg vs sumatriptan 25 mg and 50 mg in migraine. Headache 1998;38: 737–747.
9   Lines C, Visser WH, Vandormael K, Reines SA: Rizatriptan 5 mg versus sumatriptan 50 mg in the acute treatment of migraine. Headache 1997;37:319–320.
10 Block GA, Goldstein J, Polis A, Reines SA, Smith ME: Efficacy and safety of rizatriptan versus standard care during long-term treatment for migraine. Headache 1998;38:764–771.
11 IHS Committee on Clinical Trials in Migraine: Guidelines for controlled trials of drugs in migraine. Cephalalgia 1991;11:1–12.
12 Headache Classification Committee of the IHS: Classification and diagnostic criteria for headache disorders, cranial neuralgias and facial pain. Cephalalgia 1988;8(suppl 7):1–96.
13 Dahlöf C: The consistency of response to oral sumatriptan in the acute treatment of migraine. Poster presented at the 2nd International Conference of the European Headache Federation, Belgium, 1994.
14 Pfaffenrath V, Cunin G, Sjonell G, Prendergast S: Efficacy and safety of sumatriptan tablets (25 mg, 50 mg, and 100 mg) in the acute treatment of migraine: Defining the optimum doses of oral sumatriptan. Headache 1998;38:184–190.
15 Ferrari MD, James MH, Bates D, Pilgrim A, Ashford E, Anderson BA, Nappi G: Oral sumatriptan: Effect of a second dose, and incidence and treatment of recurrences. Cephalalgia 1994;14:330–338.

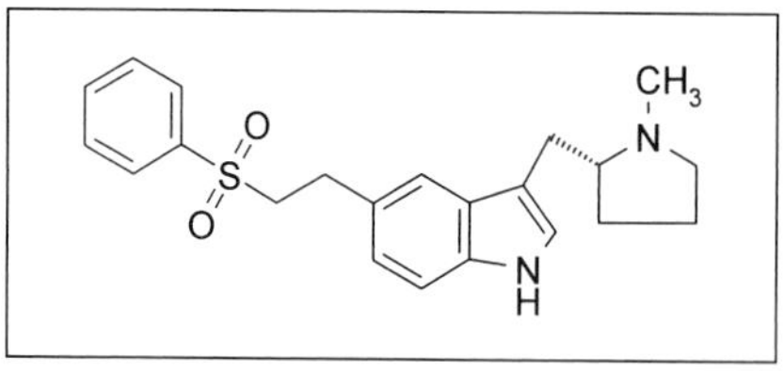

Fig. 1. Chemical structure of eletriptan.

- Rapid and complete oral absorption.
- Good oral bioavailability.
- Potential for longer duration of action that may result in a reduced headache recurrence in migraineurs.

Eletriptan (fig. 1), a new indole derivative was the outcome of research based on the above objectives. The preclinical pharmacology and pharmacokinetic profile of eletriptan is described in this review. By design, this 5-HT$_{1B/1D}$ receptor agonist possesses pharmacological and pharmacokinetic properties in animals which are likely to result in an effective oral treatment for migraine in humans with a rapid onset of action, potential for a long duration of action and a low propensity to produce adverse cardiovascular effects. Sumatriptan is the comparator compound referred to throughout this review since at the time of our discovery programme, this was the only 5-HT$_{1B/1D}$ agonist approved for the acute treatment of migraine.

5-HT$_{1B/1D}$ Agonist Potency and Selectivity

Radioligand binding studies have demonstrated that eletriptan has high affinity for the human recombinant 5-HT$_{1B}$ (pK$_1$ = 8.0) and 5-HT$_{1D}$ (pK$_1$ = 8.9) and 5-ht$_{1F}$ (pK$_i$ = 8.0) receptors. With the exception of a modest affinity for 5-HT$_{1A}$, 5-ht$_{1E}$, 5-HT$_{2B}$ and 5-HT$_7$ subtypes (pK$_1 \leq 7.4$), eletriptan shows no significant activity (pK$_1 \leq 6.0$) at a range of other receptors and ion channels [10]. The receptor selectivity profile of eletriptan is qualitatively similar to that of sumatriptan (table 1) albeit that eletriptan has higher affinity (4- and 8-fold, respectively) for the 5-HT$_{1B}$ and 5-HT$_{1D}$ receptors. Consistent with the high affinity at the human recombinant 5-HT$_{1B}$ and 5-HT$_{1D}$ receptors, eletriptan is also a potent agonist at these receptors (pEC$_{50}$s of 7.71 and 9.17, respectively).

The anti-migraine property of sumatriptan has been partly attributed to its ability to constrict intracranial arteries via the 5-HT$_{1B}$ receptor. The functional activity of eletriptan has, therefore, been assessed at this receptor in both canine

Table 1. Binding affinities (pK$_i$) of eletriptan and sumatriptan at a range of 5-HT receptors

Receptor	Eletriptan	Sumatriptan
Human 5-HT$_{1A}$	7.4	6.0
Human 5-HT$_{1B}$	8.0	7.4
Human 5-HT$_{1D}$	8.9	8.0
Human 5-ht$_{1E}$	7.2	5.8
Human 5-ht$_{1F}$	8.0	7.9
Human 5-HT$_{2A}$	<5.5	<5.5
Human 5-HT$_{2B}$	6.9	6.6
Human 5-HT$_{2C}$	<5.5	<5.5
Mouse 5-HT$_3$	<5.5	<5.5
Guinea pig 5-HT$_4$	<5.5	<5.5
Human 5-ht$_{5A}$	6.0	<5.5
Human 5-ht$_6$	6.3	<5.5
Human 5-HT$_7$	6.7	5.9

and human vascular tissue. Eletriptan, like sumatriptan, caused concentration-dependent contractions of the dog isolated saphenous vein (pEC$_{50}$s 6.3 and 6.1, respectively) and basilar artery (pEC$_{50}$s 7.2 and 6.8, respectively). However, unlike sumatriptan, the maximum responses evoked by eletriptan were significantly lower than that evoked by 5-HT (intrinsic activity, saphenous vein: eletriptan 0.57, 5-HT 1.0, sumatriptan 0.85; basilar artery: eletriptan 0.77, 5-HT 0.98, sumatriptan 0.89). Following the determination of agonist dissociation constants for eletriptan [12] and 5-HT, and sumatriptan [13], comparison of the respective receptor occupancy-response relationships indicated that eletriptan occupies 4.4 times more receptors than 5-HT in order to evoke an equivalent contraction in the dog isolated saphenous vein [10]. Thus, eletriptan is a potent partial agonist at the canine vascular 5-HT$_{1B}$ receptor.

Eletriptan, like sumatriptan, also evoked contractile responses in the human isolated middle meningeal artery. Eletriptan was equipotent with sumatriptan in contracting the human isolated middle meningeal artery and each agonist caused a similar maximum contraction in these preparations (fig. 2, tables 2, 3).

Onset and Offset Receptor Kinetics

Radioligand binding studies were also undertaken to compare the association and dissociation rates of radiolabelled eletriptan compared to sumatrip-

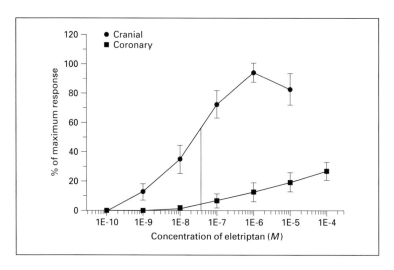

Fig. 2. Effect of eletriptan on the human isolated meningeal and coronary artery. The vertical line represents the free plasma concentration (32 nM) achieved after an oral dose of 40 mg of eletriptan in man.

Table 2. Summary of the potency (pEC$_{50}$) and maximal responses (E$_{max}$) produced by eletriptan, sumatriptan and 5-HT in the human isolated middle meningeal artery

Compound	pEC$_{50}$	E$_{max}$
Eletriptan	7.6±0.2 (5)	98±6
Sumatriptan	7.4±0.1 (5)	103±13
5-HT	7.9±0.2 (5)	124±7

Data represent the mean pEC$_{50}$ and E$_{max}$ values, ±S.E.M.

Number in parenthesis (n)=number of experiments performed in tissues from individual subjects; pEC$_{50}$=negative logarithm$_{10}$ of the mean EC$_{50}$ (concentration of agonist required to produce 50% of the maximum response attainable for that particular agonist); E$_{max}$=mean maximum response achieved by that agonist expressed as a percentage of the response to 1 μM PGF$_{2alpha}$.

ANOVA showed no significant differences in either pEC$_{50}$ (F$_{3,15}$=1.8, p>0.2) or E$_{max}$ (F$_{3,15}$=2.4, p>0.12).

tan at the human recombinant 5-HT$_{1D}$ receptor. These studies demonstrated that [^{3}H]-eletriptan had a significantly faster on-rate constant (K$_{on}$: eletriptan 0.254 min^{-1} · nM^{-1}, sumatriptan 0.026 min^{-1} · nM^{-1}) and a slower off-rate constant compared to [^{3}H]-sumatriptan (K$_{off}$: eletriptan 0.027 min^{-1}, sumatriptan 0.037 min^{-1}). In addition, washout experiments in the dog isolated basilar

Table 3. Summary of the potency (pEC_{50}) and maximal responses (E_{max}) produced by eletriptan, sumatriptan and 5-HT in the human isolated coronary artery

Compound	pEC_{50}	E_{max}
Eletriptan	5.69 ± 0.24 (9)[a, b]	27 ± 6.1[b]
Sumatriptan	6.05 ± 0.20 (9)[b]	35 ± 18[b]
5-HT	6.46 ± 0.15 (9)	83 ± 9.3

Data represent the mean pEC_{50} and E_{max} values, $\pm$ S.E.M.

Number in parenthesis (n) = number of experiments performed in tissues from individual subjects; pEC_{50} = negative logarithm$_{10}$ of the mean EC_{50} (concentration of agonist required to produce 50% of the maximum response attainable for that particular agonist); E_{max} = mean maximum response achieved by that agonist expressed as a percentage of the response to 100 mM KCl.

[a] Significance of difference when compared to sumatriptan, $p < 0.05$.

[b] Significance of difference when compared to 5-HT, $p < 0.05$.

artery measuring the reversal of $5-HT_{1B}$ receptor-mediated contractions, indicated that eletriptan was significantly slower (3-fold) to washout than sumatriptan, for an equivalent size of contraction [unpubl. observ.].

Animal Models: Vascular and Neurogenic Mechanisms Implicated in Migraine Pathology

Activation of $5-HT_{1B}$ receptors present on cranial arterio-venous anastomoses produces a flow-limiting vasoconstriction resulting in a decrease in total common carotid arterialy blood flow. In anaesthetized dog studies, measurement of this parameter has been used widely as a marker of potential clinical efficacy. Eletriptan (1–1,000 µg/kg i.v.) produced a dose-dependent reduction in carotid arterial blood flow with a similar potency and maximum effect to those of sumatriptan (fig. 3, table 4). At doses that produced a maximal reduction in carotid arterial blood flow, no changes in heart rate or blood pressure were observed.

In the now well-characterized rodent model of trigeminovascular inflammation, several $5-HT_{1B/1D}$ receptor agonists have been shown to inhibit trigeminal nerve-mediated plasma protein extravasation (PPE) in the dura mater [15, 16] by activation of inhibitory prejunctional $5-HT_{1D}$ receptors. Administration of eletriptan (30–300 µg/kg i.v.) prior to the activation of trigeminal afferents prevented neurogenic inflammation with a potency and maximum

---

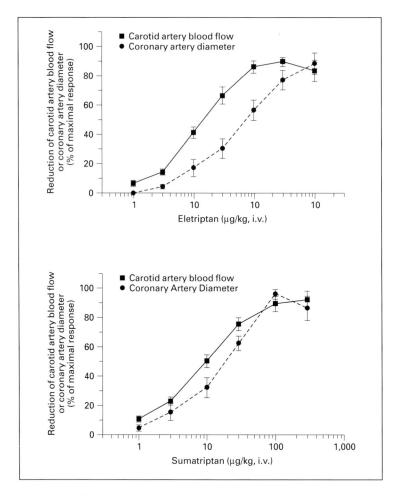

Fig. 3. Effect of eletriptan and sumatriptan on carotid arterial blood flow and coronary artery diameter in the anaesthetized dog.

effect equivalent to those of sumatriptan (dural PPE ratio: control, 1.90; minimum effective dose of eletriptan 100 μg/kg i.v., 1.04; p < 0.05) [14]. Using a modification of the original experimental protocol [14, 17] eletriptan was administered during a period of continual firing of the trigeminal nerve, when the nerve-driven PPE response was well established. Under these conditions, eletriptan (100 μg/kg i.v.), like sumatriptan [17], still produced complete inhibition of neurogenic inflammation [14]. If neurogenically-mediated inflammation of intracranial blood vessels is important in the maintenance of a migraine attack, these data support the contention that eletriptan could be used as an abortive treatment.

Table 4. Vasoconstrictor potency of eletriptan and sumatriptan in vascular beds of the anaesthetized dog

| | ED$_{50}$ [95% CI] (µg/kg i.v.) | |
	Eletriptan	Sumatriptan
Carotid	12 [7–11]	9 [8–16]
Coronary	63 [37–107][a]	19 [11–31]
Femoral	NE[b]	29 [17–49]
n	9	10

[a] <0.05 compared with sumaptrin.
[b] NE = No significant effect.
[95% CI] = 95% confidence interval.

Selectivity for the Intracranial Blood Vessels

In addition, to being the predominant 5-HT receptor present on the intracranial vasculature, the 5-HT$_{1B}$ receptor is also present on peripheral blood vessels, such as the coronary artery. Studies were, therefore, undertaken to determine if eletriptan demonstrated selectivity for the intracranial vasculature vs. other extracranial blood vessels.

Eletriptan and sumatriptan exhibited an apparent selectivity for contracting the human isolated middle meningeal artery relative to the coronary artery (tables 2, 3) albeit that this was greater for eletriptan (81-fold compared to 22-fold for sumatriptan). These studies therefore suggest that eletriptan exhibits an improved cranial/coronary selectivity compared to sumatriptan. In addition, based on free peak plasma levels of eletriptan achieved after the recommended oral dose of 40 mg (32 nM, fig. 2), these data would predict that constriction of pain-sensitive intracranial vasculature would occur in the absence of any effect on coronary artery diameter. This prediction was borne out by a study examining the effect of infused eletriptan (the dose was chosen to mimic the plasma levels after an oral dose of 40 mg) in man which demonstrated that eletriptan produced no significant changes in mean proximal, mid or distal coronary artery diameters [18].

In anaesthetized dog studies, eletriptan also exhibited significantly lower potency than sumatriptan in reducing coronary artery diameter, measured using sonomicrometry [16] (ED$_{50}$ values: eletriptan 63 µg/kg i.v.; sumatriptan 19 µg/kg i.v.; p < 0.05) (fig. 3, table 4) [14]. Neither compound altered coronary arterial blood flow. In addition, in the femoral circulation, eletriptan (1–1,000 µg/kg i.v.) had no significant effect on arterial blood flow, whereas sumatriptan

Table 5. Mean values for pharmacokinetic parameters of unchanged eletriptan in the rat and dog

Parameter	Rat	Dog
Intravenous		
Dose (mg/kg)	3	1
$t_{1/2}$ (h)	1.4	3.9
AUC[a] (ng · h/ml)	152	577
Plasma clearance (ml/min/kg)	110	29
V_d (l/kg)	10.9	7.9
Oral		
Dose (mg/kg)	10	1
C_{max}[b] (ng/ml)	17	35
T_{max} (ng/ml)	0.5	1
AUC[a] (ng · h/ml)	19	292
Estimated oral bioavailability	13	51

[a] AUC is the area under the plasma concentration time profile extrapolated to infinity.
[b] Data normalized to 1 mg/kg dose.

produced a significant vasoconstrictor effect (ED_{50} 29 µg/kg i.v.; table 3) [14]. These results clearly indicate that eletriptan has a different regional vasoconstrictor profile from sumatriptan; specifically eletriptan exhibits a greater selectivity for the carotid vascular bed. The mechanism(s) responsible for the different haemodynamic profile is unknown.

Oral Absorption

The pharmacokinetics of eletriptan have been determined following administration of single oral and intravenous doses to the rat and dog. It has been demonstrated that the absorption profile of eletriptan has two key characteristics (table 5). Firstly, eletriptan is rapidly absorbed following oral dosing with a rapid rise to peak plasma concentration in both rat (T_{max} 0.5 h) and dog (T_{max} 1 h) [19]. Secondly, eletriptan is almost completely absorbed by both rat and dog, as indicated by the similar drug-derived radioactivity in urine after oral and intravenous dosing of [14C]-labelled drug, and by the recovery of only low amounts of an oral dose (8.5% for dog; 14% for rat) of unchanged eletriptan in the faeces [19].

Thus eletriptan is absorbed more rapidly and completely than sumatriptan which has been shown to have variable and incomplete absorption in animals and man [20]. This favourable absorption profile of eletriptan compared with that of sumatriptan, is a reflection of the greater lipophilicity of eletriptan. The measured log $D_{7.4}$ distribution coefficient for eletriptan between octanol and a pH 7.4-buffered aqueous phase was $+1.1$. In contrast, the lipophilicity of sumatriptan (log $D_{7.4}$ distribution coefficient -1.6) is at least two orders of magnitude lower. This difference is primarily due to the greater lipophilicity afforded by the 2-(phenyl sulphonyl)ethyl substituent at the C_5 position of the indole moiety in eletriptan (fig. 1). Since lipophilicity is one of the key determinants of a compound's ability to cross biological membranes, the greater lipophilicity of eletriptan means that its potential for oral absorption is greatly enhanced in comparison with sumatriptan and other hydrophilic 5-$HT_{1B/1D}$ agonists.

Oral Bioavailability and Half-Life

Oral bioavailability of unchanged eletriptan was higher and elimination half-life was longer in dog than in rat (table 5). Oral bioavailability and elimination half-life in humans for eletriptan are more similar to dog than rat [21]. The differences in eletriptan bioavailability, total plasma clearance and half-life are due to species differences in the rate of metabolic clearance. The terminal elimination half-life of eletriptan of 4–5 h in the dog (table 5) and man compares favourably with sumatriptan (2 h) in this these species [20]. This difference is primarily due to the larger volume of distribution of eletriptan compared to sumatriptan, which is a consequence of the greater lipophilicity of eletriptan.

Metabolism

Eletriptan is primarily eliminated by metabolism in both the rat and dog, with only 26% and 13% of the dose recovered unchanged in the urine and faeces of rat and dog, respectively [19]. In vitro metabolic studies using microsomal fractions prepared from rat, dog and human liver have revealed that eletriptan metabolism is mediated predominantly by the hepatic cytochrome P450 enzyme system [19, 22]. Separate metabolism studies with human liver fractions have established that eletriptan is not a substrate for monoamine oxidase (MAO) (unpubl. results), unlike sumatriptan whose metabolism in animals and man primarily involves by MAO-mediated oxidative deamination [20]. Therefore, eletriptan will not be subject to drug interactions due to MAO metabolism.

Conclusions

Preclinical studies on the novel indole-derivative eletriptan reveal a pharmacological and pharmacokinetic profile which would predict that this agent should be an effective oral treatment for migraine. The key features of the preclinical profile are as follows:

• In human isolated vascular preparations eletriptan selectively constricted meningeal vs. coronary arteries and these data are consistent with the observation that efficacious clinical plasma levels of eletriptan lack coronary arterial constriction in man [18]. Consistent with these findings, studies in the anaesthetized dog also demonstrated that eletriptan has a distinct haemodynamic profile being more selective than sumatriptan for the carotid over other vascular beds. These data suggest that anti-migraine doses of eletriptan in man are less likely to cause changes in coronary artery diameter than sumatriptan.

• The preclinical pharmacokinetic profile of eletriptan indicates a compound suitable for use as an oral therapy. The moderate lipophilicity of eletriptan compared with the more hydrophilic sumatriptan means that it is more rapidly absorbed following oral dosing in the rat and dog. Rapid absorption of eletriptan occurs in man as well resulting in a rapid onset of action which is an important feature of the clinical profile of eletriptan.

• A slower rate of dissociation from human recombinant 5-HT_{1D} receptor and canine 5-HT_{1B} receptor in the basilar artery, along with the longer terminal elimination half-life of eletriptan compared to sumatriptan in dog and man suggests that eletriptan could have a longer duration of action. These data may, in part, explain the lower rate of headache recurrence in migraineurs after an oral dose of 80 mg (placebo 40 vs. 21%, $p < 0.01$) [23].

In conclusion, the rational design of eletriptan in preclinical drug testing has resulted in an effective oral treatment for migraine with a rapid onset of action, low recurrence rate and reduced propensity to produce coronary artery constriction at efficacious doses.

References

1 Ferrari MD, Haan J: Acute treatment of migraine attacks. Curr Opin Neurol 1995;8:237–242.
2 Goadsby PJ, Olesen J: Diagnosis and management of migraine. BMJ 1996;312:1279–1282.
3 Bouchelet I, Cohen Z, Case B, Seguela P, Hamel E: Differential expression of sumatriptan-sensitive 5-hydroxytryptamine receptors in human trigeminal ganglia and cerebral blood vessels. Mol Pharmacol 1996;50:219–223.
4 Saxena P, Ferrari M: Pharmacology of antimigraine 5-HT_{1D} receptor agonists. Exp Opin Invest Drugs 1996;5:581–593.

5   Adham N, Kao H-T, Scechter E, Bard J, Olsen M, Urquhart D, Durkin M, Hartig PR, Weinshank RL, Branchek TA: Cloning of another human serotonin receptor (5-HT$_{1F}$): A fifth 5-HT$_1$ receptor subtype coupled to the inhibition of adenylate cyclase. Proc Natl Acad Sci USA 1993;90:408–412.

6   Plosker GL, McTavish D: Sumatriptan: A reappraisal of its pharmacology and therapeutic efficacy in the acute treatment of migraine and cluster headache. Drugs 1994;47:622–651.

7   Ottervanger JP, van Witsen TB, Valkenburg HA, Grobbee DE, Stricker BH: Adverse reactions attributed to sumatriptan. A postmarketing study in general practice. Eur J Clin Pharmacol 1994; 47:305–309.

8   Kaumann AJ, Parson AA, Brown AM: Human arterial constrictor serotonin receptors. Cardiovasc Res 1993;27:2094–2103.

9   Lacey LF, Hussey EK, Fowler PA: Single dose pharmacokinetics of sumatriptan in healthy volunteers. Eur J Pharmacol 1995;47:543–548.

10   Gupta P, Scatchard J, Shepperson NB, Wallis RM, Wythes MJ: In vitro pharmacology of eletriptan (UK-116,044), a potent and selective partial agonist at the '5-HT$_{1D}$-like' receptor in the dog saphenous vein. Cephalalgia 1996;16:386.

11   Bouchelet I, Case B, Hamel E: Expression of mRNA for serotonin (5-HT) receptors in human coronary arteries. American Neuroscience Abstract 1996;22:1578 (abstract no. 621.1).

12   Stephenson RP: A modification of receptor theory. Br J Pharmacol 1956;11:379–393.

13   Furchgott RF, Burzstyn P: Comparison of dissociation constants and of relative efficacies of selected agonists acting on parasympathetic receptors. Ann NY Acad Sci 1967;144:882–899.

14   Gupta P, Brown D, Butler P, Closier MD, Dickinson RP, Ellis P, James K, Macor JE, Rigby JW, Shepperson NB, Wythes MJ: Preclinical in vivo pharmacology of eletriptan (UK-116,044): a potent and selective partial agonist at '5-HT$_{1D}$-like' receptors. Cephalalgia 1996;16:386.

15   Saito K, Markowitz S, Moskowitz MA: Ergot alkaloids block neurogenic extravasation in dura mater: Proposed action in vascular headache. Ann Neurol 1988;24:732–737.

16   Buzzi MG, Moskowitz MA, Peroutka SJ, Byun B: Further characterisation of the putative 5-HT receptor which mediates blockade of neurogenic plasma extravasation rat dura mater. Br J Pharmacol 1991;103:1421–1428.

17   Huang Z, Byan B, Matsubara T, Moskowitz MA: Time-dependent blockade of neurogenic plasma extravasation in dura mater by 5-HT$_{1B/1D}$ agonists and endopeptidase 24.11. Br J Pharmacol 1993; 108:331–335.

18   Muir DF, McCann GP, Swan L, Clark AL, Hillis WS: Haemodynamic and coronary effects of intravenous eletriptan, a 5-HT$_{1B/1D}$ receptor agonist. Clin Pharmacol Ther 1999;66:85–90.

19   Rance DJ, Atkinson FM, James GC, McDevitt HJ, Morgan P: The pharmacokinetics of eletriptan (UK-116,044) in rat and dog. Cephalalgia 1996;16:387.

20   Dixon CM, Saynor DA, Andrew PD, Oxford J, Bradbury A, Tarbit MH: Disposition of sumatriptan in laboratory animals and humans. Drug Metab Disp 1993;21:761.

21   Milton KA, Allen MJ, Abel S, James GC, Rance DJ: The safety, tolerability and pharmacokinetics of intravenous eletriptan, a new potent and selective 5-HT$_{1D}$ receptor agonist. Cephalalgia 1996; 16:385.

22   Hyland R, Jones BC, McCleverty P, Mitchell RJ, Morgan P: In vitro metabolism of eletriptan in human liver microsomes. Cephalalgia (in press).

23   Jackson NC for the Eletriptan Steering Committee: A comparison of oral eletriptan (UK-116,044) (20–80 mg) and oral sumatriptan (100 mg) in the acute treatment of migraine. Cephalalgia 1996; 16:368.

24   Steiner TJ on behalf of the Eletriptan Steering Committee: Efficacy, safety and tolerability of oral eletriptan (40 mg and 80 mg) in the acute treatment of migraine: Results of a phase III study. Cephalalgia 1998;18:385.

Dr. Aileen D. McHarg, Candidate Research Group IPC 155, Discovery Biology III,
Pfizer Central Research, Sandwich, Kent CT13 9NJ (UK)
Tel. +44 1304 648 202, Fax +44 1304 658 444, E-Mail AILEEN-McHARG@sandwich.pfizer.com

Diener HC (ed): Drug Treatment of Migraine and Other Headaches.
Monogr Clin Neurosci. Basel, Karger, 2000, vol 17, pp 184–189

....

Eletriptan – Therapy

H.C. Diener

Department of Neurology, University of Essen, Essen, Germany

Eletriptan underwent the normal development programme with dose-finding studies, large phase III trials with a comparison to placebo and finally a direct comparison with sumatriptan.

In an initial dose finding double-blind parallel-group study [1] 365 patients were treated with eletriptan 5 mg, 20 mg, 30 mg or placebo. At 2 h post-dose, headache response showed a dose response (5 mg 38%, 20 mg 46%, 40 mg 47%) but failed to show statistical superiority to placebo (34%) for individual doses. The incidence of all treatment emergent adverse events was similar for all three doses (5 mg 38%, 20 mg 34%, 30 mg 39%). Following the results of this study, two major dose-finding and efficacy trials were performed in the development of oral eletriptan. The first study 314 compared eletriptan 20–80 mg with sumatriptan (100 mg) and placebo [2, 3] and the second, study 305 compared eletriptan 40 and 80 mg with placebo [4].

The 314 study was a randomized, double-blind, parallel-group study that was conducted on outpatients who met the IHS criteria for migraine with and without aura. The primary endpoint was the improvement of headache from severe or moderate to mild or headache free (called headache response). A total of 692 patients were treated with 20 mg, 40 mg or 80 mg eletriptan, 100 mg sumatriptan or placebo. In the five treatment groups 80–85% of the patients were female with a mean age of 40–41 years. 11–13% suffered from migraine with aura, 66–73% from migraine without aura and 16–22% from migraine with and without aura. 42–46% of the treated migraine attacks were severe and 50–58% moderate.

Eletriptan showed a dose-response for headache improvement and number of patients who were headache free after 2 hours (fig. 1). All three doses of eletriptan were statistically superior to placebo for headache response and headache-free patients. The 80 mg dose of eletriptan was also superior to

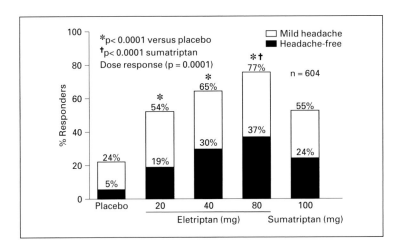

Fig. 1. Percentage of patients with improvement of headache from severe or moderate to mild or no headache ('mild headache') and patients who were headache free after 2 hours for placebo, eletriptan 20, 40 and 80 mg and sumatriptan 100 mg.

sumatriptan 100 mg. At 1-h post-dose, all three doses of eletriptan were statistically superior to placebo for headache response and eletriptan 40 and 80 mg doses were superior to sumatriptan 100 mg (response rates for eletriptan 40 mg, 80 mg, sumatriptan 100 mg and placebo were: 37.9, 40.6, 19.8 and 12.1%). Eletriptan significantly improved nausea compared to placebo. The highest dose of eletriptan was also superior to sumatriptan. Patients were asked at baseline and after 2 h about their overall ability to function. The percentage of patients who were initially bedridden or severely impaired, and improved to normal or reduced function was 29% for placebo, 53% for sumatriptan and 54, 64 and 74% with 20, 40 and 80 mg eletriptan, respectively.

Headache recurrence defined as return of moderate or severe headache within 24 h of dosing and following a headache response at 2 h after initial dosing, occurred in 33% of the patients following 100 mg sumatriptan and 28, 34 and 32% after 20, 40 and 80 mg eletriptan.

More than half (57%) of the patients in this study had taken sumatriptan previously and most had responded to it. There was no difference in efficacy or reporting of side effects between the sumatriptan-naive and sumatriptan-exposed patients.

Treatment-related side effects are shown in table 1. Eletriptan may cross the blood-brain barrier which might explain the somewhat higher incidence of asthenia. The frequency of chest tightness was not different from sumatriptan.

Table 1. Treatment-related adverse events (patients %)

	Placebo n = 142	Sumatripan 100 mg n = 129	Eletriptan 20 mg n = 144	Eletriptan 40 mg n = 138	Eletriptan 80 mg n = 141
Total incidence	8	29	26	24	38
Asthenia	0	3	2	3	10
Somnolence	1	5	2	1	4
Nausea	1	3	3	2	7
Dizziness	1	4	2	3	4
Paresthesia	1	5	4	2	8
Throat, neck, chest and shoulder symptoms	0.7	7.2	4.2	6.7	6.5

A subgroup analysis in 454 women showed that (25%) 114 attacks were treated during menstruation [5]. A similar headache response was recorded in women who were menstruating, and in those who were not.

The question whether the short T_{max} of eletriptan translates into a faster onset of action was addressed in large double-blind, placebo-controlled, parallel-group trial (study 305) comparing oral eletriptan in doses of 40 and 80 mg with placebo. Patients were instructed to take study medication within 6 h of the onset of the migraine attack. Patients could take up to two doses per attack. In total, 1,153 patients treated a migraine attack with study medication. Across the three treatment arms the percentage of females was 81–85%, the percentage of migraine with aura was 7–9%, migraine without aura 64–67% and migraine with and without aura 24–29%. Between 69% and 72% of the patients had prior exposure to sumatriptan. The pretreatment headache severity was severe in 39–42% and moderate in 58–61% of the attacks.

The study found a significant improvement in headache response within 30 min for eletriptan 40 and 80 mg compared to placebo (fig. 2). Significantly more patients were headache free at 1, 2 and 4 h compared to placebo (fig. 3). The rate of headache response after 2 h was 62% for 40 mg and 65% for 80 mg eletriptan, compared to 19% with placebo. The resulting therapeutic gain [6, 7] is 43% for 40 mg and 46% for 80 mg eletriptan. Headache free were 32% and 34%, respectively of the patients compared with 3% in the placebo group.

Eletriptan had also a significant effect on the improvement of nausea, photophobia and phonophobia. A total of 625 patients experienced headache recurrence within 24 h after initial benefit. The recurrence rate was 40% for placebo, 30% for 40 mg and 21% for 80 mg eletriptan. The time to recurrence was 5 h with placebo, 16.7 h with 40 mg and 19.0 h after 80 mg eletriptan.

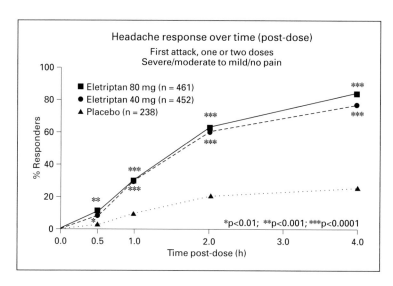

Fig. 2. Headache response over time for eletriptan 40 and 80 mg compared to palcebo.

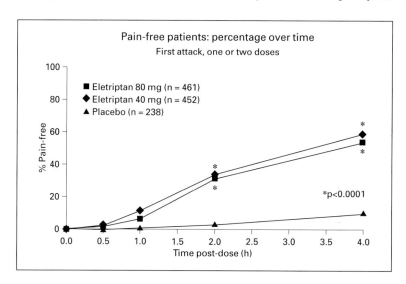

Fig. 3. Percentage of headache free patients 2 and 4 hours after 40 and 80 mg eletriptan compared to placebo.

Treatment-related adverse events for those taking one dose of eletriptan 40 and 80 mg are shown in table 2. The higher efficacy of 80 mg eletriptan results also in a higher rate of side effects. Only 0.9% (40 mg) and 2.5% (80 mg) of the patients discontinued due to side effects of eletriptan compared with 1.3% following placebo.

Table 2. Treatment-related adverse events profile (events experienced by > 5% patients (n = 712))

	Placebo n = 238 (%)	Eletriptan 40 mg n = 219 (%)	Eletriptan 80 mg n = 255 (%)
Total	21	34	53
Asthenia	0.8	5.9	16.1
Dizziness	3.4	4.1	6.7
Somnolence	1.7	4.1	7.1
Nausea	3.4	4.6	5.5
Paresthesia	1.3	3.2	6.3
Chest symptoms	0.4	1.4	6.3

The efficacy of eletriptan against sumatriptan was further confirmed in a subsequent double-blind parallel-group study (study 318) in 774 sumatriptan naive patients, who took eletriptan 40 mg, 80 mg, sumatriptan 50 mg and 100 mg and placebo in the ratio of 2:2:2:2:1 [8]. In this study, headache response rates were significantly higher for both doses of eletriptan (64% for 40 mg and 67% for 80 mg) than for both doses of sumatriptan (50% for 50 mg and 53% for 100 mg). Headache response rate was significantly higher for eletriptan 80 mg vs. sumatriptan 50 mg (37% vs. 24%) at 1 h post-dose. Dizziness, asthenia and nausea were the most common treatment-related adverse events reported for each active treatment group. Patients rated acceptability of both doses of eletriptan was higher than either dose of sumatriptan.

The comparative efficacy and tolerability of eletriptan and Cafergot (2 mg ergotamine and 200 mg caffeine) were assessed in a double-blind parallel-group study (study 307) in 733 patients who took eletriptan 40 mg, 80 mg, Cafergot or placebo in the ratio of 2:2:2:1 [9]. In this study at 2 h after treatment, a significantly higher proportion of patients in the eletriptan groups had a headache response compared to Cafergot (54, 68 vs. 33% for eletriptan 40 mg, 80 mg vs. Cafergot). At 1 h following treatment, significantly more patients had headache response compared to Cafergot (29% eletriptan 40 mg, 39% eletriptan 80 mg vs. 13% Cafergot). Both doses of eletriptan were significantly more effective than Cafergot in reducing the incidence of nausea, phonophobia, photophobia and functional impairment at 2 h post-dose. Asthenia, dizziness, and nausea were the most common adverse events following treatment with eletriptan, and asthenia and nausea were the most common adverse events after Cafergot.

In summary, eletriptan is a highly effective and fast acting drug for the treatment of acute migraine attack. Eletriptan 80 mg has the highest efficacy and lowest recurrence rate; eletriptan 40 mg is also effective and has fewer side effects. Clinical practice will show whether patients are willing to accept the slightly higher rate of side effects in the light of the better efficacy.

References

1   Färkkilä M, Diener HC, Dahlöf C, Steuber TJ, on behalf of the Eletriptan Steering Committee: A dose-finding study of eletriptan (5–30 mg) for the acute treatment of migraine. Cephalalgia 1996; 16:387.
2   Jackson NC, on behalf of the Eletriptan Steering Committee: Clinical measures of efficacy, safety and tolerability for the acute treatment of migraine: A comparison of eletriptan (20–80 mg), sumatriptan (100 mg) and placebo. Neurology 1998;50(suppl 4):A376.
3   The Eletriptan Steering Committee: Clinical measures of efficacy, safety and tolerability for the acute treatment of migraine: A comparison of eletriptan (20–80 mg), sumatriptan (100 mg) and placebo. Abstract; 50th Meeting of the American Academy of Neurology 1998.
4   Steiner TJ, on behalf of the Eletriptan Steering Committee: The efficacy, safety and tolerability of oral eletriptan (40 mg and 80 mg) for the acute treatment of migraine: Results of a double-blind, placebo-controlled, parallel group clinical trial. Migraine Trust, London 1998.
5   MacGregor EA: Migraine during menstruation and the efficacy of oral eletriptan; Neurology 1998; 50(suppl 4):A377.
6   Tfelt-Hansen P: Efficacy and adverse events of subcutaneous, oral, and intranasal sumatriptan used for migraine treatment: A systematic review based on numbers needed to treat. Cephalalgia 1998; 18:532–538.
7   Goadsby PJ: A triptan too far? J Neurol Neurosurg Psychiatry 1998;64:143–147.
8   Pryse-Philips W, on behalf of the Eletriptan Steering Committee: Comparison of oral eletriptan (Relpax^{TM}) (40–80 mg) and oral sumatriptan (50–100 mg) for the treatment of acute migraine. A randomised, placebo-controlled study in sumatriptan-naive patients. 9th Congress of the International Headache Society, 1999, Barcelona.
9   Reeches A, on behalf of the Eletriptan Steering Committee: Comparison of the efficacy, safety and tolerability of oral eletriptan (Relpax^{TM}) and Cafergot for the acute treatment of migraine. 9th Congress of the International Headache Society, 1999, Barcelona.

Prof. Dr. H.C. Diener, Neurologische Universitäts-Klinik,
Hufelandstr. 55, D–45122 Essen (Germany)
Tel. +49 201 723 2460, Fax +49 201 723 5901, E-Mail h.diener@uni-essen.de

Diener HC (ed): Drug Treatment of Migraine and Other Headaches.
Monogr Clin Neurosci. Basel, Karger, 2000, vol 17, pp 190–196

....

Pharmacology of Some Other Triptans in Development

Pramod R. Saxena, Peter De Vries

Department of Pharmacology, Dutch Migraine Research Group and
Cardiovascular Research Institute 'COEUR', Erasmus University Medical Centre
Rotterdam 'EMCR', Rotterdam, The Netherlands

The triptans belong to a class of compounds known as $5\text{-HT}_{1B/1D}$ (previously 5-HT_1-like/5-HT_{1D} [1]) receptor agonists. The first of this class, sumatriptan [2], has undoubtedly been a great advance in migraine treatment, but it has certain limitations (e.g. low oral bioavailability, high headache recurrence, possibly due to a short $t_{1/2}$ and contra-indication in patients with coronary artery disease (see chapters by Connor, and Diener). Therefore, a number of pharmaceutical companies decided to develop newer triptans having agonist activity at $5\text{-HT}_{1B/1D}$ receptors; see chapters by Edmeads, and Connor and Beattie, Dahlöf and Lines, and Diener for zolmitriptan, naratriptan, rizatriptan and eletriptan. In this paper, we will discuss frovatriptan, almotriptan and F11356, which are in different stages of development (for chemical structures, see fig. 1). Since avitriptan, BMS181885 and the non-triptan alniditan are no longer in clinical development [3, 4], these compounds will not be considered here.

Receptor Binding Profile

Like sumatriptan [5], almotriptan [6], frovatriptan [7] and F11356 [8] have a high affinity for 5-HT_{1B} and 5-HT_{1D} receptors (table 1). There are no profound differences, although F11356 is clearly the most potent at these receptors, while sumatriptan is the weakest at the 5-HT_{1B} receptor. Sumatriptan and frovatriptan also interact with the 5-HT_{1F} receptor, but F11356 has little affinity for this receptor. These compounds display a μM affinity (perhaps not clinical relevant) at the 5-HT_7 receptor, which mediates smooth muscle relaxation [1].

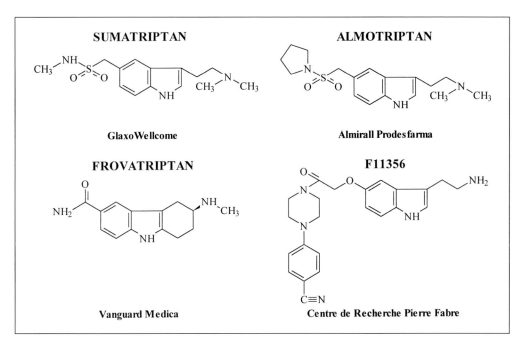

Fig. 1. Chemical structures of sumatriptan, almotriptan, F11356 and frovatriptan.

Table 1. pK$_i$ values of sumatriptan, almotriptan, frovatriptan and F11356 at 5-HT receptors

Receptor	Sumatriptan	Almotriptan	Frovatriptan	F11356
5-HT$_{1A}$	6.43 [5]	6.3 [6]	7.3 [7]	7.60 [8]
5-HT$_{1B}$	7.82 [5]	8.0 [6]	8.6 [7]	9.44 [8]
5-HT$_{1D}$	8.46 [5]	8.0 [6]	8.4 [7]	9.32 [8]
5-ht$_{1E}$	5.80 [5]		<6.0 [7]	5.94 [8]
5-HT$_{1F}$	7.86 [5]		7.0 [7]	5.47 [8]
5-HT$_{2A}$	<5.0 (pEC$_{50}$) [5]		<5.3 [7]	6.74 [8]
M5-HT$_3$	<5.0 (pEC$_{50}$) [5]		<6.0 [7]	<5.0 [8]
Gp5-HT$_4$	<5.0 (pEC$_{50}$) [5]			5.70 [8]
5-ht$_{5A}$	5.50^a			6.09 [8]
5-ht$_6$	5.31^a			5.63 [8]
5-HT$_7$	6.51^a	<6.5 [6]	6.70 [7]	6.43 [8]

^{a} P.J. Pauwels, pers. commun.

Table 2. pEC_{50} values of sumatriptan, almotriptan, frovatriptan and F11356 in producing contraction of isolated blood vessels. If known, the intrinsic activity relative to 5-HT (5-HT = 1) is given between brackets

	Sumatriptan	Almotriptan	Frovatriptan	F11356
Human basilar artery	6.93 (1.11) [18]	5.46 [6]	7.86 (1.25) [18]	
Rabbit basilar artery	6.00 [7]		7.20 [7]	
Human middle meningeal artery	7.15 (0.66) [19]	7.52 [6]		
Rabbit saphenous vein	6.48 (0.97) [20]			7.10 (0.84) [21]
Human coronary artery	6.10 (0.24) [23]		7.38 (0.42) [18]	

Pharmacodynamics

Systemic Haemodynamics

No clinically relevant changes in systemic haemodynamics are observed, but human volunteers studies show that sumatriptan [9] and frovatriptan [10] slightly increase arterial blood pressure. This is most probably a class effect associated with $5\text{-HT}_{1B/1D}$ receptor agonists.

Carotid Haemodynamics

All triptan so far studied decrease carotid blood flow in anaesthetized animals. The decrease in carotid blood flow is confined to cephalic arterio-venous anastomoses; capillary blood flow to extracerebral as well as cerebral structures either does not change or may even increase (see [11]). Sumatriptan has also been shown to decrease forearm blood flow in human volunteers by constricting on arteriovenous anastomoses [12]. This effect of the triptans, which most likely involves the 5-HT_{1B} rather than 5-HT_{1D} receptor [13], seems to be in agreement with the hypothesis that cephalic arteriovenous anastomoses dilate during the headache phase of migraine [14, 15].

No studies have been undertaken with almotriptan, frovatriptan or F11356 with regard to their effects of cephalic arteriovenous anastomoses, but these drugs do decrease total carotid blood flow [6, 16, 17].

Constriction of Isolated Blood Vessels

As shown in table 2, almotriptan and frovatriptan contract human and rabbit isolated cranial arteries [6, 7, 18, 19]. Extensive studies are not yet available with F11356, but like sumatriptan [20], F11356 also contracts the rabbit isolated saphenous vein [21].

Coronary Vascular Effects

In the human coronary artery, 5-HT$_2$ receptors are more important, but about 20–30% response is mediated by 5-HT$_1$ receptors [22]. Accordingly, sumatriptan moderately constricts the human coronary artery, both in vivo [9] and in vitro [23]. All second-generation triptans for which data are available contract the human isolated coronary artery (table 2, [18, 23]). Compared to cranial arteries, the effects of triptans is relatively weaker on the coronary artery [19]. Thus, the triptans are expected to cause only a little coronary constriction upon therapeutic doses in migraine patients *without* any coronary artery affliction, but in patients *with* coronary artery disease (stenosis or hyper-reactivity), the triptans may still cause myocardial ischaemia (for details, see [23]).

Trigeminal Inhibitory Effects

Given that cranial vasoconstriction is the most important therapeutic mechanism, it implies that agonist action at the 5-HT$_{1D}$ (and 5-HT$_{1F}$) receptor is not required for the anti-migraine action. However, several other mechanisms, which do not seem to be mediated solely by the 5-HT$_{1B}$ receptor, have also been implicated in migraine relief. These mechanisms include inhibition of the trigeminovascular system either peripherally [24] or centrally [4].

No data are available with frovatriptan and F11356, but almotriptan has only been reported to be effective in inhibiting plasma protein extravasation following trigeminal ganglion stimulation in the guinea pig [6]. It should, however, be noted that inhibition of plasma protein extravasation alone is probably not relevant to antimigraine activity (see [25]).

Pharmacokinetics

The pharmacokinetic characteristics of sumatriptan, frovatriptan and almotriptan are presented in table 3 [10, 26–29]. Compared to sumatriptan, the oral bioavailability of almotriptan (14 and 80%, respectively) is substantially high and the plasma half-life of frovatriptan (2 h and ~25 h, respectively) is particularly long. Interestingly, the t_{max} after oral administrations of almotriptan or frovatriptan is not much better than that of sumatriptan. In view of the putative relation of plasma half-life with headache recurrence, the results of clinical trials with frovatriptan are awaited with interest.

Table 3. Pharmacokinetic parameters of sumatriptan, almotriptan and frovatriptan

Drug	Dose and route of administration	T_{max} h	C_{max} ng ml^{-1}	Bioavaila-bility %	$T_{1/2}$ h	Area under curve ng h ml^{-1}	Renal clearance ml min^{-1}	References
Sumatriptan	100 mg, p.o.	1.5	54	14	2	158	260	[10, 26]
Almotriptan	12.5 mg, p.o.	2.5	49.5	80	3.1	266		[27, 28]
Frovatriptan	2.5 mg, p.o.	3.0	7.0	29.6	25.7	94		[29]
	40 mg, p.o.	5.0	53.4	17.5	29.7	881		
	0.8 mg, i.v.	–	24.4	100	23.6	104	132	

Sumatriptan does not have any active metabolite and its protein binding is between 14–21%; such data for almotriptan and frovatriptan are not available to the authors. Similarly, pharmacokinetic data are available for F11356.

Beyond the Second-Generation Triptans

It is undeniable that cranial vasoconstrictor activity of sumatriptan and other triptans, which is mediated by the 5-HT$_{1B}$ receptor [19, 25], is associated with their efficacy in the acute treatment of migraine. Unfortunately, the 5-HT$_{1B}$ receptor is most likely also responsible for the moderate hypertension and coronary constriction noticed with these drugs. Therefore, in an attempt to avoid vasoconstriction different avenues are being explored. These include selective 5-HT$_{1D}$ receptor (PNU-109291 [30]) and 5-HT$_{1F}$ (LY334370 [31]) receptor agonists and compounds that block cranial vasodilatation following cortical spreading depression (SB220453 [32]). The results of clinical trials with these compounds may determine future migraine therapy.

Conclusion

In conclusion, almotriptan, frovatriptan and F11356 resemble sumatriptan in their pharmacology. With respect to the pharmacokinetics, almotriptan has a high bioavailability and frovatriptan a longer plasma half-life than sumatriptan; F11356 has not yet been studied. We do not know whether the high bioavailability of the almotriptan or the longer plasma half-life of frovatriptan offers clinical advantage over sumatriptan.

References

1   Saxena PR, De Vries P, Villalón CM: 5-HT1-like receptors: A time to bid goodbye. Trends Pharmacol Sci 1998;19:311–316.

2   Humphrey PPA, Apperley E, Feniuk W, Perren MJ: A rational approach to identifying a fundamentally new drug for the treatment of migraine; in Saxena PR, Wallis DI, Wouters W, Bevan P (eds): Cardiovascular Pharmacology of 5-Hydroxytryptamine: Prospective Therapeutic Applications. Dordrecht, Kluwer Academic Publishers, 1990, pp 416–431.

3   Ferrari MD: Migraine. Lancet 1998;351:1043–1051.

4   Goadsby PJ: Serotonin 5-HT1B/1D receptor agonists in migraine. Comparative pharmacology and its therapeutic implications. CNS Drugs 1998;10:271–286.

5   Leysen JE, Gommeren W, Heylen L, Luyten WH, Van de Weyer I, Vanhoenacker P, Haegeman G, Schotte A, Van Gompel P, Wouters R, Lesage AS: Alniditan, a new 5-hydroxytryptamine1D agonist and migraine-abortive agent: Ligand-binding properties of human 5-hydroxytryptamine1Dα, human 5-hydroxytryptamine1Dβ, and calf 5-hydroxytryptamine1D receptors investigated with [3H]5-hydroxytryptamine and [3H]alniditan. Mol Pharmacol 1996;50:1567–1580.

6   Bou J, Domenech T, Gras J, Beleta J, Llenas J, Fernandez AG, Palacios JM: Pharmacological profile of almotriptan, a novel antimigraine agent. Cephalalgia 1997;17:421.

7   Brown AM, Parsons AA, Raval P, Porter R, Tilford NS, Gager TL, Price GW, Wood MD, Kaumann AJ, Young RA, Rana K, Warrington BH, King FD: SB 209509 (VML 251), a potent constrictor of rabbit basilar artery with high affinity and selectivity for human 5-HT1D receptors. Br J Pharmacol 1996;119:110P.

8   Pauwels PJ, Palmier C, Tardif S, Wurch T, Perez M, John GW, Halazy S, Colpaert FC: F11356, a new 5-HT derivative, with selective, potent and highly efficacious agonist properties at 5-HT1B/1D receptors. Naunyn-Schmiedeberg's Arch Pharmacol 1998;358:R523.

9   MacIntyre PD, Bhargava B, Hogg KJ, Gemmill JD, Hillis WS: Effect of subcutaneous sumatriptan, a selective 5HT1 agonist, on the systemic, pulmonary, and coronary circulation. Circulation 1993; 87:401–405.

10 Lacey LF, Hussey EK, Fowler PA: Single dose pharmacokinetics of sumatriptan in healthy volunteers. Eur J Clin Pharmacol 1995;47:543–548.

11 De Vries P, Willems EW, Heiligers JPC, Villalón CM, Saxena PR: Constriction of porcine carotid arteriovenous anastomoses as indicator of antimigraine activity: The role of 5-HT1B/1D, as well as unidentified receptors; in Edvinsson L (ed): Migraine & Headache Pathophysiology. London, Martin Dunitz Ltd, 1999, pp 119–132.

12 Van Es NM, Bruning TA, Camps J, Chang PC, Blauw GJ, Ferrari MD, Saxena PR, Van Zwieten PA: Assessment of peripheral vascular effects of antimigraine drugs in humans. Cephalalgia 1995; 15:288–291.

13 De Vries P, Sánchez-López A, Centurión D, Heiligers JPC, Saxena PR, Villalón CM: The canine external carotid vasoconstrictor 5-HT1 receptor: Blockade by 5-HT1B (SB224289), but not by 5-HT1D (BRL15572) receptor antagonists. Eur J Pharmacol 1998;362:69–72.

14 Heyck H: Pathogenesis of migraine. Res Clin Stud Headache 1969;2:1–28.

15 Saxena PR: Cranial arteriovenous shunting, an in vivo animal model for migraine; in Olesen J, Moskowitz MA (eds): Experimental Headache Models. Philadelphia, Lippincott-Raven Publishers, 1995, vol 5, pp 189–198.

16 Parsons AA, Parker SG, Raval P, Campbell CA, Lewis VA, Griffiths R, Hunter AJ, Hamilton TC, King FD: Comparison of the cardiovascular effects of the novel 5-HT(1B/1D) receptor agonist, SB 209509 (VML251), and sumatriptan in dogs. J Cardiovasc Pharmacol 1997;30:136–141.

17 John GW, Pauwels PJ, Perez M, Halazy S, Le Grand B, Verscheure Y, Valentin JP, Palmier C, Wurch T, Chopin P, Marien M, Kleven MS, Koek W, Assie MB, Carilla-Durand E, Tarayre JP, Colpeart FC: F11356, a novel 5-HT derivative with potent, selective and unique high intrinsic activity at 5-HT$_{1B/1D}$ receptors in models relevant to migraine. J Pharmacol Exp Ther 1999;290:83–95.

18 Parsons AA, Raval P, Smith S, Tilford N, King FD, Kaumann AJ, Hunter J: Effects of the novel high-affinity 5-HT(1B/1D)-receptor ligand frovatriptan in human isolated basilar and coronary arteries. J Cardiovasc Pharmacol 1998;32:220–224.

19 Longmore J, Razzaque Z, Shaw D, Davenport AP, Maguire J, Pickard JD, Schofield WN, Hill RG: Comparison of the vasoconstrictor effects of rizatriptan and sumatriptan in human isolated cranial arteries: Immunohistological demonstration of the involvement of 5-HT1B-receptors. Br J Clin Pharmacol 1998;46:577–582.

20 Martin GR, Robertson AD, MacLennan SJ, Prentice DJ, Barrett VJ, Buckingham J, Honey AC, Giles H, Moncada S: Receptor specificity and trigemino-vascular inhibitory actions of a novel 5-HT1B/1D receptor partial agonist, 311C90 (zolmitriptan). Br J Pharmacol 1997;121:157–164.

21 John GW, Valentin JP, LeGrand B, Bonnafous R, Panissie A, Vie B, Perez M, Halazy S, Pauwels PJ, Colpaert FC: In vitro vascular and neuronal actions of F11356, a novel high efficacy 5-HT1B/D receptor agonist, in models relevant to migraine. Naunyn-Schmiedeberg's Arch Pharmacol 1998; 358:R523.

22 Connor HE, Feniuk W, Humphrey PPA: 5-Hydroxytryptamine contracts human coronary arteries predominantly via 5-HT2 receptor activation. Eur J Pharmacol 1989;161:91–94.

23 MaassenvandenBrink A, Reekers M, Bax WA, Ferrari MD, Saxena PR: Coronary side-effect potential of current and prospective antimigraine drugs. Circulation 1998;98:25–30.

24 Moskowitz MA: Neurogenic versus vascular mechanisms of sumatriptan and ergot alkaloids in migraine. Trends Pharmacol Sci 1992;13:307–311.

25 De Vries P, Villalón CM, Saxena PR: Pharmacological aspects of experimental headache models in relation to acute antimigraine therapy. Eur J Pharmacol 1999;375:61–74.

26 Fowler PA, Lacey LF, Thomas M, Keene ON, Tanner RJ, Baber NS: The clinical pharmacology, pharmacokinetics and metabolism of sumatriptan. Eur Neurol 1991;31:291–294.

27 Robert M, Warrington SJ, Zayas JM, Cabarrocas X, Fernandez FJ, Ferrer P: Electrocardiographic effects and pharmacokinetics of oral almotriptan in healthy subjects. Cephalalgia 1998;18:406.

28 Cabaroccas X, Salva M: Pharmacokinetic and metabolic data on almotriptan, a new antimigraine drug. Cephalalgia 1997;17:421.

29 Buchan P, Keywood C, Ward C: The pharmacokinetics of frovatriptan (VML 251/SB 209509), a potent, selective 5-HT1B/1D agonist, following single dose administration by oral and intravenous routes to healthy male and female volunteers. Presented at the Annual Meeting of the American Association for the Study of Headache, San Francisco, USA 1998.

30 Ennis MD, Ghazal NB, Hoffman RL, Smith MW, Schlachter SK, Lawson CF, Im WB, Pregenzer JF, Svensson KA, Lewis RA, Hall ED, Sutter DM, Harris LT, McCall RB: Isochroman-6-carboxamides as highly selective 5-HT1D agonists: Potential new treatment for migraine without cardiovascular side effects. J Med Chem 1998;41:2180–2183.

31 Johnson KW, Schaus JM, Durkin MM, Audia JE, Kaldor SW, Flaugh ME, Adham N, Zgombick JM, Cohen ML, Branchek TA, Phebus LA: 5-HT1F receptor agonists inhibit neurogenic dural inflammation in guinea pigs. Neuroreport 1997;8:2237–2240.

32 Chan WN, Evans JN, Hadley MS, Herdon HJ, Jerman JC, Parsons AA, Read SJ, Stean TO, Thompson M, Upton N: Identification of (-)-cis-6-acetyl-4S-(3-chloro-4-fluoro-benzoylamino)3,4-dihydro-2,2-dimethyl-2H-benzo[b]pyran-3S-ol as a potential antimigraine agent. Bioorg Med Chem Lett 1999;9:285–290.

Pramod R. Saxena, MD, PhD, Department of Pharmacology,
Dutch Migraine Research Group and Cardiovascular Research Institute 'COEUR',
Erasmus University Medical Centre Rotterdam 'EMCR',
NL–3000 DR Rotterdam (The Netherlands)
Tel. +31 10 408 7537/47, Fax +31 10 408 9458, E-Mail saxena@farma.fgg.eur.nl

Diener HC (ed): Drug Treatment of Migraine and Other Headaches.
Monogr Clin Neurosci. Basel, Karger, 2000, vol 17, pp 197–205

....

Therapy with Other Triptans: Almotriptan

Julio Pascual

Service of Neurology, University Hospital Marqués de Valdecilla, Santander, Spain

Currently available anti-migraine 5-HT1B/D agonists 'triptans' are not ideal at least for 20–30% of patients due to both response failure and side effects, usually minor but occasionally troublesome. Almotriptan is a novel 5-HT1B/D receptor agonist with a favourable oral bioavailability developed by Almirall-Prodesfarma and Pharmacia-Upjohn for the acute treatment of migraine with and without aura. The efficacy and safety of oral almotriptan have been tested in four completed controlled clinical trials (table 1). All included a placebo control and were performed under double-blind conditions using a parallel-group design. In a fifth placebo-controlled trial, almotriptan was administered by the subcutaneous route. A total of 2,611 patients have been studied in these trials; 1,999 receiving almotriptan. In a further recently finished open label study, an additional 480 patients have treated their migraine attacks with almotriptan over a period of 12 months. Inclusion and exclusion criteria for these clinical trials did not differ from those required with other triptans. Briefly, migraine patients had to fulfil IHS diagnostic criteria, be between 18 and 65 years old and refer 1 to 6 attacks per month. The main efficacy parameter was the percentage of patients having pain relief two hours after the test drug administration, even though other current efficacy and safety and tolerability measures in these clinical trials were also studied.

Subcutaneous Administration

This was the first study performed in migraine patients with the aim of exploring the efficacy and safety of this drug. According to previous phase I results, efficacy and safety of placebo, and of 2, 6 and 10 mg almotriptan were assessed by subcutaneous route in 123 migraine inpatients who treated one

Table 1. Summary of placebo-controlled clinical trials in migraine patients with almotriptan

Trial no.	Route	No. patients	Dosage mg	Therapeutic gain at 2 h		Recurrence	Therapeutic penalty
				Response	Pain-free		
10	Subc	123	2	11	1	10	−9
			6	47	34	7	0
			10	40	14	10	1
11	Oral	169	5	24	24	30	2
			25	38	32	7	2
			100	28	33	44	17
			150	44	24	7	27
12	Oral	742	2	−3	6	26	2
			6.25	23	18	29	1
			12.5	29	27	27	3
			25	34	34	25	11
13	Oral	668	12.5	16	13	18	1
			25	18	15	15	11
			Sumatriptan 100	22	19	25	14
14	Oral	722	6.25	22	15	30	0
			12.5	32	23	30	4

single attack. Almotriptan 10 and 6 mg was associated with significantly greater rates of headache response at 2 h than almotriptan 2 mg and placebo (90 and 97% vs. 61 and 50%, respectively). The proportion of patients experiencing headache response 1 h after subcutaneous injection of placebo, almotriptan 2, 6 and 10 mg were 38, 39, 75 and 52%, respectively. Within almotriptan 6 mg recipients, 17% were pain-free at 1 h and 59% had no pain at 2 h, while 3 and 25% of patients in the placebo group were pain-free at 1 and 2 h. These numbers for 6 mg almotriptan are at least comparable to those obtained with 6 mg subcutaneous sumatriptan [1]. Patients receiving 6 and 10 mg subcutaneous almotriptan had significantly improved migraine-associated symptoms as compared with placebo [2].

Efficacy of Oral Almotriptan

Dose-Finding Studies and Phase III Comparisons with Placebo
The first clinical trial in migraine patients by the oral route assessed the efficacy and safety of 5, 25, 100 and 150 mg of almotriptan in comparison

with placebo in a single attack in 169 inpatients [3]. Headache response within 2 h occurred in 86, 70, 80, 66 and 42% with almotriptan 150, 100, 25, 5 mg and placebo, respectively. Pain-free rate at 2 h was 43, 52, 51 and 43% for almotriptan 150, 100, 25 and 5 mg and 19% in the placebo arm. At doses of 25 to 150 mg, almotriptan also significantly reduced use of rescue medication, nausea, vomiting, photophobia and phonophobia. Adverse event incidence increased significantly after 100 and 150 mg, without there being such an increase in terms of efficacy parameters.

This clinical trial confirmed the efficacy of oral almotriptan for the acute treatment of migraine attacks and suggested 25 mg as the superior margin of therapeutic doses, with the 5 mg dose having just a slight efficacy, not statistically significant, over placebo. Thus, these data showed the need for new clinical trials exploring the dose range between 5 and 25 mg. To determine the maximum and minimum effective and non-effective dose, the next clinical trial by the oral route assessed the efficacy and safety of almotriptan at doses of 2, 6.25, 12.5 and 25 mg as compared with placebo as a single dose in 742 patients. Two hours after treatment, 67, 59, 56, 30 and 33% of attacks were relieved with almotriptan 25, 12.5, 6.25 and 2 mg and with placebo, respectively. At 2 h, 45, 38, 29, 17 and 11% of patients were pain-free with almotriptan 25, 12.5, 6.25 and 2 mg and placebo, respectively. There were no significant differences between placebo and almotriptan 2 mg, while all the differences between placebo and the remaining doses of almotriptan (6.25, 12.5 and 25 mg) were significant. Even though it was clear that the decrease in pain intensity increased dose-dependently, as did the relief of migraine related symptoms, the differences between 6.25, 12.5 and 25 mg almotriptan were not statistically significant. These data show a clear dose-response relationship for almotriptan, with 2 mg not exhibiting significant efficacy, 6.25 mg being the minimum effective dose. Considering both the incidence of adverse events and efficacy parameters in this study, the 12.5 mg dose showed the most favourable ratio between tolerability and efficacy, with a significant superiority over placebo at 30 min in the overall meta-analysis (fig. 1) ([4], Almirall Prodesfarma, data on file).

Comparative Trials with Other Substances

In a placebo-controlled trial, oral almotriptan 12.5 and 25 mg was compared with oral sumatriptan 100 mg [5]. This randomized, double-blind, parallel study involved 668 migraine outpatients. After adjusting for between-group differences in baseline headache pain, it was found that the two almotriptan doses were statistically equivalent to sumatriptan 100 mg, in relieving migraine pain and migraine-associated symptoms. Headache response at 2 h occurred in a significantly higher proportion of patients receiving almotriptan 25 mg

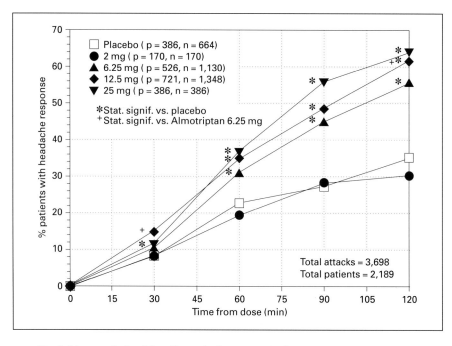

Fig. 1. Meta-analysis of the efficacy (pain response) of oral almotriptan in the treatment of migraine in double-blind trials. Notice that almotriptan 12.5 mg was statistically significant over placebo after 30 min, and that 6.25, 12.5 and 25 mg almotriptan showed statistical superiority over placebo at 1 h and onwards. Results for 2 mg almotriptan were very similar to those for placebo (Almirall-Prodesfarma, data on file). p = Number of patients treated, n = number of attacks treated.

(60%), 12.5 mg (58%) and sumatriptan 100 mg (64%) than placebo (42%); 35, 28, 34 and 15% being pain-free after 2 h, respectively. Up to now, no data have been available comparing almotriptan with either other triptans or other antimigraine symptomatic treatments, such as ergots or non-steroidal anti-inflammatory agents.

Multiple Dose and Long-Term Studies

The multiple migraine attack clinical trial studied the efficacy and tolerability of almotriptan in the treatment of three migraine episodes ([6], Almirall Prodesfarma, data on file). The aim of this study was to assess the consistency of response. Eligible patients were randomized 1:2:2 to receive placebo (131 evaluable patients), almotriptan 6.25 (287) or almotriptan 12.5 (302) mg in parallel groups during three consecutive migraine attacks. The percentages of attacks with pain response at 2 h for patients having three attacks were 38,

60 and 70% in the placebo, 6.25 and 12.5 mg groups, respectively. This dose-dependent percentage increase was statistically significant, both for pain response and pain free at 2 h, not only after the two doses of almotriptan as compared to placebo but also between the 6.25 mg and 12.5 mg doses. Statistically significant differences were found between almotriptan 12.5 and 6.25 mg and placebo, but not between the two almotriptan groups, for the number of attacks that were relieved at 1 h. The number of attacks in which patients were pain-free at 1 h after treatment showed statistically significant differences between almotriptan 12.5 mg and placebo and between almotriptan 6.25 mg and 12.5 mg. Migraine-related symptoms including nausea, vomiting, photophobia and phonophobia were ameliorated also in a dose-dependent manner by treatment with almotriptan compared with placebo. A consistent response was achieved, as shown by the very similar percentages of first and third attacks relieved at 2 h, and by the percentages of patients having headache response at 2 h in 2 out of 3 attacks: 36, 64 and 75% in the placebo, 6.25 and 12.5 mg groups, respectively. While almost 50% of patients in the 12.5 mg group had 3 out of three attacks relieved at 2 h, only 16% of placebo recipients achieved this.

Prolonged use of almotriptan has not been associated with reduced efficacy and does not lead to patients exceeding the recommended dose, according to the results of one multicentre non-comparative trial in which 806 patients (762 evaluable) could treat all their migraine attacks for one year with 12.5 mg almotriptan tablets (Almirall Prodesfarma, data on file). The percentage of attacks relieved at 1 and 2 h was 51 and 84%, respectively. Pain-free state 1 and 2 h after administration was achieved in 13 and 58% of the attacks, respectively. Escape medication was taken in only 10% of all the attacks. Complete response (pain response 2 h after administration, no rescue medication and plus no relapse for the next 24 h) was achieved in 49% of attacks, while 38% were pain free at 2 h and without the presence of relapse.

Recurrence

In the three trials exploring therapeutic doses, patients took study medication when having a recurrence within 24 h. This relapse was studied only in responders who did not take rescue medication. In all these trials the relapse treatment was always the same as patients had taken before [3–7]. The recurrence rates were 15 to 25% for 25 mg almotriptan, 18 to 30% for 12.5 mg almotriptan, 29 to 30% for 6.25 mg almotriptan and 20 to 27% for placebo. In the comparative trial against 100 mg sumatriptan, 20, 25, 18 and 15% of the responders had a relapse during the first 24 h with placebo, sumatriptan, and 12.5 and 25 mg almotriptan, respectively. Even though there was a numerical difference between the recurrence rate for almotriptan vs. sumatriptan, this difference did not reach statistical significance. The subcutaneous study showed a very low recurrence rate, between 7 and 10%, for all almotriptan-studied doses, but such data must be interpreted with caution since the recurrence rate for placebo was also very low (3%), and due to the low numbers in each treatment arm in this clinical trial [2]. In any case, and taken as a whole, these data suggest that the recurrence rate of almotriptan, 25% for 12.5 mg as an average (table 1), can be lower than that reported for other triptans, such as sumatriptan (see chapter by Diener, Sumatriptan–Therapy). Whether this will be true in clinical practice and whether this can be due in part to the relatively long half-life, almost double than that for sumatriptan, remains to be clarified.

Side Effects

In controlled trials by the oral route, a total of 1, 919 patients taking different doses of almotriptan, as well as 386 patients on placebo, were evaluated in terms of safety and tolerability [3–6]. In general, the incidence of adverse events increased with the dose. The overall incidence of drug-related adverse experiences with the recommended dose of 12.5 mg and placebo was 16 and 14% in these clinical trials. The most frequent adverse experiences after the administration of 12.5 mg almotriptan and placebo were dizziness (2.2 vs. 2.5%), paraesthesia (2.2 vs. 0.8%), nausea (2.1 vs. 0.8%), somnolence (1.7 vs. 1.3%) and fatigue (1.2 vs. 1%). The incidence of chest pain in these clinical trials was very low (0.1%, only in one case, after 12.5 mg, 1.8% after 25 mg and 0.3% after placebo).

In the comparative study against sumatriptan, the incidence of adverse events for both almotriptan doses was lower than that of sumatriptan 100 mg (fig. 2) [5]. Leaving local reactions aside, the other adverse experiences most frequently reported in almotriptan recipients were dizziness (incidence 3.2 to 6.4%), nausea (3.2 to 6.4%), vomiting (0 to 6.8%), burning sensation (3.2 to 6.4%) and flushing (3.2 to 6.4%) [2].

In all controlled clinical trials in which almotriptan has been administered, both orally and subcutaneously and including patients and healthy volunteers, only 13 serious adverse events were recorded in 10 patients. Twelve of them occurred with placebo, before drug administration or were not considered as drug related. The remaining occurred to a woman aged 47 who, 27 h after taking the third dose of 6.25 mg almotriptan in the multiple dose study, experienced an episode of epigastric discomfort and vomiting. The patient

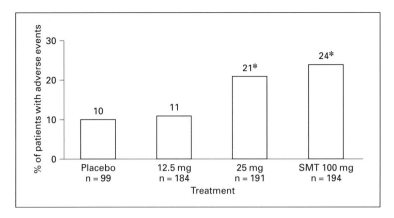

Fig. 2. Incidence of adverse events in the comparative study vs. sumatriptan 100 mg. In this clinical trial the incidence of adverse events for placebo and 12.5 mg almotriptan were comparable, while both 25 mg almotriptan and 100 mg sumatriptan showed a statistically higher incidence of adverse events [5].

went to bed normally that night, but on her routine final treatment visit the following day the ECG was found to be abnormal for repolarization changes. She was hospitalized, although she remained asymptomatic. A control ECG performed two days after the admission was normal, as well as a coronary angiogram. In spite of her age, she was found to have taken oral contraceptives for the previous three years without a doctor's supervision.

In the long-term study, in which 806 migraine patients could treat their migraine attacks (and migraine recurrence) for one year with 12.5 mg almotriptan tablets, the primary variable was the nature and incidence of adverse events. A total of 51% of patients experienced adverse events; only 29% of these, however, were considered as almotriptan-related. The intake of the two tablets during the migraine attack did not increase the adverse event incidence. Only two patients suffered from possibly drug-related serious adverse events: one case of transient chest pain with no ECG changes and one case of vagal syncope. Only 24 patients (3% of all evaluable cases) withdrew due to an adverse event. Most of them were unrelated to the study medication. There was only one ECG abnormality considered to be related to the study medication (one case of 1st degree AV-block) (Almirall Prodesfarma, data on file).

In all these clinical trials, there were no clinically significant interactions with the current anti-migraine preventive medications and with other habitual medications taken by these patients, such as oral contraceptives. Five further trials have been designed to evaluate possible interactions of almotriptan with other compounds which may be used concommitantly, such as a propranolol, verapamil, ergotamine, fluoxetine and moclobemide, and are metabolized via the same routes (CYP3A4, CYP2D6 and MAO-A). Concomitant administration of almotriptan and any of these medications did not induce clinically relevant pharmacokinetic alterations and was well-tolerated (Almirall Prodesfarma, data on file). As almotriptan is eliminated mainly unchanged by the urine, a clinical trial evaluated the pharmacokinetic profile and the safety and tolerability of a single oral 12.5 mg dose of almotriptan in subjects with renal impairment. This dose was well-tolerated independently of the degree of renal impairment. Pharmacokinetic data showed that no adjustment is necessary in patients with slight or moderate renal impairment, while those patients with severe renal impairment should take a single dose of 12.5 mg over 24 h (Almirall Prodesfarma, data on file).

Practical Advice

Almotriptan is a new 5-HT1B/D agonist that is in late phase clinical trials for the symptomatic treatment of migraine. The optimal dose of this drug in terms of efficacy and safety seems to be 12.5 mg. Double-blind, placebo-controlled trials have shown that almotriptan is effective in relief of migraine and associated symptoms, both by the oral and subcutaneous routes. From the results of just one comparative trial, the efficacy and consistency of the recommended dose appear to be comparable to those of 100 mg sumatriptan. In the opinion of this author, the encouraging recurrence numbers need to be confirmed in future comparative trials with other triptans. Perhaps the clinically specific advantage of this drug could be its very satisfactory tolerability profile. Even though almotriptan seems to resemble naratriptan in this last measurement, almotriptan is faster acting than naratriptan. Taking all available data into account, almotriptan can be considered a safe drug for the treatment of migraine. As other drugs within this therapeutic class, however, almotriptan is contraindicated in patients with known or suspected cardiovascular disease [8].

References

1   Subcutaneous Sumatriptan International Study Group: Treatment of migraine attacks with sumatriptan. N Engl J Med 1991;325:316–321.
2   Cabarrocas X for and on behalf of the Almotriptan Subcutaneous Study Group: First efficacy data on subcutaneous almotriptan, a novel 5-HT$_{1D}$ agonist. Cephalalgia 1997;17:420.
3   Cabarrocas X for and on behalf of the Almotriptan Oral Study Group: Efficacy of oral almotriptan, a novel 5-HT$_{1D}$ agonist in migraine. Cephalalgia 1997;17:421.
4   Martínez E, Cabarrocas X, Peris F, Ferrer P, Luria X: Meta-analysis on the efficacy and safety of almotriptan in the treatment of migraine. Cephalalgia 1999;19:362.

5   Cabarrocas X, Zayas JM: Advantageous tolerability of almotriptan 12.5 mg compared with sumatriptan 100 mg. Headache 1999;39:347.
6   Robert M, Cabarrocas X, Zayas JM, Ferrer P, Luria X: Overall response of oral almotriptan in the treatment of three migraine attacks. Cephalalgia 1999;19:363.
7   Cabarrocas X, Zayas JM, Surís M: Efficacy of oral almotriptan in the treatment of migraine. Headache 1998;38:377–378.
8   Holm KJ, Spencer CM: Almotriptan. CNS Drugs 1999;11:159–165.

Dr. Julio Pascual, Servicio de Neurología, Hospital Universitario Marqués de Valdecilla,
E–39008 Santander (Spain)
Tel. +34 942 202 507, Fax +34 942 202 655, E-Mail pascualj@medi.unican.es

Diener HC (ed): Drug Treatment of Migraine and Other Headaches.
Monogr Clin Neurosci. Basel, Karger, 2000, vol 17, pp 206–215

The Acute Treatment of Migraine with Frovatriptan

Gilles Géraud

Service de Neurologie, Hôpital de Rangueil, Toulouse, France

Frovatriptan is a new 5-HT$_1$ agonist being developed for the acute treatment of migraine. Frovatriptan has a high affinity for 5-HT$_{1D/1B}$ receptors [1], especially for the 5-HT$_{1B}$ receptor subtype where it appears to have the highest affinity of any compound in the triptan class [2]. In addition, data from preclinical studies suggest that frovatriptan has a distinctive pharmacological profile, different from the currently available triptans, particularly with respect to its selectivity for the cerebral vasculature [3, 4].

Frovatriptan has a considerably longer elimination half-life, $t_{1/2}$ (about 25 h) [5] than the other triptans (2–6 h) [6]. The kinetics of frovatriptan were not significantly altered in patients with renal or hepatic disease and it appears that each organ has sufficient capacity to compensate for impairment of the other [7]. An explanation for these observations and the longer $t_{1/2}$ is that the blood cell binding properties of frovatriptan play an important, determinant role in the elimination of frovatriptan [8]. The $t_{1/2}$ of frovatriptan is independent of dose, age, sex, renal impairment, hepatic impairment, use of oral contraceptives, and co-administration with ergotamine, propanolol or moclobemide [5, 7–11]. The lack of interaction with moclobemide is consistent with the observation that frovatriptan is not a substrate for monoamine oxidase [12] and therefore, unlike some other triptans is not subject to interactions with monoamine oxidase [13–15]. The pharmacokinetics of frovatriptan are unaffected during a migraine attack [16]. Thus, from a pharmacokinetic viewpoint, frovatriptan appears to be suitable for a wide range of patients.

A summary of whole blood pharmacokinetic parameters for frovatriptan is given in table 1.

Table 1. Pharmacokinetic profile of oral frovatriptan 2.5 mg, in healthy subjects

C_{max} (ng · ml^{-1})[1]	7.0 (females); 4.2 (males)
T_{max} (hours)[1]	2–3
Bioavailability[1]	30% (females); 22% (males)
$t_{1/2}$ (hours)[1]	25
Renal excretion	33% of total elimination
Metabolism	CYP 1A2

[1] Based on whole blood data.

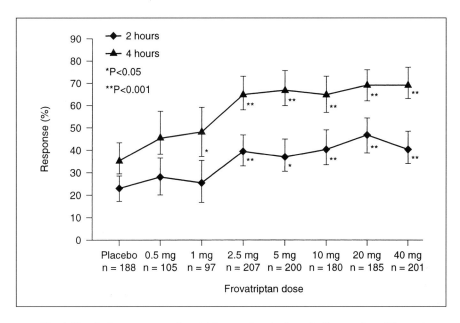

Fig. 1. Headache response at 2 and 4 h post-dose in dose-finding studies of frovatriptan 0.5–40 mg.

Frovatriptan Dose-Finding Studies

Frovatriptan was shown to be effective and well tolerated across a broad dose range of 0.5-40 mg, in two, large, placebo-controlled studies involving, in total, over 1,600 patients [17, 18]. Headache response at 2 and 4 h post-dose (change in headache severity from Grade 3 or 2 to Grade 1 or 0 [19]) was statistically superior at 2 and 4 h in the groups receiving frovatriptan 2.5–40 mg when compared with those receiving placebo (p < 0.05) (fig. 1).

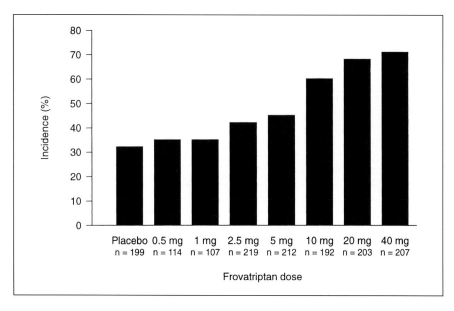

Fig. 2. The incidence of treatment-emergent adverse events reported in dose-finding studies of frovatriptan 0.5–40 mg.

Doses of 0.5 and 1 mg were not effective when compared with placebo at 2 h. There was no dose-response relationship at doses above 2.5 mg, indicating that increasing the dose of frovatriptan beyond this level does not confer any additional efficacy.

The 24-h headache recurrence in patients who had a headache response at 4 h was low across all frovatriptan groups and no dose relationship was apparent. In patients treated with frovatriptan, 9–16% experienced recurrence, compared with 27% of patients in the placebo group. This finding is consistent with the long elimination half-life $t_{1/2}$ of frovatriptan.

A dose relationship for the incidence of adverse events was observed, particularly with doses of 10 mg and greater. However, the vast majority of adverse events were described as mild or moderate in all dose groups (fig. 2).

Thus, frovatriptan 2.5 mg represented the optimal combination of efficacy and tolerability for the acute treatment of migraine and was formally evaluated as the proposed dose for the acute treatment of migraine.

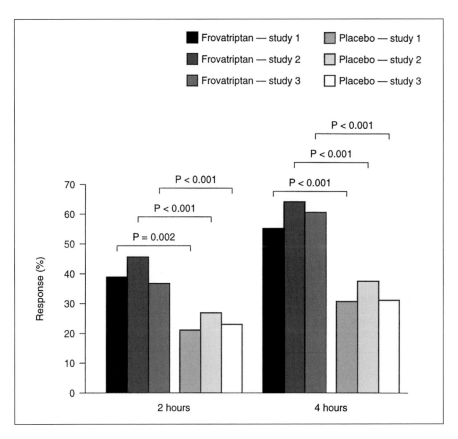

Fig. 3. The proportion of patients responding to frovatriptan 2.5 mg, at 2 and 4 h post-dose, in phase III studies.

Clinical Efficacy of Frovatriptan

The efficacy of frovatriptan 2.5 mg in the treatment of migraine was investigated in three, short-term, placebo-controlled studies in which a total of 1,632 patients took frovatriptan 2.5 mg and 811 patients took placebo [20].

Frovatriptan 2.5 mg, proved an effective treatment for migraine headache and accompanying symptoms. In each study, the proportion of patients with headache response (Grade 3 or 2 becoming Grade 1 or 0) at both 2 and 4 h after taking frovatriptan was significantly ($p \leq 0.002$) greater than with placebo (fig. 3). Overall, there was an approximately 2-fold higher headache response with frovatriptan than with placebo. In addition, the exact time of headache response as documented by patients using their wristwatch was shorter in patients taking frovatriptan (median 3.3 h) than with placebo (median 6.2 h) (fig. 4).

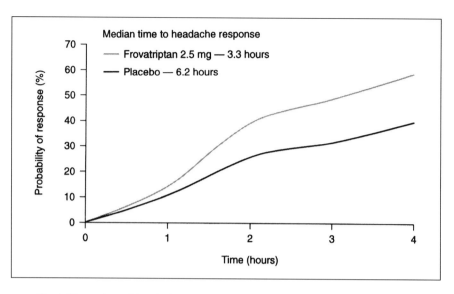

Fig. 4. Exact time of headache response using wristwatch.

The incidence of 24-h headache recurrence in patients responding at 4 h who had not used rescue medication was significantly lower with frovatriptan (range 8 to 24%) than placebo (range 24 to 40%); (p < 0.05). The incidence of headache recurrence in these studies was similar to that observed for the frovatriptan doses in the dose-finding studies.

As well as providing effective and prolonged relief of migraine headache, frovatriptan demonstrated consistent benefits on the accompanying migraine symptoms (i.e. nausea, photophobia and phonophobia). This resulted in a more rapid return to normal function. At 2 and 4 h after dosing, more patients had no or mild functional impairment in the frovatriptan group than in the placebo group (39–50% for frovatriptan vs. 26–36% for placebo at 2 h; 57–64% for frovatriptan vs. 36–43% for placebo at 4 h) (fig. 5).

Overall, frovatriptan 2.5 mg provided consistently effective relief of migraine attacks with consistent efficacy across studies [21].

Tolerability of Frovatriptan

Frovatriptan has a broad therapeutic index, with single doses of up to 100 mg being well tolerated in healthy subjects [22] and 40 mg being well tolerated in patients [18]. A comparison of the most frequently reported adverse

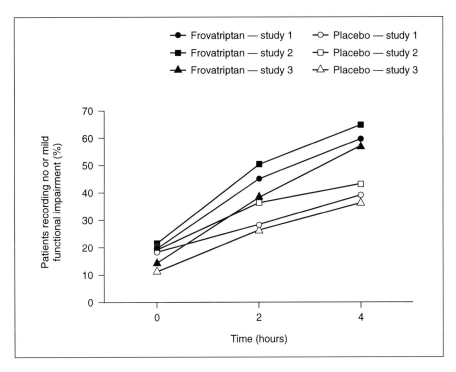

Fig. 5. The proportion of patients recording no or mild functional impairment at 0, 2 and 4 h following frovatriptan 2.5 mg or placebo.

events in patients taking frovatriptan or placebo showed that, while the incidence of adverse events was slightly higher than with placebo, the types of adverse events were similar in the frovatriptan- and placebo-treated groups [23]. The most commonly reported adverse events in both the frovatriptan and placebo groups were dizziness, nausea, headache and fatigue, all of which are commonly experienced during a migraine attack.

Importantly, the incidence of cardiovascular-type adverse events in the frovatriptan group was low and very similar to that in the placebo group (table 2). In both treatment groups, 90% of adverse events were described as mild or moderate, and less than 1% of patients withdrew from the studies due to poor tolerability of the treatment.

Long-term use of frovatriptan for the acute treatment of migraine was also well tolerated. The tolerability profile of frovatriptan 2.5 mg, observed in a 12-month, open-label study, in which patients could take up to three 2.5 mg doses in 24 h, was similar to that observed in the short-term, placebo-controlled studies [17, 18, 21]. In the long-term study, 496 patients treated a

Table 2. Treatment-emergent adverse events reported by at least 2% of patients in four placebo-controlled migraine trials

Adverse events	Frovatriptan 2.5 mg (n = 1,554)	Placebo (n = 838)
Central and peripheral nervous system		
Dizziness	8%	5%
Headache	4%	3%
Paraesthesia	4%	2%
Gastrointestinal system disorders		
Nausea	6%	6%
Mouth dry	3%	1%
Dyspepsia	2%	1%
Body as a whole – general disorders		
Fatigue	5%	2%
Temperature-change sensation	3%	2%
Chest pain	2%	1%
Psychiatric disorders		
Somnolence	4%	4%
Musculo-skeletal		
Skeletal pain	3%	2%
Vascular		
Flushing	4%	2%

total of 13,878 attacks. Again, the most common events were mild or moderate, and were dizziness, nausea, fatigue, headache, paraesthesia and somnolence. Neither prolonged use of frovatriptan nor use of up to 7.5 mg in 24 h resulted in the occurrence of undesirable effects not previously observed in short-term studies.

In a specifically designed, intensively monitored, placebo-controlled study, administration of frovatriptan, 2.5 mg, to patients at high risk of coronary artery disease (CAD) (Framingham Heart Study Risk Prediction score ≥ 14), or with known CAD, during a migraine attack was well tolerated and was not associated with an increase in cardiovascular monitoring abnormalities [24].

Furthermore, no clinically significant changes in heart rate or blood pressure were seen in either frovatriptan- or placebo-treated patients in this study

Table 3. Incidence of ischaemic episodes and type of arrhythmic episode in patients with CAD or risk factors for CAD during a migraine attack

	Frovatriptan 2.5 mg (n = 37)[1]	Placebo (n = 38)[1]
Incidence of ischaemia, n (%)	4 (11%)	5 (13%)
Mean duration of ischaemic episodes, minutes (SD)	12.2 (28.18)	14.1 (30.3)
Incidence of arrhythmic episodes, n (%)	1 (3%)	4 (11%)
Mean duration of arrhythmic episodes, seconds (SD)	2.8 (0.84)	7.1 (10.1)
Type of arrhythmic episode [2]		
Ventricular tachycardia		1
Ventricular tachycardia and supraventricular tachycardia		1
Supraventricular tachycardia		1
Sinus arrest	1	1

[1] n = 72 with risk factors, n = 3 with known CAD.
[2] Patients could have more than one type of arrhythmic episode.
SD = Standard deviation.

[24]. There was a higher incidence of clinically significant changes in 12-lead ECG at all time points post-dosing in the placebo group when compared with the frovatriptan group, and this difference reached statistical significance at 4 h post-dose (40 vs. 19%; p = 0.026). The incidence of ischaemic episodes on 24-h Holter monitoring was comparable between the frovatriptan and placebo groups. By contrast, the proportion of patients with arrhythmic episodes was higher with placebo than with frovatriptan (table 3). Chest pain was only reported by patients in the placebo group, and was not accompanied by ECG or Holter monitor changes.

Conclusions

The findings of the clinical studies of frovatriptan in the acute treatment of migraine are consistent with its pharmacological and pharmacokinetic profile. Frovatriptan is a potent 5-HT$_{1B/1D}$ agonist and it is consistently effective at a low dose of 2.5 mg with both long- and short-term use. Frovatriptan has the longest elimination half-life of the triptans and the 24-h headache recurrence observed following use of frovatriptan is lower than that reported for the other triptans. The selective effect of frovatriptan seen in pharmacology studies is supported by its excellent safety and tolerability profile in a wide variety of migraine patients, including those with cardiovascular risk factors. Hence, frovatriptan offers a new choice for migraine patients troubled by headache recurrence and side effects with other treatments.

References

1   Brown AM, Parsons AA, Raval P, Porter R, Tilford NS, Gager TL, Price GW, Wood MD, Kaumann AJ, Young RA, Rana K, Warrington BH, King FD: SB 209509 (VML 251), a potent constrictor of rabbit basilar artery with high affinity and selectivity for human 5-HT$_{1D}$ receptors. Br J Pharmacol 1996;119(suppl) (abstract 110 pp).

2   Stewart M, Napier CM, Katagampola SD, McHarg AD, Wallis RM: The binding affinity and functional activity of eletriptan and other 5-HT1$_{B/1D}$ agonists at human recombinant 5-HT$_{1B}$ and 5-HT$_{1D}$ receptors. Br J Pharmacol 1999 (in press).

3   Parsons AA, Raval P, Smith S, Tilford N, King FD, Kaumann AJ, Hunter J: Effects of the novel antimigraine agent, frovatriptan, in human isolated basilar and coronary arteries. J Cardiovasc Pharmacol 1998;32:220–224.

4   Parsons AA, Parker SG, Raval P, Campbell CA, Lewis VA, Griffiths R, Hunter AJ, Hamilton TC, King FD: Comparison of the cardiovascular effects of the novel 5-HT$_{1B/1D}$ receptor agonist, SB 209509 (VML251), and sumatriptan in dogs. J Cardiovasc Pharmacol 1997;30:136–141.

5   Buchan P, Keywood C, Ward C: Pharmacokinetics of frovatriptan (VML 251/SB 209509) in male and female subjects. Funct Neurol 1998;13:BC3,177.

6   Rose A: Facing migraine in the new millennium. Inpharma 1997;1101:3–4.

7   Cohen SAF, van der Post J, Sacks S, Marsh J, Keywood C, Buchan P: Pharmacokinetics of frovatriptan in patients with renal impairment. Cephalalgia 1999;19:II-G1-33.

8   Buchan P, Keywood C, Ward C: Pharmacokinetics of frovatriptan (VML 251/SB 209509) in healthy young and elderly male and female subjects. Cephalalgia 1998;18:P52,410.

9   Buchan P, Keywood, Ward C, Oliver SD: Lack of clinically significant interactions between frovatriptan and ergotamine. Cephalalgia 1999;19:II-G1-31.

10   Buchan P, Ward C, Stewart AJ: The effect of propranolol on the pharmacokinetic and safety profiles of frovatriptan. Cephalalgia 1999;19:II-G1-32.

11   Buchan P, Ward C, Freestone S: Lack of interaction between frovatriptan and the monoamine oxidase inhibitor, moclobemide. Cephalalgia 1999;19:II-G1-30.

12   Buchan P, Davey G, Tipton K, Motherway M: Interactions of frovatriptan and its desmethyl derivative with monoamine oxidase. Abstract 4th EFNS Congress, Lisbon, Portugal, September 7–11, 1999.

13   Dixon CM, Park GR, Tarbit MH: Characterization of the enzyme responsible for the metabolism of sumatriptan in human liver. Biochem Pharmacol 1994;47:1253–1257.

14   Seaber E, On N, Dixon RM, Gibbens M, Leavens WJ, Liptrot J, Chittick G, Posner J, Rolan PE, Pack RW: The absolute bioavailability and metabolic disposition of the novel antimigraine compound zolmitriptan (311C90). Br J Clin Pharmacol 1997;43:579–587.

15   Rogers JD, Lee Y, Goldberg MR, Olah TV, Musson DG, Birk KM, McGloughlin DA, Beer M, Slaughter D, Halpin RA, Vyas KP: Human pharmacokinetics of rizatriptan, a 5-HT$_{1B/1D}$ receptor agonist. Functional Neurology 1998;13:179.

16   Buchan P, Ward C, Zeig S: Frovatriptan pharmacokinetics are unaffected during a migraine attack. Cephalalgia 1999;19:II-G1-34.

17   Goldstein J, Keywood C: A low dose range finding study of frovatriptan (VML251) a potent cerebroselective 5-HT$_{1B/1D}$ agonist for the acute treatment of migraine. Funct Neurol 1998:13:BC7, 178.

18   Ryan R, Keywood C: A preliminary study of VML 251 (SB209509): a novel 5-HT$_{1B/1D}$ agonist for the acute treatment of migraine. Eur J Neurol 1998;5 (suppl 3):S46.

19   Headache Classification Committee of the International Headache Society. Classification and diag-
      nostic criteria for headache disorders, cranial neuralgias and facial pain. Cephalalgia 1988;8(suppl 7):
      1–96.
20   McDaris HL, Hutchison J on behalf of the frovatriptan Phase III investigators: Frovatriptan – A
      review of overall clinical efficacy. Cephalalgia 1999;19:II-G1-29.
21   Spierings EHL, Keywood C: Consistent relief with frovatriptan, a novel 5-HT$_{1B/1D}$ agonist. Cephalal-
      gia 1999;19:II-G1-40.
22   Keywood C: The effects of ascending doses of oral frovatriptan (VML 251/SB209509), a potent
      selective 5HT$_{1B/1D}$ agonist, for the acute treatment of migraine on the cardiovascular system of
      healthy male volunteers. Headache 1998;38:388.
23   Spierings EHL, Hutchison J on behalf of the frovatriptan Phase III Investigators: Frovatriptan –
      A review of safety and tolerability. Cephalalgia 1999;19:II-G1-41.
24   Elkind A, McDaris HL, Satin L, Keywood C: The cardiovascular safety of frovatriptan in patients
      at high risk of or with known coronary artery disease during a migraine attack. Cephalalgia 1999;
      19:II-G1-35.

Prof. Gilles Géraud, Service de Neurologie, Hôpital de Rangueil,
1 Avenue Jean Poulheis, F–31403 Toulouse (France)
Tel. +33 5 61 32 26 42, Fax +33 5 61 32 29 26, E-Mail geraud.g@chu-toulouse.fr

Diener HC (ed): Drug Treatment of Migraine and Other Headaches.
Monogr Clin Neurosci. Basel, Karger, 2000, vol 17, pp 216–221

....

Which Oral Triptan to Choose?

Michel D. Ferrari

Leiden University Medical Centre, Leiden, The Netherlands

The decision to choose for a specific drug is influenced by both drug- and patient-related factors. For the acute treatment of migraine, the most important drug-related factors are [1]:

i) speed of onset of action (which is primarily determined by the T_{max} of the drug, i.e. the time-to-peak plasma levels);

ii) the degree of pain relief, i.e. obtaining complete freedom of pain (possibly determined, among other pharmacokinetic factors, by the capacity of a drug to penetrate the brainstem and centrally inhibit the trigeminal nuclear complex);

iii) the duration of pain relief (i.e. whether the pain relief is sustained throughout the attack without experiencing a recurrence); this sustained effect is usually, but incorrectly, believed to be related to the $T_{1/2}$, i.e. the plasma half-life of the drug; the mechanism of recurrence is however unknown (see also below);

iv) consistency of the effect in each attack treated (this property is among other factors determined by the bioavailability of a drug; the higher the bio-availability, the greater the likelihood of a consistent response over multiple attacks);

v) tolerability, i.e. the incidence and severity of adverse events (primarily determined by the receptor binding and pharmacokinetic profiles of the drug);

vi) safety, i.e. the risk of life-threatening side effects, which in the case of triptans mainly are cardiovascular events (primarily determined by its pharmacological profile);

vii) convenience, which is mainly dependent on the flexibility in dosing, the range of available formulations, and lack of interactions with other drugs;

viii) overall long-term experience with the drug, i.e. how long is a drug already on the market and how many patients and attacks have been treated with it, and what are the experiences;

ix) personal experience of the prescribing physician with the drug and the manufacturer.

The most important patient-related factors for the selection of a specific drug are:

i) personal wishes of the patients, e.g. whether they prefer a faster onset of action or a more sustained effect;

ii) personal experience of the patient, which may bias the patients towards or away from specific drugs;

iii) individual contra-indications related to comorbid conditions and con-comitant use of medication, potentially interacting with specific drugs;

iv) issues related to reimbursement of the drug;

v) acceptance of specific adverse events and disadvantages of e.g. the subcutaneous route of administration.

Comparison of the drug-related factors should preferentially be based on the results of double blind, placebo-controlled, head-to-head comparator trials, preferably involving use of the drugs in multiple attacks. It is, however, unlikely that we will have each triptan compared with one other in such trials in the near future. We therefore should also attempt to compare the results obtained in placebo controlled trials without active comparators. As the vast majority of triptan trials have been conducted applying the same standard guidelines resulting in highly comparable study designs, study populations, and results across the different trials and triptans, this seems an acceptable and useful approach. The conclusions below will therefore be based on the results from an ongoing meta-analysis of all head-to-head-comparator and placebo-controlled triptan trials (Ferrari et al., in preparation). This meta-analysis includes both published and as yet unpublished data; an interim analysis was published recently [1].

A number of pitfalls in the clinical evaluation of acute migraine treatments deserve special attention as they might impact on the interpretation of clinical trial data. These will be discussed in the next paragraphs.

Endpoints in Clinical Trials

Firstly, improvement from moderate or severe pain at baseline to pain free by 2 h is now considered to be the preferred primary clinical endpoint.

It reflects both speed of onset and complete freedom of pain, the two most important attributes (according to the patient) of an acute migraine treatment. Patients improving only from moderate to mild pain may confound the traditional endpoint of 'response by 2 hours' (i.e. improvement to mild or no pain). It should also be emphasized that sometimes only the efficacy data at 4 h are presented which may mislead the reader when comparing with historical 2-h results for other triptans.

Recurrence

Secondly, recurrence of the headache within 24–48 h after initial relief is a major problem common to all acute migraine treatments, including ergots, analgesics, NSAIDs, and triptans. Isolated comparison of recurrence rates is misleading and technically not allowed. Recurrence can only occur in patients who have responded to the treatment and thus the population at risk for recurrence is not randomized. Because of possible differential initial responder rates and use of escape medication, there may be an imbalance of the patient characteristics at risk for recurrence. As recurrence is clearly conditional on the initial response and possible use of escape medication these factors must be included in a composite sustained relief measure in order to evaluate these effects correctly. Sustained response is defined as improvement to mild or no pain by 2 h and no recurrence and no use of additional medication within the subsequent 24 h. Sustained pain free is defined as pain free by 2 h and no recurrence and no use of additional medication within the subsequent 24 h. In simple clinical words this means: the proportion of patients requiring only a single tablet to abort the attack by 2 h and for at least 24 h. The sustained pain-free measure seems to correlate best with the patients' wishes. It should be emphasized that, contrary to earlier belief, risk of recurrence is not related to plasma half-life of the drug. Thus, a longer half-life will not reduce the incidence of recurrence. Other, as yet unknown mechanisms must be involved.

Consistency

Thirdly, intra-individual consistency of the efficacy in multiple attacks is often confused with population consistency over multiple attacks. In both cases a group of patients is treated during a number of attacks. Frequently the results of such a trial are presented as the proportion of patients who responded in each attack; i.e. x% in attack 1, y% in attack 2, z% in attack

3, and so on. This however represents a population response without any information whether patients who responded in attack 1 also had a response in attacks 2 and 3. Although response in all treated attacks (i.e. 100% consistency) would be desirable, response in at least 2/3 of the treated attacks is arbitrarily considered to represent a good consistency. Thus, intra-individual consistency of a drug can be expressed as the proportion of patients who showed a response in at least 2/3 of the treated attacks.

Prior Experience

Another problem is whether the inclusion of patients with a history of previous use of a particular triptan will introduce a bias against that particular triptan in a comparator trial against a new triptan? The argument is that such patients may enter a trial with a new triptan because they were unhappy with the 'old' triptan due to lack of efficacy. However, it appears that the majority of patients enter such a trial, not because of lack of initial response, but because they experienced recurrence with the 'old' triptan. When the response and pain-free endpoints are used as primary endpoints the results will not be affected, as by definition such patients are responders to the 'old' triptan. Comparing efficacy in 'triptan-experienced' and 'triptan-naive' patients confirmed this.

Adverse Events

Finally, how should one compare adverse event profiles of different triptans and how should one balance adverse profiles with efficacy? Adverse events are being collected differently by different companies, using different criteria and categories, making comparison between trials virtually impossible. Furthermore, some adverse events may be bothering to one patient whilst not at all to others. So, just counting the incidence of adverse events, irrespective of their impact on the patient, may not be clinically relevant. All available triptans are safe (i.e. no life-threatening side effects) when used in the appropriate patient population (no cardiovascular disease or risk factors), but may differ with respect to tolerability, i.e. incidence of bothersome or significant adverse events. Due to the limited number of direct comparison trials, only limited conclusions can be drawn to what extent triptans differ in their adverse event profiles. Preference trials over multiple attacks, which assess patient preference and thus a combination of efficacy, consistency, predictability, convenience and adverse events, may provide us with more useful information.

With respect to their pharmacology, the new triptans have, compared to sumatriptan, similar receptor profiles with only slightly different receptor affinities, and only slightly prolonged plasma half-lives which differences do not seem to be of any clinical relevance. Major differences however are that the new triptans have greater brain penetration, which may or may not provide additional therapeutic benefit, increased bioavailability predicting greater within-patient consistency over multiple attacks, and shorter time to peak plasma levels during attacks (especially rizatriptan) predicting faster onset of action.

Conclusions

Applying all these considerations to the oral triptans, the following preliminary conclusions can be drawn. Compared to the benchmark sumatriptan, the new triptans all have an improved oral pharmacokinetic profile. Rizatriptan and eletriptan show better efficacy whereas naratriptan is inferior in this respect. Rizatriptan shows very good consistency, which seems better than that for sumatriptan (although the comparison is complicated by the different designs of the studies in which this was tested for these drugs). Naratriptan and eletriptan show lower recurrence rates but especially in the case of naratriptan this may not be a clinical relevant difference as the initial response is also lower. Eletriptan however appears to show both high initial response and low recurrence rates. Comparing sustained relief data (which include both initial response and recurrence rates and looks at efficacy over a 24-h period) show the best results for rizatriptan and eletriptan whereas naratriptan is still inferior despite its apparent recurrence advantage. The latter triptan does however provide a very good side effect profile, probably because of the recommended low dose, which is a trade off with the lower efficacy.

Because of the still limited comparative data, one should be cautious in drawing any firm and final conclusion. We clearly need more and better comparative data, preferentially based on head-to-head comparator preference trials over multiple attacks. As patients characteristics and needs differ, and responses to triptans differ among patients, physicians need more than one triptan to individualize and optimalize the acute treatment of migraine attacks. Finally, it should be emphasized that the above comparison is only among the oral triptans. Subcutaneous sumatriptan undoubtedly is by far the fastest and most complete abortive drug currently available for migraine. The subcutaneous route of administration is however also associated with the disadvantage of injecting oneself and of a higher incidence and severity of the side effects.

References

1   Ferrari MD: Migraine. Lancet 1998;351:1043–1052.
2   Ferrari MD, Roon KI: The triptan war anno 1999. Education Program at the 51st Annual Meeting of the American Academy of Neurology 1999; 5TP.001: pp 6–21.

Michel D. Ferrari, MD, PhD, Leiden University Medical Centre,
NL–2300 Leiden (The Netherlands)
Tel. +31 71 5262134, Fax +31 71 5248253, E-Mail mferrari@neurology.AZL.NL

Diener HC (ed): Drug Treatment of Migraine and Other Headaches.
Monogr Clin Neurosci. Basel, Karger, 2000, vol 17, pp 222–236

••••••••••••••••••••••••

Opioids

Stephen D. Silberstein[a], *Douglas C. McCrory*[b]

[a] Jefferson Headache Center, Thomas Jefferson University, Philadelphia, Pa., USA, and
[b] Evidence-Based Practice Center, Duke University Medical Center, Center for
  Clinical Health Policy Research, Durham, N.C., USA

Pain is an unpleasant, subjective, sensory and emotional experience usually
associated with actual or potential tissue damage. The pain experience involves
a series of complex processes: transduction, transmission, modulation, and
perception. Transduction is the conversion of a noxious stimulus into a coded
electrical message at the nerve terminal. Transmission of the message, modulation, and perception occur within the CNS. This review specifically examines
the chemistry, biology, and effectiveness in clinical use of the opioids in the
treatment of head pain.

Opioids

Opium is the Greek term for the juice of the poppy plant. *Opiates* are
drugs derived from opium. They can be chemically divided into two groups:
phenanthrene (morphine, codeine, and thebaine) and benzylisoquinolines (pa-
paverine and noscapine, which both lack morphine-like properties) [1]. *Opioid*
is a more inclusive term, applying to all agonists or antagonists with morphine-
like activity such as derivatives of opium (opiates) or endogenous or synthetic
opioid peptides [2]. The term *narcotic* is derived from the Greek word for
stupor, but it is no longer used pharmacologically because of its legal meaning.
Three families of endogenous opioid peptides, each derived from a different
polypeptide precursor, have been identified: the enkephalins (from proen-
kephalin), the endorphins (from pro-opiomelanocortin), and the dynorphins
(from prodynorphin). In addition, there is good evidence for the presence of
endogenous morphine and codeine. Morphine- and codeine-like substances
have been isolated from the brain of several species, and biosynthetic pathways

Table 1. Opioids

Receptor	Endogenous ligand	Agonist	Antagonist
Mu μ_1, μ_2, μ_3	Beta-Endorphin	Morphine	Naloxone
Delta δ_1, δ_2	Enkephalin		Naloxone
Kappa κ_1, κ_2, κ_3, κ	Dynorphin	Butorphanol	Naloxone
Orphan	OFQ/N		

for morphine production, similar to that used by the opium poppy, have been demonstrated in mammals.

Receptors

There are four distinct opioid receptor types: μ, δ, κ and the 'opioid-like orphan receptor' [3–5]. It is no longer believed that there is a sigma opioid receptor. The μ receptor, important in sensory processing, including the modulation of nociceptive stimuli, extrapyramidal functioning and in limbic and neuroendocrine regulation, has three subtypes: a high-affinity μ_1, a low-affinity μ_2, and a newly described μ_3 subtype [4]. Morphine and other morphine-like opioid agonists produce analgesia primarily through μ-receptor activation, which also produces respiratory depression, miosis, reduced gastrointestinal motility, and feelings of well-being (euphoria) [6]. The supraspinal mechanisms of analgesia produced by μ-opioid agonist drugs are thought to involve the μ_1 receptor, whereas spinal analgesia, respiratory depression, and the effects of opioids on gastrointestinal function are associated with the μ_2 receptor [2]. The μ_3 receptor binds opioid alkaloids such as morphine, but has exceedingly low or no affinity for the naturally occurring endogenous opioid peptides. The μ_3 receptor occurs in macrophages, astrocytes, and endothelial cells and may be involved in immune processes. The endogenous ligand for this receptor may be morphine or codeine [4].

There are three κ receptor subtypes (table 1). The κ_3 receptor is the dominant brain opioid receptor. Instead of euphoria, κ agonists produce dysphoric, psychotomimetic effects (disoriented and/or depersonalized feelings) [2, 7]. Two subtypes of the δ receptor, whose natural ligand is the enkephalins, have been identified. The novel opioid-like orphan receptor is coded by a gene (LC132, ORL1, XOR, ROR-6, or KOR3) that was originally identified because of its extensive nucleotide sequence homology with the δ receptor [5]. The natural ligand for this receptor, an endogenous peptide [orphanin FQ/nociceptin (ORQ/N)] has been identified as a part of a larger protein (preORQ/N), whose gene maps to human chromosome 8p21 [5].

Opioid receptors have seven transmembrane-spanning domains and three extra- and three intracellular loops. They couple to a pertussis toxin-sensitive G protein (G/G_0) to influence one or more second messenger pathways: cytoplasmic-free Ca^{2+} $[Ca^{2+}]_I$, the phosphatidylinositol-$[Ca^{2+}]_I$ system and the cyclic nucleotide cAMP [3, 4]. Opioids are primarily inhibitory. They close N-type voltage-operated calcium channels and open calcium-dependent inwardly rectifying potassium channels resulting in hyperpolarization and a reduced neuronal excitability. κ receptors may act only on calcium channels. P/Q type Ca^{2+} channels may be inhibited by μ, but not by δ-receptor opioids. Opioids inhibit adenylyl cyclase decreasing cAMP concentration.

The opioids have been divided into three groups: morphine and related opioid agonists; opioids with mixed actions, such as nalorphine and pentazocine, which are agonists at some receptors and antagonists or very weak partial agonists at others; and opioid antagonists, such as naloxone. Mixed agonist/antagonists, such as pentazocine and nalorphine, can produce disturbing psychotomimetic effects that are not effectively blocked by naloxone [2, 6].

Opioid-Induced Analgesia

Opioid-induced analgesia occurs at multiple spinal and supraspinal sites [2, 8]. μ-opioid agonists selectively inhibit nociceptive reflexes and induce profound analgesia when administered intrathecally or instilled locally into the dorsal horn of the spinal cord; other sensory modalities usually are unaffected [2, 8]. Opioids modulate sensation carried by slowly conducting, unmyelinated C fibers in the dorsal horn. Pain transmission involves the release of substance P, neurokinine A, and glutamate. Release of these transmitters is inhibited by presynaptic activation of μ, δ, and κ receptors. Opioids also directly hyperpolarize and inhibit postsynaptic dorsal horn and nucleus caudalis neurons, decreasing the output of the spino- and quintothalamic tract neurons that convey nociceptive information to higher brain centers.

Clinical Studies in Migraine and Tension-Type Headache

Duke University and the American Academy of Neurology under contract to the Agency for Healthcare Policy and Research (AHCPR) identified and summarized evidence from controlled trials on the efficacy and tolerability of drug treatments for acute migraine headache. The use of opioids is a subset of that analysis. The results and methods have been published elsewhere.

Data collection and analysis was based on the number of patients obtaining headache relief according to an a priori definition of at least a 50% reduction in pain severity. Results were recorded and used to calculate odds ratios for headache relief. Measures of pain severity reported as group means (and standard deviations) were used to calculate standardized mean differences (or effect sizes). Where similar trials provided data, meta-analysis of efficacy measures was performed. The identity and rates of adverse events were recorded and statistically compared.

Oral Opioids

Codeine-containing combination agents have been studied in both migraine and tension-type headache. Among patients with migraine, seven placebo-controlled randomized trials tested the efficacy of a variety of oral codeine-containing agents, including acetaminophen + codeine and proprietary combinations of acetaminophen and codeine. Two studies compared acetaminophen + codeine with placebo [9, 10]. The two trials used slightly different formulations (400 mg + 25 mg for [9] and 650 mg + 16 mg for [10]).

Boureau et al. [9] compared acetaminophen + codeine to placebo. Two different 2-h pain outcomes for analysis were used to calculate an odds ratio of 2.3 (95% confidence interval = CI 1.5 to 3.5) for 'complete or almost complete' relief at 2 h, which confirms the study's finding of a statistically significant difference in favor of acetaminophen + codeine for this outcome. The 20% difference in response rate between the active drug and placebo suggests that the difference between the two treatments is also clinically significant. The comparison of patients experiencing complete relief at 2 h yielded an odds ratio of 1.8 (95% CI 1 to 3.2), which is just statistically significant.

Gawel et al. [10] compared acetaminophen + codeine with placebo for the treatment of several types of headache and reported only limited separate results for migraine patients. The most appropriate outcome was the sum of pain intensity differences (SPID) measured over 5 h. There was no significant difference between acetaminophen + codeine and placebo as far as this outcome was concerned, but no SPID scores and no p-value for the comparison were reported.

Two studies included comparisons of combinations of acetaminophen + codeine + doxylamine succinate (Mersyndol®) with placebo [10, 11]. Gawel et al. [10], described above, also compared acetaminophen + codeine +

doxylamine succinate with placebo. There was no significant difference between acetaminophen + codeine + doxylamine succinate and placebo, using the SPID.

Somerville [11] reported the percentage of patients reporting 'partial or complete' headache relief. An odds ratio of 5.2 (95% CI 0.99 to 27) for complete relief of headache was calculated, which is not statistically significant. The investigators' analysis, which may have been more powerful, found that Mer-syndol® was statistically superior to placebo for this outcome (p < 0.05). The 22% difference in response rate is clinically significant.

Three studies compared acetaminophen + codeine phosphate + buclizine hydrochloride + dioctyl sodium sulfosuccinate (Migraleve®) to placebo [12]. The headache duration data showed an effect size of 0.41 (95% CI –0.07 to 0.89), which confirms the study's finding that there was no significant difference between Migraleve® and placebo [12].

Carasso and Yehuda [13] calculated an odds ratio of 31 (95% CI 5.6 to 171) for 'complete or considerable' relief of migraine symptoms. This confirms the study's finding that Migraleve® was statistically superior to placebo and, together with the 64% difference in response rates, suggests a very large clinical difference between the two treatments. However, these results may be prone to bias because the study was not double-blinded and did not describe dropouts from the trial [13].

Two pain outcomes were reported (mean headache severity and headache index) in the study by Uzogara et al. [14], but no firm conclusions could be drawn about them. Mean headache severity was actually lower for attacks treated with placebo than for attacks treated with Migraleve® in periods one (4.2 vs. 4.7) and two (3.1 vs. 4.2). The treatment term in the investigators' ANOVA analysis was significant for this outcome (p = 0.022), but a carry-over effect (treatment-period interaction) was present (p = 0.016), which made interpretation of the treatment effect difficult.

Opioids were compared to other agents in a number of trials. Boureau et al. [9] compared acetaminophen + codeine with aspirin. An odds ratio of 0.90 (95% CI 0.61 to 1.3) for 'complete or almost complete' relief was calculated at 2 h, which confirms the study's finding that there was no significant difference between the two treatments for this outcome. Acetaminophen + codeine was compared with Fioricet® for the treatment of tension-type headache in one trial [15]. Investigators found significantly better complete relief with Fioricet® at 4 h, but no difference at 2 h.

The General Practitioner Research Group [16] compared Migraleve® with Migril® (ergotamine tartrate 2 mg + cyclizine 50 mg + caffeine 100 mg). There was no significant difference between the two treatments. Hakkarainen et al. [17] compared the combination drug Doleron Novum® with aspirin

500 mg. The only efficacy outcome reported (in terms of rank sums) was complete relief within 30 min. The investigators' analysis showed that Doleron Novum® was significantly better than aspirin for this outcome (p < 0.01) [17].

Hakkarainen et al. [17] also compared the combination drug Doleron Novum® with ergotamine tartrate 1 mg. The investigators' analysis showed that there was no significant difference between Doleron Novum® and ergotamine for this outcome (no p-value reported).

The literature review identified three placebo-controlled trials of Fiorinal with Codeine® including primarily patients with tension-type headache [18–20]. No placebo-controlled trials of these agents have been conducted among patients with migraine. All three trials reported significantly better pain intensity difference (PID) scores with Fiorinal® with codeine than with placebo at both 2 and 4 h. Friedman et al. (1988) also reported that > 50% headache relief was experienced at 4 h by 82% of patients treated with Fiorinal® with codeine, compared to 56% of patients treated with placebo, a difference that is statistically significant (odds ratio 3.7; 95% CI, 1.3 to 10) [19].

Direct comparisons between Fiorinal® with Codeine and Fiorinal® (without codeine) were permitted by the three studies discussed above [18–20]. Pain intensity difference scores were significantly better for the codeine-containing compound in two of the three studies at 2 h [18, 19], and in one of the three studies at 4 h [18]. At 4 h, the remaining two studies [19, 20] showed statistical trends (0.05 < p < 0.10) toward better PID for Fiorinal® with codeine.

A single trial compared Fiorinal® with codeine vs. butorphanol nasal spray (Stadol®) [21]. It was the only study of Fiorinal® with codeine conducted among patients with migraine and the only trial to use the IHS diagnostic criteria. It was also the largest of all the clinical trials of opioid drugs for headache (n = 275). At 2 h, investigators reported that butorphanol was significantly better than Fiorinal® with codeine for mean headache relief scores and for the percentage of patients reporting headache relief (defined as a reduction in headache severity from moderate or severe to mild or none). There was no significant difference between the two interventions for mean PID scores at this time-point. Headache relief was achieved at 2 h by 47% of patients treated with Fiorinal® with codeine and by 60% of patients treated with butorphanol (odds ratio, 0.58; 95% CI, 0.36 to 0.93).

At 4 h, there was still no significant difference between the two interventions for PID and no significant difference between them for mean headache relief or percentage of patients reporting headache relief. Pain intensity plotted over time showed that pain relief occurred more quickly with butorphanol than with Fiorinal® with codeine, thus accounting for the significant differences at early time-points.

Transnasal Opioids

Butorphanol nasal spray was superior to placebo in two trials. In one of them [22] treatment was administered in a clinical setting; in the other [23] patients treated themselves at home. Both provided measures of headache relief at 2 h. Diamond et al. [22] compared butorphanol nasal spray (1 mg IN) to methadone (10 mg IM) and placebo in a double-blind trial of 96 outpatients in a headache clinic. Using PID both active treatments were superior to placebo and butorphanol was superior to methadone.

In a double-blind, placebo-controlled, parallel group trial, Hoffert et al. [23] compared butorphanol (1 mg IN) to placebo in migraine patients treated at home. At 2 h, 60% of patients using butorphanol, compared to 18% of patients using placebo, had relief. This study reported data on the percentage of patients whose headache pain was reduced from moderate or severe to slight or none within 2 h. From this data an odds ratio of 6.8 (95% CI 3 to 15) was calculated, which confirms the study's finding that butorphanol is statistically significantly better than placebo at providing headache relief at 2 h. The 42% difference in response rates suggests that the difference is also clinically significant and large in magnitude.

Goldstein et al. [21] compared Fiorinal® with codeine (butalbital + aspirin + caffeine + codeine) to butorphanol, administered as a nasal spray (Stadol NS). Butorphanol was superior in efficacy to Fiorinal® with codeine at 2 h, but differences between the two treatments were not significant at 4 h.

Adverse Events

The orally administered opiate compounds were associated with only slightly higher rates of adverse events than was placebo, and were comparable to aspirin and better than ergotamine. The most commonly reported adverse events with the opiate analgesics were dizziness, fatigue, nausea, and drowsiness. Adverse events were much more frequently reported with intranasal butorphanol than with placebo or with oral opiate analgesics and most frequently involved dizziness, nausea/vomiting, drowsiness, and confusion. Complaints of an unpleasant taste and nasal irritation were also common and were probably related to the intranasal route of administration.

Parenteral Opioids

Parenteral opioid analgesics are frequently used for the treatment of acute migraine in the emergency department (ED). Opioid analgesics are associated with well-known side effects that may affect the functional status of patients (e.g. drowsiness) and reduce the drugs' effectiveness for migraine (e.g. nausea). The AHCPR literature review identified 15 publications reporting on 12 separate controlled trials of opioid analgesics for the treatment of acute migraine. Analyses included 11 published reports on 10 separate trials. Only three studies cited the International Headache Society (IHS) diagnostic criteria for migraine.

Diamond et al. [22] compared methadone IM, administered as a single 10 mg injection, to placebo. The TOTPAR scores at 2 h were analyzed. At 2 h, TOTPAR scores were 2.54 for methadone and 1.10 for placebo. Based on these numbers, the effect size was 0.36 (95% CI −0.13 to 0.85), which is not statistically significant. However, the authors' analysis of the primary data showed a statistically significant benefit of methadone over placebo ($p \leq 0.05$).

Elenbaas et al. [24] studied three single doses of butorphanol IM (1, 2 and 3 mg) in patients presenting to the ED. A parenteral antinauseant was permitted if vomiting persisted. Pain intensity and relief data were reported from immediately before treatment and after 15, 30, 45 and 60 min. Effect sizes for the various dose comparisons were: 1.1 (0.36 to 1.8) for 3 mg vs. 1 mg; 1.1 (0.32 to 1.8) for 2 mg vs. 1 mg; and 0.09 (−0.57 to 0.74) for 3 mg vs. 2 mg. Both the 3 mg and 2 mg dose were significantly better than the 1 mg dose, but there was no significant difference between the two higher doses.

Belgrade et al. [25] compared single doses of butorphanol 2 mg IM to meperidine 75 mg + hydroxyzine 50 mg IM. Results were reported for 30 min only in a blinded study. On the basis of the continuous data, an effect size of 0.62 (−0.27 to 1.5) compared butorphanol with meperidine + hydroxyzine. This effect size was not statistically significant.

Diamond et al. [22] investigated a single 10 mg injection of methadone IM to butorphanol IN administered initially in a 1 mg dose followed by a second dose at 1 h. At 2 h, TOTPAR scores were 2.54 for methadone and 3.57 for butorphanol. A not statistically significant effect size of −0.26 (−0.75 to 0.23) was calculated. The investigators' more powerful analysis found that the difference was statistically significant in favor of butorphanol ($p < 0.05$). Any difference between the two treatments is not likely to have been clinically significant.

Two trials compared meperidine plus dimenhydrinate IV with different antinauseants. Lane et al. [26] compared meperidine 0.4-mg/kg, repeated at 15 min intervals up to a maximum of three doses, plus dimenhydrinate IV to chlorpromazine IV 0.1 mg/kg, repeated at 15 min intervals up to a maximum of three doses. Dimenhydrinate 25 mg was administered along with only the first dose of meperidine. Pain intensity was evaluated on a 10 cm visual analog scale. The primary outcome was the change in mean pain intensity scores from time zero to a final time-point, defined as 45 min. An effect size of –1.1 (–1.7 to –0.49) was calculated, which supports the study's finding that chlorpromazine was significantly better than meperidine + dimenhydrinate (p < 0.001).

Stiell et al. [27] compared intramuscular meperidine + dimenhydrinate with methotrimeprazine. Patients received a single dose of either meperidine 75 mg + dimenhydrinate 50 mg or methotrimeprazine 37.5 mg. Patients measured headache relief at 1 h on a 10 cm visual analog scale. Mean pain relief scores for the meperidine + dimenhydrinate and methotrimeprazine groups were 6.63 (±3.43) and 5.84 (±2.90), respectively. The effect size corresponding to these figures was 0.25 (–0.21 to 0.71), which confirms the study's finding that the difference between the two groups for this outcome was not statistically significant (p = 0.29).

Three trials compared meperidine ± an antinauseant with the NSAID, ketorolac [28–30]. Larkin and Prescott [30] compared a single dose of intramuscular meperidine 75 mg to ketorolac 30 mg. Pain relief was measured on a verbal analog scale that ranged from 'no relief' to 'complete relief'. Meperidine was significantly better than ketorolac at providing headache relief at 1 h (p = 0.02, Wilcoxon rank sum test). An odds ratio for this outcome could not be calculated.

Duarte et al. [29] compared single doses of meperidine (100 mg) + hydroxyzine (50 mg IM) to ketorolac (60 mg IM). Both continuous data on headache intensity and dichotomous data on headache relief were analyzed. Headache pain intensity was graded before treatment and again at 60 min on a visual analog scale of 0 to 10. Pretreatment mean headache intensity scores were 8.28 (±1.65) for the meperidine plus hydroxyzine group and 7.74 (±1.84) for the ketorolac group (no p-value reported). At 60 min, mean scores were 3.37 (±3.40) and 3.35 (±2.92), respectively (p = 0.76). A statistically significant effect size for the change in headache intensity from 0 to 60 min 0.006 (–0.55 to 0.56) was calculated.

Headache relief was measured on a five-point scale. A score of 'complete relief' or 'great deal of relief' was considered a treatment success. At 60 min, this level of relief had been achieved in 14/25 cases (56%) treated with meperidine + hydroxyzine and 15/25 cases (60%) treated with ketorolac, generating an odds ratio of 0.85 (0.28 to 2.6), which supports the study's finding that there was no significant difference between the two interventions for this outcome (p = 0.77).

Davis et al. [28] compared a single dose of meperidine 75 mg + promethazine 25 mg IM to ketorolac 60 mg IM. Headache relief was defined as a reduction of four or more units on a scale of 0 to 10. At 1 h, there was no significant difference between the two interventions for this outcome (p=0.372).

Belgrade et al. [25] compared single doses of butorphanol 2 mg IM to DHE 1 mg + metoclopramide 10 mg IV. Headache pain was measured before and after treatment on a scale of 0 to 100. An effect size of –0.14 (95% CI –0.76 to 0.48) comparing butorphanol with DHE + metoclopramide for this outcome was calculated, which is not statistically significant. Three of 19 patients (16%) treated with butorphanol and 8/21 (38%) treated with DHE + metoclopramide achieved a >90% reduction in headache severity from 0 to 30 min. These numbers yielded statistically significant odds ratio of 0.30 (95% CI 0.67 to 1.4) in favor of DHE + metoclopramide.

Belgrade et al. [25] also compared single doses of meperidine 75 mg + hydroxyzine 50 mg IM and DHE 1 mg + metoclopramide 10 mg IV. Results were reported for 30 min only. A statistically significant odds ratio was calculated in favor of DHE + metoclopramide of 0.010 (<0.001 to 0.91).

Klapper and Stanton [31] compared a higher dose of hydroxyzine (75 mg vs. 50 mg); otherwise, the doses used were the same as in Belgrade et al. [25]. Both treatment groups experienced significant improvement in mean headache severity scores from 0 to 60 min. An effect size of –1.02 (–1.8 to –0.23) was calculated, which confirms the study's finding that DHE + metoclopramide was significantly more effective than meperidine + hydroxyzine at reducing headache pain (p=0.006). The difference was clinically significant as well.

Scherl and Wilson [32] compared meperidine (75 mg with promethazine 25 mg) to DHE (0.5 mg), only half the dose used in the preceding two trials. Metoclopramide 10 mg was given along with the DHE. The mean percent of pain relief for each group was 77.2% for meperidine + promethazine vs. 86.2% for DHE + metoclopramide. A not statistically significant effect size of –0.13 (–0.88 to 0.63) was calculated.

Summary of Clinical Trials
The clinical trials available with which to examine the use of opioid drug in clinical practice do support the effectiveness of several agents for episodic treatment of acute migraine and tension-type headache. However, they fall short in several respects. The available trials do not address one role in which opioid drugs are often used, that is as rescue medications after other treatments have failed. Clinical trials of opioid drugs are all conducted over short time frames. By focusing on pain relief of acute headache attacks, these studies do not address clinically important questions about frequent or prolonged use of opioid analgesics, such as rebound headache, tolerance, and dependence.

Table 2. Doses of opioids equivalent to 10 mg parenteral morphine

Drug	Oral dose (mg)	Oral-to-parenteral dose ratio	Parenteral dose (mg)
Butorphanol	NA	NA	2
Codeine	200	1.5:1	130
Hydromorphone	7.5	5:1	1.5
Meperidine	300	4:1	75
Methadone	20	2:1	10
Morphine			
Single dose	60	6:1	10
Repeated dose	30	3:1	10
Oxycodone	15	2:1	30

Headache Treatment with Opioids

The choice of acute medication depends on headache frequency and severity, the time to peak onset of pain, the presence of associated symptoms, the presence of coexistent illnesses, and the patient's treatment response profile. Opioids may be considered for patients who have infrequent, moderate-to-severe headache that does not respond to standard medication. Opioids are particularly useful in patients who cannot use specific headache medications because of coexisting disease or the lack of a diagnosis (such as the patient presenting to the ED with a new headache). They are one of the safest treatments for the pregnant patient when given in limited amounts. They are useful for severe middle-of-the-night headache and as a rescue medication. A self-administered rescue medication should be prescribed for severe migraine since most treatments do not always work. In fact, the triptans may not work at all in as many as 20 to 30% of attacks. While rescue medications often do not maintain normal function, they permit the patient to achieve relief of pain and suffering without the discomfort and expense of a visit to the physician's office or ED. Rescue medications include opioids and neuroleptics.

Opioids can be used in patients who have not overused or abused medication or violated treatment recommendations. They should be avoided or used cautiously and restrictively in patients who have demonstrated addictive tendencies or have a family history of addictive disease. Strict limits should be set and small amounts of medication should be prescribed to avoid the risk of excessive use to patients otherwise resistant to treatment [33]. The limits can be relaxed in migraineurs who are menstruating and in pregnant women. Meperidine, for example, is often useful in the pregnant patient, and occasional

Table 3. Clinical trials of opioids

Drug	Population	Findings
APAP/Codeine	Migraine	Better HA relief than placebo (2 of 3 trials)
		No better than aspirin (1 trial)
	Tension-type	No better complete relief than Fioricet® @ 2 h (1 trial)
		Less complete relief than Fioricet® @ 4 h (1 trial)
APAP/codeine/doxylamine	Migraine	No better (HA complete relief, SPID) than placebo (2 of 2 trials)
		No better SPID than APAP/codeine (1 trial)
APAP/codeine/buclizine	Migraine	Better HA relief than placebo (1 of 3 trials)
		No better HA severity than ergotamine/cyclizine/caffeine (Migril®)
Butorphanol (IM)	Migraine	No better HA relief than meperidine/hydroxyzine (IM) (1 trial)
		No better HA relief than dihydroergotamine/metoclopramide (IV) (1 trial)
Butorphanol (IN)	Migraine	Better HA severity than placebo (2 of 2 trials)
Doleron®	Migraine	Better HA relief than aspirin (1 of 1 trial)
		No better HA relief than ergotamine tartrate
Doleron novum®	Migraine	Better HA relief than aspirin (1 of 1 trial)
		No better HA relief than ergotamine tartrate
Fiorinal® with codeine	Tension-type	Better PID than placebo (3 of 3 trials)
		Better PID than Fiorinal® (1 of 3 trials)
		Less HA relief than butorphanol (1 trial)
Meperidine (IV)	Migraine	No better than ketorolac (IM) (1 trial)
Meperidine/promethazine (IV)	Migraine	No better than placebo (1 trial)
		No better than ketorolac (IM) (2 of 2 trials)
		No better HA relief than dihydroergotamine/metoclopramide (IV) (1 trial)
Meperidine/dimenhydrinate (IV)	Migraine	Less reduction in HA severity than chlorpromazine (IV) (1 trial)
		No beHA severity than methotrimeprazine (IV) (1 trial)
Meperidine/hydroxyzine IM	Migraine	No better HA relief than butorphanol (IM)
		Less HA relief than dihydroergotamine/metoclopramide (IV) (2 trials)
		No better HA relief than ketorolac (IM) (1 trial)

opioid use in the patient who cannot tolerate or does not respond to ergots, triptans, or other symptomatic medications is appropriate.

Opioid dosages should be adjusted to account for the difference in bioavailability between the oral, parenteral, and rectal routes of administration (table 2). The selection of a specific drug should be based on its route of administration, adverse effect profile, time to peak drug levels, and bioavailability. A nonoral route should be considered when there is severe nausea or vomiting. The agonist-antagonist opioids such as butorphanol and nalbuphine have lower abuse potential than the pure agonists. Parenteral butorphanol (2 to 3 mg) produces analgesia and respiratory depression equal to that of 10 mg of morphine (with similar onset, peak, and duration of action) or 80 mg of meperidine. Butorphanol's plasma half-life is about 3 h; higher values are observed in the elderly. Like other κ receptor agonists, there is much less of an increase in respiratory depression with higher doses compared to morphine and other μ-receptor agonists.

Opioids should be limited to one or two doses a week. Although admittedly controversial, some pain authorities have argued that the liberal use of opioids in intractable headache (e.g. intractable menstrual migraine) or special circumstances (e.g. elderly patients in whom the otherwise standard treatment of ergotamine is contraindicated) is justifiable.

Based on the evidence reports (table 3), the following recommendations can be made. Opioids (nasal): Butorphanol is a treatment option for migraine and headache patients when other medications cannot be used or for use as a rescue medication when significant sedation would not jeopardize the patient. As with all opioids and most acute headache treatments, overuse and dependency limits the usefulness of butorphanol for acute migraine treatment. The major side effects of butorphanol are drowsiness, weakness, sweating, feelings of floating, and nausea. The incidence of psychotomimetic side effects is lower than that with equi-analgesic doses of pentazocine, but qualitatively similar.

Oral opioid combinations (e.g. aspirin or acetaminophen + codeine) may be considered for use in acute migraine when sedation side effects will not put the patient at risk and/or the risk for abuse has been addressed. Parenteral opioids may be considered as a choice for rescue therapy in a supervised setting for acute migraine when sedation side effects will not put the patient at risk and/or the risk for abuse has been addressed.

References

1   Ferrante FM: Principles of opioid pharmacotherapy: practical implications of basic mechanisms. J Pain Symptom Mgt 1996;11:265–273.
2   Reisine T, Pasternak G: Opioid analgesics and antagonists; in Hardman JG, Limbird LE, Molinoff PB, Ruddon RW, Gilman AG (eds): Goodman & Gilman's The Pharmacological Basis of Therapeutics, ed 9. New York, McGraw-Hill, 1996, pp 521–556.
3   Piros ET, Hales TG, Evans CJ: Functional analysis of cloned opioid receptors in transfected cell lines. Neurochem Res 1996;21:1277–1285.
4   Bovill JG: Mechanisms of actions of opioids and nonsteroidal antiinflammatory drugs. Eur J Anesthesiol 1997;14:9–15.
5   Darland T, Heinricher MM, Grandy DK: Orphanin FQ/nociceptin: A role in pain and analgesia, but so much more. TINS 1998;21:215–221.
6   Pasternak GW: Review: Pharmacological mechanisms of opioid analgesics. Clin Neuropharmacol 1993;16:1–18.

7   Pfeiffer A, Brantl V, Herz A, Emrich HM: Psychotomimesis mediated by κ opiate receptors. Science 1986;233:774–776.

8   Yaksh TL: Pharmacology and mechanisms of opioid analgesic activity. Acta Anesthesiol Scand 1997;41:94–111.

9   Boureau F, Joubert JM, Lasserre V, Prum B, Delecoeuillerie G: Double-blind comparison of an acetaminophen 400 mg-codeine 25 mg combination versus aspirin 1,000 mg and placebo in acute migraine attack. Cephalalgia 1994;14:156–161.

10   Gawel MJ, Szalai JF, Stiglick A, Aimola N, Weiner M: Evaluation of analgesic agents in recurring headache compared with other clinical pain models. Clin Pharmacol Ther 1990;47:504–508.

11   Somerville BW: Treatment of migraine attacks with an analgesic combination (Mersyndol). Med J Aust 1976;1:865–866.

12   Adam EI: A treatment for the acute migraine attack. J Int Med Res 1987;15:71–75.

13   Carasso RL, Yehuda S: The prevention and treatment of migraine with an analgesic combination. Br J Clin Pract 1984;38:25–27.

14   Uzogara E, Sheehan DV, Manschreck TC, Jones KJ: A combination drug treatment for acute common migraine. Headache 1986;26:231–236.

15   Friedman AP, Diserio FJ: Symptomatic treatment of chronically recurring tension headache: A placebo-controlled, multicenter investigation of Fioricet and acetaminophen with codeine. Clin Ther 1987;10:69–81.

16   General Practitioner Research Group: Migraine treated with an antihistamine-analgesic combination. Practitioner 1973;211:357–361.

17   Hakkarainen H, Quiding H, Stockman O: Mild analgesics as an alternative to ergotamine in migraine. A comparative trail with acetylsalicylic acid, ergotamine tartrate, and dextropropoxyphene compound. J Clin Pharmacol 1980;20:590–595.

18   Friedman AP: Assessment of Fiorinal with codeine in the treatment of tension headache. Clin Ther 1986;8:703–721.

19   Friedman AP, Boyles WF, Elkind AH, Fillingim J, Ford RG, Gallagher RM, Hobbs D, Rapoport A, Richards BA, Sheftell FD: Fiorinal with codeine in the treatment of tension headache – The contribution of components to the combination drug. Clin Ther 1988;10:303–315.

20   Hwang DS, Mietlowski MJ, Friedman AP: Fiorinal with codeine in the management of tension headache: Impact of placebo response. Clin Ther 1987;9:201–222.

21   Goldstein J, Gawel MJ, Winner P, Diamond S, Reich L, Davidson WJ, Sussman NM: Comparison of butorphanol nasal spray and Fiorinal with codeine in the treatment of migraine. Headache 1988; 38:516–522.

22   Diamond S, Freitag FG, Diamond ML, Urban G: Transnasal butorphanol in the treatment of migraine headache pain. Headache Quarterly 1992;3:164–171.

23   Hoffert MJ, Couch JR, Diamond S, Elkind AH, Goldstein J, Kohlerman NJ, Saper JR, Solomon S: Transnasal butorphanol in the treatment of acute migraine. Headache 1995;35:65–69.

24   Elenbaas RM, Iacono CU, Koellner KJ, Pribble JP, Gratton M, Racz G, Evens RP: Dose effectiveness and safety of butorphanol in acute migraine headache. Pharmacother 1991;11:56–63.

25   Belgrade MJ, Ling LJ, Schleevogt MB, Ettinger MG, Ruiz E: Comparison of single-dose meperidine, butorphanol, and dihydroergotamine in the treatment of vascular headache. Neurology 1989;39: 590–592.

26   Lane PL, McLellan BA, Boggoley CJ: Comparative efficacy of chlorpromazine and meperidine with dimenhydrinate in migraine headache. Ann Emerg Med 1989;18:360–365.

27   Stiell IG, Dufour DG, Moher D, Yen M, Beilby WJ, Smith NA: Methotrimeprazine versus meperidine and dimenhydrinate in the treatment of severe migraine: A randomized, controlled trial. Ann Emerg Med 1991;20:1201–1205.

28   Davis CP, Torre PR, Williams C, Gray C, Barrett K, Krucke G, Peake D, Bass B: Ketorolac versus meperidine-plus-promethazine treatment of migraine headache: Evaluations by patients. Am J Emerg Med 1995;13:146–150.

29   Duarte C, Dunaway F, Turner L, Aldag J, Frederick R: Ketorolac versus meperidine and hydroxyzine in the treatment of acute migraine headache: A randomized, prospective, double-blind trial. Ann Emerg Med 1992;21:1116–1121.

30 Larkin GL, Prescott JE: A randomized, double-blind, comparative study of the efficacy of ketorolac tromethamine versus meperidine in the treatment of severe migraine. Ann Emerg Med 1992;21: 919–924.

31 Klapper JA, Stanton J. Current emergency treatment of severe migraine headaches. Headache 1993; 33:560–562.

32 Scherl ER, Wilson JF: Comparison of dihydroergotamine with metoclopramide versus meperidine with promethazine in the treatment of acute migraine. Headache 1995;35:256–259.

33 Portenoy RK, Foley KM, Inturrisi CE: The nature of opioid responsiveness and its implications for neuropathic pain: New hypotheses derived from studies of opioid infusions. Pain 1990;43: 273–286.

Stephen D. Silberstein, MD, FACP, Professor of Neurology, Director, Jefferson Headache Center, Thomas Jefferson University, Philadelphia, PA 19107 (USA)
Tel. +1 215 955 7734, Fax +1 215 955 6682, E-Mail stephen.silberstein@mail.tju.edu

Diener HC (ed): Drug Treatment of Migraine and Other Headaches.
Monogr Clin Neurosci. Basel, Karger, 2000, vol 17, pp 237–242

....

Miscellaneous Drugs in Acute Migraine Therapy

Ninan T. Mathew

Houston Headache Clinic, Houston, Tex., USA

Apart from the three major classes of drugs used in the acute treatment of migraine, namely 5-HT$_1$ agonists, dopamine antagonists and prokinetic agents and prostaglandin inhibitors several alternative drugs for treatment of migraine attacks deserve mention. These are drugs in common use despite limited evidence of its efficacy in controlled double-blind trials (isometheptene combinations, analgesic combinations containing butalbital/aspirin/acetaminophen/caffeine and combinations or analgesic with anti-istamines and dextropropoxyphene combinations). Other drugs commonly used without any evidence of efficacy from controlled trials include opioids, and corticosteroids.

Isometheptene

Isometheptene is a sympathomimetic amine widely used in the United States in combination with dichloralphenazone and acetaminophen. Isometheptene is a mild vasoconstrictive agent, which in combination with a mild sedative dichloralphenazone, and mild analgesic acetaminophen, is moderately efficacious in the treatment of mild to moderate migraine. It should be noted that there is no evidence from controlled trials that combination is better than isometheptene alone [1].

Pharmacology

Isometheptene is an indirectly acting sympathomimetic, which causes vasoconstriction and stimulation of heart [2]. It has an antispasmodic action on structures normally inhibited by sympathetic stimulation and was previously used in the treatment of gastrointestinal disorders [2]. Isometheptene is believed to exert its efficacy in migraine through vasoconstriction in the head. In cats, isometheptene caused a decrease in the carotid flow and greatly reduced fraction of carotid blood flow shunted through the arteriovenous anastomosis, similar to the effect reported by ergotamine and dihydroergotamine [2]. Since the early 1980s there have been no further investigations as to the possible mechanisms of action of isometheptene in migraine. Pharmacokinetic data is not available.

Controlled Double-Blind Trials with Isometheptene and Isometheptene Combination Agents

There have been five controlled clinical trials with isometheptene combination (65 mg isometheptene mucate, 100 mg dichloralphenazone, and 325 mg of acetaminophen) or 130 mg of isometheptene alone [1, 3–6]. In two trials, the isometheptene combination was found to be superior [1] or marginally superior [4] to placebo. In one of these trials, isometheptene alone was found to be superior to placebo [5], and in another study to be comparable to isometheptene combination [1].

Two studies examined the clinical efficacy of isometheptene combination in comparison with one of its constituents (acetaminophen and isometheptene, respectively) and found no significant advantage to the combination product [1, 4]. One trial showed isometheptene combination to be significantly more effective than ergotamine plus caffeine in reducing headache intensity [6]. Combination was also associated with significant less nausea and vomiting. On the other hand, isometheptene combination was found to be marginally inferior to a combination of ergotamine and caffeine in another trial [3].

Adverse events associated with isometheptene and combinations were not significantly more frequent than placebo or with comparative medications. Side effects, mainly nausea, vomiting occurred less frequently with isometheptene combination than with ergotamine in both comparative [3, 6] studies. The conclusion from controlled trials demonstrates some efficacy of isometheptene combination in the treatment of migraine attacks, but the combination has not been shown to be better than isometheptene alone. The combination seems to induce fewer side effects than oral ergotamine, but relative efficacy of these treatments remain uncertain.

Clinical Use

Isometheptene combination has a role in the acute treatment of mild to moderate migraine. It is also indicated in patients with side effects or contraindications to triptans, ergotamine and non-steroidal anti-inflammatory agents. In migraine patients with coronary artery disease, isometheptene combination is a safer and better choice than triptans or ergotamines. Two capsules can be given at the onset of attack followed by one capsule every half hour if necessary for a maximum of four or five capsules in 24 hours.

The side effects include dizziness and some circulatory disturbance. Caution is advised in patients with frequent headaches. Like many other acute agents, isometheptene can also be overused, resulting in possible rebound headache.

The contraindications for isometheptene include concomitant use of monoamino oxidase inhibitors within two weeks of treatment, glaucoma, porphyria and severe renal disease, hypertension and hepatic disease. Isometheptene being a sympathomimetic agent, if administered with monoamino oxidase inhibitors may result in severe reactions.

Barbiturate Hypnotics

Throughout the literature, ten separate controlled studies were identified that tested the efficacy of butalbital/containing agents in the treatment of headache. Only one of these trials was conducted among patients with migraine and did not include a placebo. This trial compared butalbital plus aspirin plus caffeine, plus codeine to butorphanol administered as a nasal spray. Butorphanol was superior in efficacy to butalbital combination with codeine in two hours but the difference between the two treatments were not significant at four hours. Butalbital combination with codeine was associated with significantly fewer adverse events than butorphanol nasal spray [7, 8]. The remaining nine trials identified by the literature search examined efficacy of butalbital containing agents in the treatment of episodic tension-type headache. In spite of the lack of sound clinical trial evidence of efficacy combination medications containing butalbital, it is widely used in the United States in the acute treatment of migraine and related headaches. It is one of the most overused medications, which has been shown to result in drug dependent daily headache [9].

Since there are no randomized placebo controlled studies to prove or refute efficacy for butalbital containing agents in the treatment of acute migraine headaches, it is not recommended for treatment of migraine headaches. In addition, because of the concerns of overuse, analgesic rebound headache and untoward withdrawal effects, use of butalbital containing analgesics should be limited and carefully monitored.

Lidocaine

Intravenous lidocaine demonstrated limited benefit over placebo in a small study that failed to demonstrate clinically significant benefit or harm [10].

In a second trial, intravenous lidocaine was significantly less effective than chlorpromazine IV and not more effective than intravenous DHE [11]. One study suggested that intranasal lidocaine is effective in relieving headache pain quickly within 15 min, but a high incidence of recurrence and pronounced local adverse events were also reported [12]. In a recently published abstract, intranasal lidocaine provided rapid relief; however, the previously reported high incidence of recurrence was not confirmed in this latter study [13].

Clinical Use of Lidocaine

Intranasal lidocaine does not appear to be a practical solution for patients with recurrent migraine. The intranasal lidocaine drips down the throat and makes the throat anesthetic, which is rather uncomfortable for the patient. The effect of repeated use of lidocaine in the nose on the nasal mucosa is not known. Therefore, at the present time, lidocaine is not a recommended treatment for acute migraine attacks.

Corticosteroids

Intravenous IV Dexamethasone or Hydrocortisone. Two small studies have been done, but they provide insufficient data from which to draw conclusions about the efficacy of safety of either dexamethasone IV or hydrocortisone IV for the acute treatment of migraine [14, 15].

Combination of Analgesics and Antihistamines

In order to treat head pain and nausea/vomiting simultaneously combinations of analgesics and antihistamines with anti-nausea properties were introduced. This was an alternative to ergotamine on patients experiencing nausea from the drug. Acetaminophen, small doses of codeine (8–15 mg) and histamine H_1 receptor antagonists such as buclizine and doxylamine were used. Among the five randomized studies [16–20], there were double-blind and placebo controlled [1, 19, 20] whereas the other two studies were 'semi-blind' [17, 18]. Crossover design was used in all studies except one [18].

A combination of accetaminophen 450 mg, codeine phosphate 9.75 mg, caffeine 30 mg and doxylamine succinate 5 mg per tablet was found to be superior to placebo [19]. Drowsiness was a more frequent side effect with the combination (57%) than with placebo (18%).

Two trials compared a combination of acetaminophen 550 mg, buclizine 6.25 mg, and codeine 8 mg or 15 mg with placebo [16, 20]. Careful review of these studies, found no convincing evidence that the combination is superior to placebo. This combination was reported to be comparable to ergotamine in a randomized, open, crossover trial [21].

Clinical Use

In spite of the lack of definite superiority of combination of analgesics with buclizine in controlled clinical trials, this combination is in common use in some countries such as the United Kingdom. Initial dose is two tablets containing 12.5 mg buclizine at the onset of migraine attack, followed by two tablets without buclizine but the other components every four hours if necessary, for a maximum of up to six extra tablets.

Drowsiness, fatigue and dry mouth are common side effects. Driving a car or operating dangerous equipment are to be prohibited. Glaucoma is a contraindication.

Dextropropoxyphene

Dextropropoxyphene produces analgesic and other central neuron system effects by binding primarily to μ-opioid receptors [22]. The analgesic potency of dextropropoxyphene is above 50–70% of that of codeine. Combinations of dextropropoxyphene and aspirin give a higher level of analgesia than does either agent alone [23]. T-max after oral administration of dextropropoxyphene is 1–2 h and the plasma half-life ranges from 6–12 h [22].

Two trials compared aspirin plus dextroproxophene plus phenazone combinations (dextropropoxyphene chloride 65 mg, acetylsalicylic acid 350 mg and phenazine 150 mg) with aspirin alone and ergotamine, and found that these combination agents were more significantly effective than aspirin in providing complete headache relief in 30 min [24, 25]. The same two trials found no significant difference between combination dextropropoxyphene and ergotamine. In both studies, 25 female patients treated seven attacks with each treatment at the very onset of attack, main efficacy parameter being prevention of the attacks. The dextropropoxyphene combination prevented 37 to 41% of attacks and was comparable to ergotamine (47–51%) and superior to aspirin 16–18%. However, the combination was significantly better than ergotamine in controlling nausea and vomiting [25].

References

1   Ryan R: A study of midrin in the symptomatic relief of migraine headache. Headache 1974;14:
    33–42.
2   Spierings ELH, Saxena PR: Effect of isometheptene on the distribution and shunting of 15 μm
    microspheres throughout the cephalic circulation of the cat. Headache 1980;20:103–106.

3   Adams M, Aikman P, Allardyce K: General practitioner clinical trials: Treatment of migraine. Practitioner 1971;206:551–554.

4   Diamond S: Treatment of migraine with isometheptene, acetaminophen, and dichloralphenazone combination: A double-blind crossover trial. Headache 1976;15:282–287.

5   Diamond S, Medina J: Isometheptene – A non-ergot drug in the treatment of migraine. Headache 1975;15:211–213.

6   Yuill G: A double-blind crossover trial of isometheptene cucate compound and ergotamine in migraine. Br J Clin Pract 1973;26:73–79.

7   Goldstein J, Gawel MJ, Winner P, Diamond S, Reich L, Davidson WJ, Sussman NM: Comparison of butorphanol nasal spray and Fiorinal with Codeine in the treatment of migraine. Headache 1998;38:516–522.

8   McCrory DC, Goslin RE, Gray RN: Evidence Report: Butalbital-containing compounds for the treatment of tension-type and migraine headache. Prepared by Duke University Center for Health Policy Research: October 6, 1998; Raleigh, NC.

9   Mathew NT, Kurman R, Perez F: Drug induced refractory headache: Clinical features and management. Headache 1990;30:634–638.

10 Reutens DC, Fatovich DM, Stewart-Wynne EG, Prentice DA: Is intravenous lidocaine clinically effective in acute migraine? Cephalalgia 1991;11:245–247.

11 Bell R, Montoya D, Shuaib A, Lee MA: A comparative trial of three agents in the treatment of acute migraine headache. Ann Emerg Med 1990;19:1079–1082.

12 Maizels M, Scott B, Cohen W, Chen W: Intranasal lidocaine for treatment of migraine: A randomized, double-blind, controlled trial. JAMA 1996;276:319–321.

13 Maizels M: Intranasal lidocaine for migraine in an outpatient population. Headache 1998;38:391.

14 Klapper J, Stanton J: The emergency treatment of acute migraine headache: a comparison of intravenous dihydroergotamine, dexamethasone, and placebo. Cephalalgia 1991;11(suppl 11):159–160.

15 Kozubski W: Methimazole and hydrocortisone for the interruption of a migraine attack – Preliminary study. Headache Quarterly 1992;3:326–328.

16 Adam EI: A treatment for the acute migraine attack. J Intern Med Res 1987;15:71–75.

17 Baird H, Barbour J, Cameron P: Clinical trials: Reports from the general practitioner clinical research group; migraine combination. Practitioner 1973;211:357–361.

18 Carasso P, Ychuda S: The prevention and treatment of migraine with an analgesic combination. Br J Clin Pract 1984;38:25–27.

19 Somerville B: Treatment of migraine attacks with an analgesic combination (mersyndol). Med J Aust 1976;1:865–866.

20 Uzogara E, Sheehan DV, Manschreek TC, Jones KJ: A combination drug for acute common migraine. Headache 1986;26:231–236.

21 Gebauer R, Hoffmann J, Kuhl E-D, Lehman H: Zur Migranetherapie. Med Welt 1985;36:550–556.

22 Jaffe JH, Martin WR: Opioid analgesics and antagonists; in Gilman AG, Rall TW, Nies AS, Taylor P (eds): Goodman and Gilman's the pharmacological basis of therapeutics, ed 8. New York, Pergamon Press, 1990, pp 485–521.

23 Beaver WT: Impact of non-narcotic oral analgesics on pain management. Am J Med 1988; 84(suppl 5A):3–15.

24 Hakkarainen H, Gustafsson B, Stockman O: A comparative trial of ergotamine tartrate, acetyl salicylic acid and a dextropropoxyphene compound in acute migraine attacks. Headache 1978;18: 35–39.

25 Hakkarainen H, Quiding H, Stockman O: Mild analgesics as an alternative to ergotamine in migraine. A comparative trial with acetylsalicylicacid, ergotamine tartrate, and a dextropropoxyphene compound. J Clin Pharmacol 1980;20:590–595.

Ninan T. Mathew, MD, Houston Headache Clinic,
1213 Hermann Drive, Suite 350, Houston, TX 77004 (USA)
Tel. +1 713 528 1916, Fax +1 713 526 6369, E-Mail ntmathew@houstonheadacheclinic.com

....
Migraine Prophylaxis

Diener HC (ed): Drug Treatment of Migraine and Other Headaches.
Monogr Clin Neurosci. Basel, Karger, 2000, vol 17, pp 244–249

••••••••••••••••••••••

Trial Design in Migraine Prophylaxis

Peer Tfelt-Hansen

Department of Neurology, Glostrup Hospital, Glostrup, Denmark

In general, the subjective nature of migraine and a high placebo effect generally invalidate open and single-blind trials. Clinical observations, however, most often with drugs used for another indication, e.g. valproate for epilepsy [1], can be hypothesis-generating and should be followed by randomized, controlled clinical trials which are the only way to demonstrate definitely the efficacy of a drug.

Firstly, it should be demonstrated in randomized, double-blind, placebo-controlled, clinical trials that a drug is more effective in migraine prophylaxis than placebo. The drug should then in the optimum dose be compared to currently established treatment for efficacy and tolerability. Whereas there are generally no problems with the comparison with placebo (the drug should be demonstrated to be better than placebo in several studies), the comparison with established drugs often poses problems. Sometimes the new drug is found better than an established drug, but in most trials the two drugs are not found to be statistically significantly different. If the results of these trials are reviewed critically [2, 3], it is often apparent that the trials are too small to demonstrate comparability. Furthermore, if both drugs are found effective by comparison with a baseline period, the improvements noted may be due to the natural history of migraine with amelioration purely with time [4]. Therefore comparative trials should also be placebo-controlled. The numbers of patients needed (see section on statistics) will therefore even in a crossover trial be so big that multi-center trials should be considered. If enough patients cannot be recruited for the trial it is better to avoid doing comparative trials with a low power.

The following is based mainly on the recommendations of the Drug Trial Committee of the International Headache Society (IHS) [5].

Selection of Patients

Migraine Definition. The operational diagnostic criteria of the IHS [6] should be strictly adhered to. In clinical practice there are patients who do not conform to the IHS criteria but, nevertheless, are diagnosed as having migraine, treated accordingly and respond appropriately to prophylactic migraine drugs. For clinical drug trials, however, requirements should be more rigid than in clinical practice. Relatively few people will be excluded by requiring IHS criteria.

Frequency of Attacks. Attacks of migraine should occur 2 to 6 times per month. The frequency of interval headaches should be no more than 6 days per month. There should be at least 24 h of freedom from headache between attacks. A minimum of 2 attacks per month is needed in order to detect a prophylactic effect within a reasonable time, and this is also generally the limit for when to use prophylactic treatment of migraine in clinical practice. An upper limit of migraine attacks is needed in order to avoid inclusion of patients with very frequent attacks because these patients often have drug abuse [7]. Interval headaches of more than 6 per month would begin to blend into attacks of migraine without aura if migraine were to occur as often as 6 per month. Twenty-four hours freedom between attacks of migraine permits identification of individual attacks.

Duration Since Onset. Migraine should have been present for more than one year. A minimum course of one year is advisable to help exclude headaches due to organic disease that may mimic migraine, and to establish a stereotyped pattern for the patient's headaches.

Trial Design

Blinding. Randomized controlled trials in migraine prophylaxis should be double-blind.

Placebo-control. Drugs used for migraine prophylaxis should be compared with placebo. When two presumably active drugs are compared, placebo control should also be included in order to test the reactivity of the patient sample.

The placebo effect in migraine prophylaxis is usually in the range of 20–40% and in some trials even higher, e.g. [8], and a drug should therefore be demonstrated to be superior to placebo. That two presumably active drugs are found equally effective in a trial is no proof of efficacy or comparability. To refer to the previous efficacy of the established drug in other trials is not enough; it is using historical controls, a method largely discouraged in medicine. Both drugs should also be shown to be superior to placebo.

Crossover/Parallel Group Comparison. Both crossover and the parallel group comparison (non-crossover) designs can be used in certain situations. The advantage of the crossover design is that it is approximately eight times more powerful than the non-crossover design in prophylactic migraine trials [9]. For certain non-crossover designs, however, the number of patients required is no more than 2 to 4 times the number required in a crossover design [10]; for further discussion see [11]. The drawbacks of the crossover design is the possibility of a carryover effect; the need for a long total period of treatment (extended by washout periods) that may cause problems with dropouts; and side effects can more easily affect blinding with this design. A period effect is not a problem in the crossover design, because suitable statistical techniques can deal with it [4].

When a drug is compared with placebo or an inferior drug both designs can be used if a carryover effect is not present. If there are indications from previous trials of a carryover effect, the non-crossover design should be used.

In the comparison of two drugs and placebo, the 3-way crossover design should be used. This design, if properly performed, is not invalidated by a possible carryover effect and will result in narrow confidence intervals.

Baseline Recording. A one-month baseline should be used. During baseline, placebo can be given to exclude placebo responders. This will, however, in some cases hinder actual observation of the placebo response later in the trial. The use of placebo during baseline is optional.

Duration of Treatment Periods. Treatment periods of at least 3 months should be used. Relatively long treatment periods are important for the power of the trial and also because the efficacy of many drugs accrues gradually (i.e needs some weeks before becoming fully established). Furthermore, only effects of sufficient duration are clinically relevant. With some drugs with long equilibration half lives [12] longer treatment periods of 4–5 months may be necessary to demonstrate the potential efficacy.

Washout Periods. In crossover trials a washout period of one month should be used. In the crossover design, the effect of treatment in one period must not affect the results in the subsequent period. Since drug effects are often slow in onset and wane gradually, a drug-free (placebo) washout period must be interposed between the trial periods. Its length must exceed the time taken to eliminate both the drug and its effect, which is often unknown. A washout period of one month is recommended as a practically feasible compromise.

Dosage. In assessing any new drug in migraine prophylaxis no assumptions should be made regarding dosage, and attempts should be made to test as wide a range as possible in different trials. As long as the pharmacological background for the efficacy of certain drugs in migraine remains unknown, the choice of doses in trials is a purely empirical compromise between efficacy and side effects. The willingness of the patients to take the drug for months depends heavily on the ratio between efficacy and side effects. The choice of dose is therefore one of the crucial factors in determining the chances for a successful completion of the trial. This compromise tends to induce the use of sub-optimal doses in prophylactic migraine trials.

Dosage can in triple-blind RCTs be adjusted to a certain plasma level of the drug, e.g. to anti-epileptic plasma concentrations with sodium valproate [13].

So far, no dose-response curve has been established for any drug used in migraine prophylaxis.

Evaluation of Results

Headache Diary. The evaluation of efficacy should be based on a headache diary, which should be consistent with what were identified as the assessment parameters, and should include no more.

Frequency of Attacks. Frequency of attacks per 4 weeks should be the main efficacy parameter. The number of migraine attacks should be recorded irrespective of their duration.

Most trials permit the inclusion of patients with interval headaches, but only if they are able to differentiate them well from migraine attacks. The headache diary should differentiate between the two types of headache by simply asking the patient: 'Is this a true migraine attack or another headache?' When identified, interval headaches may simply be recorded by the number of days per 4 weeks with interval headache.

Number of Days with Migraine. Number of days with migraine per 4 weeks can be used as an assessment parameter. This parameter, which allows the use of a more simple headache diary, where the patient for each day can indicate whether or not a migraine headache was present. In the same diary the patients can also indicate interval headaches, which possibly are migraine fragments.[1]

Severity of Headache. The severity of headache should be noted by the patient on a verbal scale: 0: no headache; 1: mild headache; 2: moderate headache; 3: severe headache. Alternatively, visual analogue scales can be used. One should be aware that patients are probably rating the maximum headache of the attack. Furthermore, acute treatment may possibly modify severity,

---

[1] In the earlier phases evaluation of a drug for migraine prophylaxis frequency of attacks should be preferred as the primary efficacy parameter, since number of days with migraine mixes up the frequency and duration of attacks, the latter being also dependent on acute treatment of attacks.

independently of the trial drug. Severity of headache should thus probably not be used as a primary efficacy parameter.

Duration in Hours. Patients should be asked to record time of start and time of end of attacks (in their view only), as raw data. Measurement of duration is difficult because of uncertainties relating to time of onset, time of offset and interaction of sleep. Duration of attacks should therefore not be chosen as a primary efficacy parameter.

Headache Index. The use of headache indices is not recommended. Conceivably the headache indices (I: frequency × severity and II: frequency × severity × duration) reflect the total suffering of the patients. There are, however, considerable problems with both severity and duration and when used in the headache indices, faulty weighting in the arbitrary numerical severity score will be increased by multiplication. Most important, the headache indices can in no meaningful way be compared among subjects, and a certain decrease in a headache index is difficult to evaluate clinically. Lastly, there is no need for headache indices, because in most cases where a decrease is found this is due to a decrease in frequency of attacks [14].

Patients' Preferences. The use of patients' preferences is not recommended. Patients' preferences for one or other treatment can be asked only in a crossover trial and is not recommended because it can endanger the blinding of patients since the design of the study has to be disclosed.

Responders (50% Effect). The number of responders can be expressed as those with a more than 50% reduction in attack frequency during treatment compared with the baseline period. The choice of more than 50% reduction is traditional and arbitrary. This parameter is insensitive, but can probably be used as a way of identifying retrospectively subgroups of responders. Number of responders can be used in meta-analysis of placebo-controlled RCTs with the same drug. Alternatively, time series analysis [15] can be used in defining responders.

Side Effects. All adverse events, not necessarily the same as side effects, occurring in the treatment periods should be recorded. Side effects are especially important in prophylactic trials since in clinical practice many patients stop such treatment because of them. So if the report of such a trial indicates that active drug and placebo give rise to similar side effect incidences the result should be treated with caution, as it is probably due either to the trial including too few patients or to an inadequate adverse events reporting system.

Statistics

Calculations of sample sizes in prophylactic crossover and non-crossover trials, based on frequency of attacks, indicate that the former has eight times more power than the latter for detecting a certain effect [9]. For practical purposes one can detect a difference with both designs. If, however, comparability between two drugs is to be demonstrated, only the crossover design will be suitable. In this case, as mentioned above, placebo should also be included, and this 3-way crossover design, if properly conducted, is not invalidated by a possible carryover effect (Tfelt-Hansen, pers. observ.).

In the non-crossover design, comparisons between groups can be made either as comparisons during the treatment periods or as comparisons of changes from baseline. The latter is conceivably more powerful, but analyses have so far only shown a marginal increase in power (Tfelt-Hansen, pers. observ.). In non-crossover trials the use of the baseline value as a covariate should also be examined.

References

1   Sørensen KV. Valproate: A new drug in migraine prophylaxis. Acta Neurol Scand 1988;78:346–348.
2   Tfelt-Hansen P: Efficacy of beta-blockers in migraine. A critical review. Cephalalgia 1986;6(suppl 5): 15–24.
3   Olesen J: The role of calcium entry blockers in the prophylaxis of migraine. Eur Neurol 1986; 25(suppl 1):72–79.
4   Olesen J, Krabbe AÆ, Tfelt-Hansen P: Methodological aspects of prophylactic drug trials in migraine. Cephalalgia 1981;1:127–141.
5   International Headache Society Committee on Clinical Trials in Migraine: Guidelines for controlled trials of drugs in migraine, ed 1. Cephalalgia 1991;11:1–12.
6   Headache Classification Committee of the International Headache Society: Classification and diagnostic criteria for headache disorders, cranial neuralgias and facial pain. Cephalalgia 1988;8(suppl 7): 1–96.
7   Diener H-C, Tfelt-Hansen P: Headache associated with chronic use of substances; in Olesen J, Tfelt-Hansen P, Welch KMA (eds): The Headaches, ed 1. New York, Raven Press, 1993, pp 721–727.
8   Migraine-Nimodipine European Study Group (MINES): European multicenter trial of nimodipine in the prophylaxis of classic migraine (migraine with aura). Headache 1989;29:639–642.
9   Tfelt-Hansen P, Nielsen SL: Patients numbers needed in prophylactic migraine trials. Neuroepidemiology 1987;6:214–219.
10 Lewis JA: Migraine trials: Crossover or parallel group. Neuroepidemiology 1987;6:198–208.
11 Olesen J, Tfelt-Hansen P: Headache; in Porter RJ, Schoenberg BS (eds): Controlled clinical trials in neurological disease. Boston, Dortrecht, London, Kluwer Academic Publishers, 1990, pp 185–201.
12 Sørensen P, Hansen K, Olesen J: A placebo-controlled, double-blind, crossover trial of flunarizine in common migraine. Cephalalgia 1986;6:7–14.
13 Jensen R, Brinck T, Olesen J: Sodium valproate has a prophylactic effect in migraine without aura: A triple-blind, placebo-controlled crossover study. Neurology 1994;44:647–651.
14 Tfelt-Hansen P, Standnes B, Kangasneimi P, Hakkarainen H, Olesen J: Timolol vs propranolol vs placebo in common migraine prophylaxis. Acta Neurol Scand 1984;69:1–8.
15 Langohr HD, Gerber WD, Koletzki E, Mayer K, Schroth G: Clomipramine and metoprolol in migraine prophylaxis – a double-blind crossover study. Headache 1985;25:107–113.

P. Tfelt-Hansen, Department of Neurology, Glostrup Hospital, DK-2600 Glostrup (Denmark)
Tel. +45 43 23 30 50, Fax +45 43 23 39 26, E-Mail tfelt@inet.uni2.dk

Diener HC (ed): Drug Treatment of Migraine and Other Headaches.
Monogr Clin Neurosci. Basel, Karger, 2000, vol 17, pp 250–255

....

Migraine Prophylaxis – Indication for Drug Therapy

James W. Lance

Institute of Neurological Sciences, Prince of Wales Hospital, Sydney, Australia

'I don't want to take pills all my life, doctor; I want to know the cause of my headaches and find the cure'. Patients may know of sufferers who have been cured of their headaches by removal of their gall bladder, uterus or some other superfluous viscus. Others seek natural remedies and attend their doctors only when disenchanted by dietary restrictions, neck manipulation, acupuncture, herbal infusions and incantations.

How do we start to explain the complexities of migraine to people who require instant and preferably permanent relief? I think that we have to confess to them at the beginning that there is no cure for migraine and that it is unlikely that there ever will be. While the genetics of migraine is slowly being unravelled, the manifestations of an hereditary susceptibility involve so many factors that are normally part of the individual's personality and emotional state, that the chance of specifically removing the headache components without disturbing the remainder seems remote indeed.

We can describe the intimate relationship between the brain and its blood vessels and portray the migrainous brain as being unduly sensitive to stress, forceful afferent stimulation (flicker, noise, smells) and a myriad other potential headache detonators. We can explain how the body's own pain control pathway normally monitors and modulates the impact that the external world has on our perception of pain and how this breaks down episodically to permit excessive discharge of central pain pathways. Most patients can understand that the enhanced excitability of the brain can then influence arteries both inside and outside the cranium to produce the throbbing component of migraine headache.

We can go further and speak of serotonin, noradrenaline and dopamine as chemical transmitters implicated in the migrainous process and that therapeutic agents have been designed to influence them. We can tell our patients how blood vessels become sensitive so that they give a throb of pain with each heart beat. We can aim to 'splint' the 'vascular end-organ' by constricting arteries and prevent the release of dilator substances that sensitize arterial walls together with the nerves that convey painful impulses from them. Alternatively, or in addition, we can endeavour to reinforce the pain control system centrally or switch off the internal clocks that can initiate migraine headache even in the absence of any external triggers. We can thus present to receptive patients a plausible mechanism for migraine with our therapeutic arrows aimed peripherally and centrally. They may therefore accept that there is a rationale for the pills we prescribe. We cannot cure migraine but, in most instances, can control it and restore confidence in the ability to lead a normal life.

To Treat or Not to Treat?

Prophylactic therapy is usually offered to those patients who experience two or more migraine headaches each month without adequate response to acute medication. There are, however, exceptions in both directions. Some patients who are subject to frequent attacks, even if they resolve rapidly after taking one of the triptans, ergotamine or other agent, may tire of the unpredictability of headache onset and the need for repeated acute medication. Others may be subject to tension-type headaches inbetween migrainous episodes and find it difficult to decide when they should take specific antimigrainous therapy. They may also be alarmed by the quantity of analgesics that they are consuming and would prefer to suppress the headache tendency entirely.

On the other hand, there are those patients whose headaches recur once a month or less but whose attacks are devastating in severity or duration. They include patients with prolonged aura, hemiparetic migraine, 'vertebrobasilar migraine' and menstrual migraine. The patient's wishes usually become apparent during the taking of the case history and should guide the clinician to the most appropriate treatment. The management of migraine is a collaborative venture between doctor and patient. The link may become fragile but must be maintained for a successful outcome. The patient must be aware that success cannot be guaranteed for any particular medication and that it is often necessary to persevere with a succession of trials until the most appropriate agent is found for each individual. It remains a mystery why patients with a seemingly identical pattern of migraine show such variable responses to any given prophylactic agent.

Which Preventive Therapy to Choose?

People are often reluctant to disclose that they are subject to frequent minor headaches requiring analgesics as well as their typical migraine which they have described in detail. Once the presence of inter-ictal headaches has been ascertained by questioning, patients should be asked about symptoms of anxiety or depression. Do they frown often? Do people comment that they look worried? Do they grind their teeth while sleeping, wake up with their jaw muscles taut or clench their jaws during the day? Are they restless sleepers? Positive answers to these questions may lead the clinician to favour tricyclics as the initial form of prophylaxis in conjunction with relaxation therapy or psychological counselling. Some patients object to taking antidepressants as they believe that this carries some sort of stigma by casting aspersions on their mental stability. They must understand that these agents block the reuptake of serotonin and noradrenaline and thereby improve the efficacy of the pain control system. Their use in the management of frequent headaches does not depend on their antidepressant action, although this may prove to be a useful side-effect, as well as restoring a sound night's sleep. The tricyclics are best given with the evening meal or just before retiring at night to minimize morning drowsiness. Dosage should start low, since patients vary more than ten-fold in their rate of metabolism. If patients are adamant in refusing tricyclic medication, pizotifen or cyproheptadine can be prescribed at night to promote sleep and, with luck, reduce the frequency and severity of headache. These agents increase appetite and are therefore best avoided for those who have a problem keeping their weight under control.

When minor inter-ictal headaches have a vascular component, β-adrenergic blocking agents are often effective, alone or in combination with one of the above medications. Even the relatively selective β-1 blockers such as metoprolol and atenolol are best avoided in asthmatics. The β-blockers are the only anti-migrainous agents that do not usually increase appetite and so become the treatment of choice for obese patients. Fatigue and sleep disturbances often limit their use.

Supposing that the headaches recur remorselessly after a trial of these medications, my next choice is methysergide, warning the patient to start cautiously with one half a pill twice daily, and work up slowly to one or two pills three times daily with meals if there are no side effects. Cutting the pill in half is made easier by resting it on a piece of sticky tape to prevent it rolling away. The conventional advice is for this medication to stop for one month, every four to six months, to minimize the possibility of retroperitoneal or pleural fibrosis, although these complications are rare and capricious.

For those patients whose headaches are suppressed by methysergide therapy and who suffer a serious recurrence of attacks after stopping treatment, I am prepared for them to continue without a rest period, providing that they report to their doctor every three months for physical examination and estimation of blood urea and creatinine levels. They should of course report to their doctor immediately if they experience pain in their abdomen or chest or if they have urinary symptoms. Intelligence and compliance are essential for those patients permitted to remain continuously on methysergide.

Many clinicians have found sodium valproate/valproic acid to be an effective prophylactic agent, particularly in patients subject to frequent headaches. Initial studies employed a dose of 400 mg twice daily, but recent experience suggests that the dose can be increased to 1,000–1,500 mg daily with advantage. I have not been as impressed with the efficacy of valproate as much as others, possibly because I have tended to prescribe it only when patients have failed to respond to other medications.

The calcium channel and dopamine blocking agent flunarizine, given as a single 10 mg dose at night can be remarkably effective in settling inter-ictal headaches and reducing the frequency and severity of migraine attacks. I have found it useful in patients with prolonged auras or those with hemiparetic migraine who are often resistant to other drugs. A close watch has to be held for the onset of depression as a side-effect – uncommon but potentially serious. I have never observed any convincing response to verapamil in migraine, contrary to my experience in cluster headache where it can be very useful.

For patients unresponsive to all of the above medications, the judicious use of the monoamine oxidase A, MAO(A) inhibitor, phenelzine can be gratifying. Written instructions about foods and drugs (especially nasal decongestants and treatments for sinusitis) to be avoided, should be provided to the patient in writing and the importance of compliance emphasized with dire threats of pressor headaches and possible cerebral haemorrhage if the rules are violated. Non-steroidal anti-inflammatory drugs (NSAIDs) have a limited application in migraine because of their propensity for gastrointestinal irritation. The newer antidepressants (the SSRIs), have an unpredictable effect and may make headaches worse, even if accompanying depression is relieved. I have not observed any beneficial result from the use of clonidine, riboflavin or magnesium.

Starting and Stopping Medication

As the agents we prescribe for the prophylaxis of migraine have potent pharmacological actions, whether or not they prove useful for a particular individual, the dosage should be increased gradually at the onset of treatment and diminished gradually at its termination. The surprising variation in toler-ance of drugs from patient to patient is partly accounted for by different rates of metabolism and resulting blood levels. Nevertheless patients may still react in different ways to the same blood level of a particular drug. It is helpful to enquire whether the patient has become unduly drowsy in the past to antihistamines, sedatives or compound analgesics. The answer may determine the size of the dose selected and the advice given about the time taken to achieve a therapeutic level. An obvious example is amitriptyline. Some patients tolerate 150 mg or more daily with equanimity while others become intolerably drowsy during the day after taking 10 mg the night before. The solution is for the patient to take half a tablet on the first night – half of a 25 mg tablet if previous experience has shown that they are not sedated easily, or half of a 10 mg tablet if they are. The dose can then be increased every second night until patients reach the point where they are having a sound night's sleep but are not still heavy headed after they have had breakfast and are ready to start the day. Dryness of the mouth is an indication that an adequate blood level has been achieved. The same principle applies to pizotifen or cyproheptadine which have similar soporific effects and are best given at night as a single dose.

The duration of treatment is another important consideration. Once the optimum dose has been achieved any prophylactic agent should be taken for at least 1 month, unless side effects make this impractical. The response to tricyclics may become apparent only after 2 weeks of treatment while valproate and flunarizine take 6–8 weeks to become fully effective. In questioning each patient about previous medication it is important to find out the dose employed and the duration of treatment. It is not uncommon for a patient to challenge the doctor by declaring at the outset, quite proudly, saying 'I have had every possible treatment for migraine and none of them have worked'. A careful enquiry may disclose that this is not the case or that drugs prescribed have been inappropriate or inadequate in dose or duration of treatment.

Effects and Side Effects

With any therapeutic regimen, the improvement achieved must be balanced against the severity of any adverse reaction. If no side effect of the medicine is perceptible it is probable that the drug is not being well absorbed or that the required blood level has not yet been reached. Drugs such as β-blockers and methysergide are best avoided in patients with peripheral vascular disease, coron-ary artery disease and uncontrolled hypertension because of their vasoconstric-tive properties. Because methysergide doubles gastric secretion of hydrochloric acid, its use in patients with a history of peptic ulcer is contra-indicated.

Other contra-indications are self evident. Beta blockers are avoided in asthmatics. Pizotifen, cyproheptadine and valproate are not suitable for overweight patients as they stimulate appetite. A history of depression would lead one away from prescribing flunarizine. An agitated insomniac patient would be more appropriately treated with tricyclics than MAO inhibitors.

The variety of medications employed in the prophylaxis of migraine indicates that no one is completely effective. Some 60% of patients improve on each of the agents available but still require acute therapy for their migraine headaches that remain. Some drugs have been considered as effective because they have proven better than placebo on the basis of the analysis of a headache index in a double-blind trial. Such a statistical triumph may leave the patient dissatisfied, still subject to frequent headaches. The only good result is freedom from headache but reduction of frequency and/or severity of attacks to less than half the previous intensity can be regarded as acceptable.

We live in hope of more effective preventive agents being introduced.

Conclusion

The development of new agents for the prophylaxis of migraine lags behind the advances in acute therapy since the introduction of the triptans. We are faced with the problem of trying one medication after another until, hopefully, we find one effective for each particular patient. Providing patients understand that we proceed largely by trial and error and they are prepared to try a variety of medications in succession, a useful result can usually be obtained. It may take patience on the part of both physician and patient for the maximum benefit to be extracted from regular prophylactic medication but the outcome is usually gratifying and may occasionally be spectacular.

Reference

Lance JW, Goadsby PJ: Mechanism and Management of Headache, Sixth Ed, Oxford, Butterworth-Heinemann, 1998, pp 116–157.

Prof. James W. Lance, Suite 5A, 66 High Street, Randwick, NSW 2031 (Australia)
Tel. +61 2 9398 7789, Fax +61 2 9398 7451, E-Mail jimlance@bigpond.com

Diener HC (ed): Drug Treatment of Migraine and Other Headaches.
Monogr Clin Neurosci. Basel, Karger, 2000, vol 17, pp 256–268

Migraine Prophylaxis: Beta-Blockers

Volker Limmroth, Petra Mummel

Department of Neurology, University of Essen, Essen, Germany

In the 1960s, beta-adrenoceptor antagonists, the so-called β-blockers, were introduced for the treatment of cardiac disorders including angina pectoris, arrhythmias and later hypertension. As with several other prophylactic acting anti-migraine drugs, the efficacy of β-blockers for the prophylaxis of migraine was discovered by chance when patients with migraine who received β-blockers for a cardiac disorder observed a significant reduction of migraine frequency [1]. Since then, β-blockers became the drugs of first choice worldwide for the prophylaxis of migraine (for reviews see [2–6]). Although several substances of this group such as metoprolol, propranolol, nadolol, atenolol, bisoprolol and timolol have been shown to be effective for this indication, other β-blockers such as acebutol, alprenolol, oxprenolol and pindolol have not been superior to placebo. Meanwhile, the mechanism of action of β-blockers in the prophylaxis of migraine remains unclear. This chapter reviews the current knowledge on β-blockers as prophylactic agents in the treatment of migraine.

Pharmacological Properties

In 1958 the first β-blocker, dicholorisoprenaline, was described but never introduced into the market, due to very high intrinsic activity. In the early 1960s, Sir J.W. Black, who later received the Nobel Prize, developed the first clinically usable β-blocker, and introduced it in 1964 into the market: propranolol. Within the following 35 years a large variety of similar substances followed and have been introduced, leading to at least 26 different commercially available β-blockers.

Adrenergic receptors can be divided in alpha (α) and beta (β) subtypes and mediate their effects mainly through noradrenaline released from sympathetic fibers. The β-adrenoceptors are further subdivided in β1- and β2-receptors.

The activation of both β1- and β2-receptors results in an activation of the adenylyl cyclase system which increases the conversion of ATP to cAMP. Beta-blockers occupy the β-adrenoceptor and competitively reduce receptor occupancy by catecholamines and other β-agonists. While β1-receptors are mainly expressed on cardial structures mediating positive inotropic and chronotropic effects through an increase of calcium influx into the myocardial cell, β2-receptors are mainly found on pulmonary structures and the skeletal musculature mediating vasodilatation and brochodilatation.

The pharmacological differences between the drugs are relatively small. Four aspects differentiate the substances:

a) subreceptor selectivity;
b) lipophilicity and penetration into the CNS;
c) intrinsic (agonistic) properties;
d) membrane stabilizing effects.

Subreceptor selectivity: Several of the β-blockers affect β1 and β2 receptors equally (e.g. propranolol, timolol, pindolol, soltalol). Beta-blockers such as metoprolol, bisoprolol and acebutol are so-called 'cardioselective' and exhibit a higher affinity to β1 receptors than β2 receptors. These substances are believed to cause less pulmonary side effects (especially vasoconstriction of the pulmonary tract). This selectivity, however, should not be overestimated and cardioselective β-blockers are contraindicated in patients with asthma as well. Since both types of β-blockers, with and without subreceptor selectivity, have been shown to be effective in migraine, this aspect does not appear to be important for their efficacy in migraine.

Lipophilicity: This is the most important factor for potential penetration into the CNS. With regard to this aspect the β-blocker family is a very heterogenic group. While propranolol, metoprolol, oxprenolol and alprenolol are very lipophilic, atenolol, nadolol, and practolol are only slightly or not at all lipophilic. Again, since β-blockers with and without high lipophilicity have been shown to be effective, this aspect does not appear to be important either.

Intrinsic activity: Aside from their effect as β-adrenoceptor antagonists, several β-blockers including pindolol and acebutol, exhibit intrinsic activity at the adrenoceptor. In other words they act as (partial) agonists. This partial agonism, however, is significantly lower than those of full agonists. Pindolol and acebutol are among the few β-blockers without proven efficacy in migraine prophylaxis. Whether this aspect is important or not is still to be determined since the clinical trials in which these two drugs have been evaluated suffered from poor trial design (see below), so that conclusion regarding the lack of efficacy cannot be made.

Membrane Stabilizing Activity: Several members of the β-blocker family, such as propranolol, alprenolol and oxprenolol, block sodium and calcium ion channels when applied in high dosages. The clinical effects are comparable with the effects of local anaesthetics. Since this effect, however, is only seen in few substances, but not others with proven efficacy and only in dosages beyond clinical usage, this aspect is unlikely to be of importance for the migraine treatment.

Possible Mode of Action in Migraine

The mode of action for most drugs used in migraine prophylaxis is not known nor are animal models for drugs used in migraine prophylaxis available. Some β-blockers have demonstrated efficacy in the prophylaxis of migraine, while other members of the same family are not considered effective at all. As discussed above, a (single) mechanism of action can not be concluded from the pharmacological properties. Neither subreceptor selectivity nor the ability to penetrate into the CNS or other aspects explain why some β-blockers are effective while others are not. Unfortunately, conclusions from pharmacological properties have to be drawn very cautiously since the evaluation of the β-blockers which seem to lack efficacy in migraine have mostly been evaluated in a single clinical trial of poor trial design (see later).

Initially, it was suggested that β-blockers act through the reduction of the vasodilatory phase during the migraine attack. This rather simple view of migraine pathophysiology was called into question for several reasons. Firstly, it became clear that vasodilatation is not the primary source of pain and headache. Secondly, and more importantly, there is a general agreement that neurotransmitters different from those affecting adrenergic receptors such as serotonin (5-HT) or calcitonin gene related peptide (CGRP), and thus their receptor-families are more likely to be involved in migraine pathophysiology and therapy [7]. In this context it is interesting to note that most members of the β-blocker family possess affinities for serotonin receptors as well. The affinity varies, however, and β-blockers such as pindolol and alprenolol, which have not shown efficacy in migraine prophylaxis, exhibit high affinities for (rat) 5-HT receptors as well. This aspect deserves further attention and investigation since 5-HT antagonists (on $5-HT_2$ receptors) such as methysergide are among the most potent drugs in migraine prophylaxis.

Clinical Trials on β-Blockers in the Prophylaxis of Migraine

The prophylactic action of β-blockers was detected incidentally in patients who were treated for hypertension and who also suffered from migraine. In the meantime, several clinical trials have proven that propranolol (for a review see [3, 8]) and metoprolol (for a review see [5]) are clearly effective in the prophylaxis of migraine. Atenolol [9], timolol [10], nadolol [11] and bisoprolol [12, 13] are very likely to be effective as prophylactic agents. Some β-blockers are considered to have no prophylactic efficacy in migraine: acebutolol, alprenolol, oxprenolol and pindolol.

Not all β-blockers, however, have been evaluated carefully. Many clinical trials were carried out in the 1970s when headache syndromes were not clearly defined by the criteria of the International Headache Society [14]. Furthermore, clinical trial design was far from being standardized. Hence, results of these mostly old clinical trials should be read and judged with caution. Especially those β-blockers considered to be ineffective in migraine prophylaxis have often been evaluated in only one single clinical trial or with a short evaluation time or very small number of participating patients:

- Oxprenolol: n = 30, evaluation time 8 weeks [15]
- Acebutol: n = 33, evaluation time 12 weeks, headache type not clearly defined [16]
- Alprenolol: n = 28, evaluation time 6 weeks [17]
- Pindolol (two trials): a) n = 24, evaluation time 4 weeks (!) [18], b) n = 26, evaluation time 4 weeks [19].

Although these β-blockers are considered in the general literature to be without efficacy in the prophylaxis of migraine, this should not be taken as a proven fact. Even β-blockers such as propranolol and metoprolol who's efficacy in the prophylactic treatment cannot be called into question did not show any efficacy in several trials [20–23]. Interestingly, all these trials share the same problem of trial design: an evaluation period of 8 weeks or less. Taken together, the critical review of the literature does not allow the conclusion that certain β-blockers are without efficacy in the prophylaxis of migraine.

Among all β-blockers, propranolol – and to a lesser extent metoprolol – underwent the most extensive clinical testing and served in many clinical trials as reference drugs when β-blockers were compared to other non-adrenergic drugs. Holroyd et al. [3] performed a meta-analysis for propranolol in the prophylaxis of migraine. The 53 studies included in the meta-analysis reported 2,403 patients who were treated with either the β-blocker (modal treatment 160 mg propranolol), a reference substance or placebo. On average, propranolol yielded a 44% reduction in migraine activity when daily headache recordings were used to assess treatment outcome, and a 65% reduction of migraine activity when clinical ratings of improvement and global patient reports were used. The drop-out rate due to side effects was 5.3%. The fact that propranolol in three clinical trials [20–22] and metoprolol in one clinical trial [23] did not perform better than placebo again emphasizes that the efficacy of a drug cannot be judged by a single trial and more important, that the trial design is crucial to prove the efficacy of a drug. If efficacy is shown, the overall performance among the group of β-blockers, however, is very similar with regard to the reduction of migraine attacks. Again, following a run-in-phase, an evaluation time of at least 3 months is necessary to receive reliable data on the potential efficacy in migraine prophylaxis. For further details of any specific drug the reader is referred to the original publications listed in tables 1 and 2 (these tables contain all clinical trials conducted later than 1980; for earlier trials see [4]).

β-Blockers in Comparison to Other Prophylactic Anti-Migraine Drugs

More recently β-blockers have been compared to other drugs used in the prophylaxis of migraine (see table 3). Meanwhile eight clinical trials [41–48] compared β-blockers (six trials used propranolol, two trials metoprolol) with flunarizine, a calcium channel blocker and a drug of first choice in migraine prophylaxis as well. In all trials the drugs tested were equally effective. The profile of adverse events was better with flunarizine in five trials, better with β-blockers in one trial and identical in two trials. Hence, β-blockers and flunarizine appear to be of comparable efficacy (but flunarizine has a different profile of adverse events). Other calcium channel blockers such as nifedipine and cyclandelate, which are not/less established in migraine prophylaxis, were each evaluated in a single clinical trial against propranolol as well. Albers et al. [49] compared propranolol (60 mg t.i.d.) vs. nifedipine (40 mg t.i.d.) and found an efficacy of 67% ('headache days' per month, improvement of > 50%) for the propranolol group but only of 30% in the nifedipine group. Furthermore, drop out rate and the reported side effects were significantly higher in the nifedipine group. In a large parallel double-blind trial [50] propranolol was evaluated against cyclandelate and placebo. Although propranolol reduced the monthly number of migraine attacks by > 50% in 42.3% of the patients this did not reach statistical significance against cyclandelate (37%) or placebo (30.9%).

Beta-blockers were evaluated against non-steroidal anti-inflammatory drugs (NSAIDs) in migraine prophylaxis as well. As early as 1983 Baldrati et al. [51] compared in a small trial including 18 patients the efficacy of propranolol (1.8 mg/kg) with ASA (13.5 mg/kg). In this trial, both drugs were equally effective and reduced frequency, duration, and intensity of the attacks to the same extent. Other studies, however, were not able to confirm these results. In a small double-blind cross-over trial, 200 mg propranolol daily were

Table 1. Controlled, double-blind clinical trials comparing β-blocking drugs with placebo in the prophylaxis of migraine

N	Drug, dosage (mg)/ study design	Follow up	Primary endpoints	Results	Comments	Reference
62	Prop 80–160/day/Co	4–8 weeks × 2	Preference, headache index, relief medication index	Prop > Pla	No run-in phase	Diamond and Medina 1982 [24]
41	Prop 20–80 q.i.d./Co	12 weeks × 2	Headache unit index, relief medication index	Prop > Pla		Nadelmann et al. (1986) [25]
31	PropLA 160/day/Co	8 weeks × 2	Reduction of migraine frequency, severity, duration	PropLa > Pla	Short evaluation period	Kuritzky and Hering (1987) [26]
41	PropLA 160/day/Pa	12 weeks	Reduction of migraine frequency	PropLa > Pla		Pradalier et al. (1989) [27]
62	MetLA 200 o.d./Pa	8 weeks	Reduction of migraine frequency and migraine days, severity score, relief medication	MetLA > Pla	Short evaluation period	Anderson et al. (1983) [28]
74	MetLA 200 o.d./Co (4 weeks wash-out)	8 weeks × 2 (4 weeks wash-out)	Reduction of migraine frequency and migraine days, global duration, relief medication	MetLa > Pla	Short evaluation period	Kangasneimi and Hedman (1984) [29]
54	Met 50–100 b.i.d./Pa	8 weeks	Reduction of migraine frequency, severity score, relief medication	Met vs. Pla; NS	Short evaluation period	Steiner et al. (1988) [23]
20	Aten 100 o.d./Co	90 days × 2 (2 weeks wash-out)	Reduction of migraine frequency	Aten > Pla	Well designed, small N	Forssman et al. (1983) [30]
63	Aten 100 o.d./Co	2 weeks × 2 (2 weeks wash-out)	Reduction of migraine days, integrated headache score	Aten > Pla		Johannsson et al. (1987) [31]
79	Nad 80–240/day/Pa	3 months	Reduction of migraine frequency, severity	Nad > Pla		Ryan et al. (1983) [32]
94	Tim 10 b.i.d./Co	8 weeks × 2	Reduction of migraine frequency, global preference	Tim > Pla	Short evaluation period	Stellar et al. (1984) [33]
226	Bis 5 o.d./Pa	12 weeks	Reduction of migraine frequency, duration, severity	Bis 5 > Pla	Well designed, large N	van de Ven et al. (1997) [13]

Aten = Atenolol; Bis = Bisoprolol; Met = Metoprolol; Nad = Nadolol; Prop = Propranolol; Tim = Timolol; La = long-acting, slow-release formulation; Pla = Placebo; o.d. = once daily; b.i.d. = twice daily; t.i.d. = three times daily; q.i.d. = four times daily; Co = crossover; Pa = parallel groups; MO = migraine without aura; MA = migraine with aura; NS = no statistically significant difference; > = more effective than.

Migraine Prophylaxis: Beta-Blockers

Table 2. Controlled, double-blind clinical trials comparing two β-blocking drugs or two doses of a β-blocking drug in migraine prophylaxis

N	Drug, dosage (mg)/ study design	Follow up	Primary endpoints	Results	Comments	Reference
28	Prop 80 b.i.d. Aten 50 b.i.d. Pla/Co	6 weeks × 2	Headache index, reduction of migraine days	Aten = Prop, Aten > Pla, Prop = Pla	Very short evaluation period	Stensrud and Sjaastad (1980) [9]
35	MetLA 200 o.d. Prop 80 b.i.d./Co	8 weeks × 2 (4 weeks wash-out)	Reduction of migraine frequency, severity, migraine days, relief medication	MetLA vs. = Prop both > Pla run-in	Short evaluation period	Kangasneimi and Hedman (1984) [29]
56	Prop 80 b.i.d. Met 50 b.i.d./Co	8 weeks × 2 (4 weeks wash-out)	Reduction of migraine frequency, migraine days, severity, relief medication	Met = Prop, Both > Pla run-in	Short evaluation period	Olsson et al. (1984) [34]
45	Prop 160/day Nad 80/day Nad 160/day/Pa	12 weeks	Reduction of migraine frequency, headache index	Suggest that both Nad and Prop reduce frequency and severity		Ryan (1984) [35]
80	Tim 10 b.i.d. Prop 80 b.i.d. Pla/Co	12 weeks × 3	Reduction of migraine frequency, headache indices	Tim = Prop, Tim > Pla Prop > Pla		Tfelt-Hansen et al. (1984) [10]
27	Nad 80–160/day Prop 80–160/day/Pa	24 weeks	Reduction of migraine frequency, relief medication, duration	Nad = Prop		Olerud et al. (1986) [36]
98	Prop 160/day Nad 80/day Nad 160/day/Pa	12 weeks	Several headache indices	Nad 160 > Prop 160, Nad 160 = Nad 80		Sudlikovsky et al. (1987) [37]
42	PropLA 80 o.d. PropLA 160 o.d./Co	12 weeks × 2 (4 weeks wash-out)	Reduction of migraine frequency, migraine days, severity	PropLA 80 = PropLA 160		Havanka-Kanniainen et al. (1988) [38]
37	PropLA 80 o.d. PropLA 160 o.d./Co	12 weeks × 2 (2 weeks wash-out)	Reduction of migraine frequency, duration, severity	PropLA 160 > PropLA 80		Carroll et al. (1990) [39]
125	Bis 5 o.d. Met 50 b.i.d./Co	12 weeks × 2	Reduction of migraine frequency	Met = Bis		Worz et al. (1992) [40]
30	PropLA 80 o.d. PropLA 160 o.d. Pla/Co	8 weeks	Reduction of headache frequency, severity, duration, Nausea frequency and severity	PropLA 80 vs. 160, NS; PropLA 80 vs. Pla, NS; PropLA 160 vs. Pla, NS	Poor trial design, evaluation period too short, no run-in phase	al-Quassab and Findley (1993) [22]

For abbreviations, see footnote to Table 1.

significantly more effective than 500 mg ASA daily [52]. In a double-blind multicenter trial including 243 patients Diener et al. [53] compared low dose acetylsalicylic acid (ASA, 300 mg/day) vs. metoprolol (200 mg/day) and placebo [53]. Both drugs were superior to placebo, but metoprolol reduced the frequency of migraine attacks significantly better than ASA (reduction of monthly attacks from 3.55 to 1.82 vs. 3.38 to 2.27 respectively). ASA, however, caused significantly less adverse events and showed a lower rate of drop outs. Kjaersgard Rasmussen et al. [54] compared propranolol (40 mg/t.i.d.) with tolfenamic acid (100 mg/t.i.d.) in 76 patients and found both drugs to be equally effective in the reduction of headache time (migraine days and hours) as well in pain intensity. Again, the NSAID caused less adverse events and less drop outs.

In two small clinical trials [55, 56] propranolol (up to 240 mg/day) was compared to valproic acid (up to 2,000 mg/day). In both trials the efficacy (reduction of attack frequency) of both drugs was identical. Although the profiles of adverse effects are different, a comparable low rate of adverse events was reported in both trials.

Adverse Effects and Contraindications

β-blockers are generally well tolerated when used carefully, dosages are slowly increased and individually adapted. The types of adverse effects and contraindications are nearly identical for the entire β-blocker family, regardless of their pharmacological properties (e.g. subreceptor selectivity) and are mostly dose-dependent. Typical adverse effects are: fatigue, tiredness, dizziness, sleep disturbances, abnormal dreaming, muscle cramps and depression). Contraindications are heart failure, AV block, insulin dependent diabetes and bronchial asthma.

Important Aspects for the Use of β-Blockers

In general, prior to the start of (any) migraine prophylaxis the patient should note frequency, duration and severity of migraine attacks in a diary. This diary may help to verify effects of therapy. The initial dosage of the β-blocker should be low (e.g. propranolol 20 mg) and must be slowly increased since adverse effects will occur prior to the prophylactic effects and could influence the compliance of drug intake. Again, as a general rule, patients must be informed of specific adverse effects of β-blockers. Patients should be told as well that the prophylactic effect will not appear until up to 2 months

Table 3. Controlled, double-blind clinical trials and post-marketing cohort study comparing different drugs in migraine prophylaxis

N	Drug, dosage (mg)/ study design	Follow up	Primary endpoints	Results	Comments	Reference
29	Met 200 o.d. Flu 10 o.d./Co	2 × 2 months	Reduction of migraine frequency	Met = Flu	Short evaluation period	Grotemeyer (1988) [41]
71	Pro 40 t.i.d. Flu 10 o.d./Pa	4 months	Reduction of number of attacks, satisfaction of patients	Prop = Flu		Ludin 1989 [42]
58	Prop 60 t.i.d. Flu 10 o.d./Pa	4 months	Reduction of migraine frequency	Prop = Flu	No difference in rate of adverse events (low)	Shimell et al. (1990) [43]
32	Pro 40 t.i.d. Flu 5 o.d./Pa	2 months	Reduction of migraine attacks	Prop = Flu	This trial included only children	Lutschg and Vassella (1990) [44]
149	Flu 10 o.d. Met 200 o.d./Pa	16 weeks	Number of migraine days/month	Met = Flu		Sorensen et al. (1991) [45]
94	Prop 80 b.i.d. Flu 10 o.d./Pa	4 months	Reduction of migraine frequency, use of rescue analgetics	Prop = Flu		Gawel et al. (1992) [46]
1601	Prop vs. Flu (different dosages) PMCS	up to 8 months	Risk/benefit	Prop = Flu		Verspeelt et al. (1996) [47]
45	Prop 60/day, Flu 10/day Prop 60 + Flu 10/day/Pa	120 days	Migraine index, mean frequency, global evaluation	Prop = Flu = Prop + Flu, All groups > baseline	Prop dosage too low	Bordini et al. (1997) [48]
38	Prop 60 t.i.d. Nife 30 t.i.d./Pa	6 months	Reduction of number of headaches per month	Prop > Nife (Nife – group difficult to analyze due to a drop out rate of 47%)	High drop out rate in Nife – group due to adverse events	Albers et al. (1989) [49]
214	Prop 40 t.i.d. Cycl 400 t.i.d. Pla t.i.d./Pa	12 weeks	Percentage of patients with reduction in number of migraine attacks > 50%	Prop = 42.3%, Cycl = 37.0%, Pla = 30.9% Differences n.s.		Diener et al. (1996) [50]

Table 3 (continued)

N	Drug, dosage (mg)/ study design	Follow up	Primary endpoints	Results	Comments	Reference
18	Prop 1.8 mg/kg/day ASA 13.5 mg/kg/day	3 months	Reduction of migraine index	Prop = ASA	Small number of patients	Baldretti et al. (1983)[51]
28	Met 200 o.d. (+pl t.i.d.) ASA 500 t.i.d./Co	3 months following 8 weeks of run-in	Reduction of migraine frequency (25%, 25–50%, >50%)	Met>ASA > baseline	Very high ASA dosage, small number of patients	Grotemeyer et al. (1990) [52]
243	Met 200 o.d. ASA 300 o.d./Pa	16 weeks	Number of responders with reduction in attack frequency >50%	Met>ASA > placebo	Significantly less adverse events in ASA group	Diener et al. (1997) [53]
56	Tolf 100 t.i.d. Prop 40 t.i.d./Co	12 weeks	Migraine hours, migraine days, migraine intensity	Prop = Tolf > run-in phase	Less adverse events in Tolf group	Kjaersgard et al. (1994) [54]
35	Val 1,000–1,500/day Prop 120–160 mg/day/Co	10 weeks	Reduction of migraine frequency, severity	Prop = Val > baseline	No difference in rate of adverse events	Kozubski and Prusinski (1995) [55]
32	Dival 1,500–2,000/day Prop 180–240/day/Co	12 weeks × 2 (4 weeks wash-out)	Reduction of migraine frequency, assessment of migraine-days	Prop = Dival >> Pla-phase	No difference in rate of adverse events	Kaniecki (1997) [56]

Flu = Flunarizine; Nife = Nifedipine; Cycl = Cyclandelate; Tolf = Tolfenamic acid; Val = Sodium valproate; Dival = Divalproex; PMCS = post-marketing cohort study. For other abbreviations, see footnote Table 1.

following the initiation of medication. The prophylaxis, however, should be maintained for a minimum of 3 months, otherwise therapeutical success cannot be clearly evaluated. When successful it should be carried out for 9–12 months until the dose of β-blockers is slowly decreased (do not terminate abruptly since this may cause tachycardia or hypertension). The natural occurrence of migraine should then be assessed for 2–3 months.

Although β-blockers are the drugs of first choice in migraine prophylaxis it is very important to remember that prophylaxis can be most successful when adverse events are smartly used to treat other symptoms from which the patient suffers. Therefore it is crucial to know the typical adverse effects in detail and inquire about other symptoms or medical problems. β-blockers are most successful if the patient, in addition to migraine, also suffers from arterial hypertension, an anxiety disorder or tremor. Beta-blockers will not be accepted, however, from patients with pre-existing orthostatic hypotension, sleep disturbances or impotence. And again, in rare cases β-blockers might cause depression or worsen pre-existing depression.

Which β-blocker should be used for which patient? As described in the section of pharmacological properties, the differences within the β-blocker family are relatively small. Only a few trials have compared the different β-blockers, and did not find significant differences in efficacy (as long as those drugs were effective for this indication) or in their profile of adverse events. Taking all trials into account it seems to be more important to use a drug the physician is familiar with, especially in determining initial dosage and subsequent gradual increases in dosage.

References

1   Rabkin R, Stables DP, Levin NW, Suzman MM: Propranolol and prophylaxis of angina pectoris. Am J Cardiol 1966;18:370–380.
2   Anderson KE, Vinge E: β-Adrenoreceptor blockers and calcium antagonists in the prophylaxis of migraine. Drugs 1990;39:355–373.
3   Holroyd KA, Penzien DB, Cordingley GE: Propranolol in the management of recurrent migraine: A meta-analytic review. Headache 1991;31:333–340.
4   Tfelt-Hansen P, Shanks RG: β-Adrenoreceptor blocking drugs; in Olesen J, Tfelt-Hansen P, Welch KMA (eds): The Headaches. New York, Raven Press, 1993, pp 263–372.
5   Diener HC, Peatfield RC: Migraine; in Brandt T, Caplan LR, Dichgans J, Diener HC, Kennard C (eds): Neurological Disorders: Course and treatment. San Diego, Academic Press, 1996, pp 1–16.
6   Limmroth V, Kaube H, Diener HC: Management and Prevention of Migraine: A practical guide; in Mallarkey G (ed): Migraine in Perspective. Auckland, ADIS Books, 1999, pp 19–33.
7   Limmroth V, Cutrer FM, Moskowitz MA: The role of neurotransmitters and neuropeptides in headache. Curr Opin Neurol 1996;9:206–210.
8   Peatfield RC, Fozard JR, Rose CF: Drug treatment of migraine; in Clifford Rose F (ed): Handbook of Clinical Neurology, vol 4 (48): Headache. Amsterdam, Elsevier Science Publishers B.V., 1986, pp 173–217.

9   Stensrud P, Sjaastad O: Comparative trial of Tenormin (atenolol) and Inderal (propranolol) in migraine. Headache 1980;20:204–207.

10 Tfelt-Hansen P, Standnes B, Kangasniemi P, Hakkarainen H, Oleson J: Timolol vs. propranolol vs. placebo in common migraine prophylaxis: A double-blind multicenter trial. Acta Neurol Scand 1984;69:1–8.

11 Freitag FG, Diamond S: Nadolol and placebo comparison study in the prophylactic treatment of migraine. J Amer Osteopath Assoc 1984;84:343–347.

12 Wörz R, Reinhardt-Benmalek B, Grotemeyer K-H, Föh M: Bisoprolol and metoprolol in the prophylactic treatment of migraine with and without aura – A randomized double-blind cross over multicenter study. Cephalalgia 1991;11(suppl 11):152–153.

13 van de Ven LLM, Franke CL, Koehler PJ: Prophylactic treatment of migraine with bisoprolol: A placebo-controlled study. Cephalalgia 1997;17:596–599.

14 Headache Classification Committee of the International Headache Society. Classification and diagnostic criteria for headache disorders, cranial neuralgias and facial pain. Cephalalgia 1988;8(suppl 7): 1–93.

15 Ekbom K, Zetterman M: Oxprenolol in the treatment of migraine. Acta Neurol Scand 1977;56: 181–184.

16 Nanda RN, Johnson RH, Gray J, Keogh HJ, Melville ID: A double-blind trial of acebutol for migraine prophylaxis. Headache 1978;18:20–22.

17 Ekbom K: Alprenolol for migraine prophylaxis. Headache 1975;15:129–132.

18 Sjastad O, Stenrud P: Clinical trial of a beta-receptor blocking agent (LB46) in migraine prophylaxis. Acta Neurol Scand 1972;48:124–128.

19 Ekbom K, Lundberg PO: Clinical trial of LB-46 (d, 1-4(2-hydroxy-3-isopropylaminopropoxy) indol). An adrenergic betareceptor blocking agent in migraine prophylaxis. Headache 1972;12:15–17.

20 Holdorff B, Sinn M, Roth G: Propranolol in der Migräneprophylaxe. Med Klin 1977;72:1115–1118.

21 Stensrud P, Sjaastad O: Comparative trial of Tenormin (atenolol) and Inderal (propranolol) in migraine. Headache 1980;20:204–207.

22 al-Quassab HK, Findley LJ: Comparison of propranolol LA 80 mg and propranolol 160 mg in migraine prophylaxis: A placebo controlled study. Cephalalgia 1993;13:128–131.

23 Steiner TJ, Joseph R, Hedman C, Rose FC: Metoprolol in the prophylaxis of migraine: Parallel-groups comparison with placebo and dose-ranging follow-up. Headache 1988;28:15–23.

24 Diamond S, Medina JL: Double-blind study of propranolol for migraine prophylaxis. Headache 1982;22:268–271.

25 Nadelmann JW, Phil M, Stevens J, Saper JR: Propranolol in the prophylaxis of migraine. Headache 1986;26:175–182.

26 Kuritzky A, Hering R: Prophylactic treatment of migraine with long acting propranolol – A comparison with placebo. Cephalalgia 1987;7:457–458.

27 Pradalier A, Serratrice G, Collard M: Long-acting propranolol in migraine prophylaxis: Results of a double-blind, placebo-controlled study. Cephalalgia 1989;9:247–253.

28 Anderson PG, Dahl S, Hansen JH: Prophylactic treatment of classical and non-classical migraine with metoprolol – A comparison with placebo. Cephalalgia 1983;3:207–212.

29 Kangasneimi P, Hedman C: Metoprolol and propranolol in the prophylactic treatment of classical and common migraine: A double-blind study. Cephalalgia 1984;4:91–96.

30 Forssman B, Lindblad CJ, Zbornikova V: Atenolol for migraine prophylaxis. Headache 1983;23: 188–190.

31 Johannsson V, Nilsson LR, Widelius T: Atenolol in migraine prophylaxis: A double-blind cross-over multicenter study. Headache 1987;27:372–374.

32 Ryan RE Sr, Ryan RE Jr, Sudilovski A: Nadolol: Its use in the prophylactic treatment of migraine. Headache 1983;23:26–31.

33 Stellar S, Ahrens SP, Meibohm AR, Reines SA: Migraine prevention with timolol. JAMA 1984; 252:2576–2579.

34 Olsson JE, Behring HC, Forssman B: Metoprolol and propranolol in migraine prophylaxis: A double-blind multicenter study. Acta Neurol Scand 1984;70:160–168.

35 Ryan RE: Comparative study of nadolol and propranolol in prophylactic treatment of migraine. Am Heart J 1984;108:1156–1159.

36 Olerud B, Gustavsson CL, Furberg B: Nadolol and propranolol in migraine management. Headache 1986;26:490–493.

37 Sudlikovski A, Elkind AH, Ryan RE Sr, Saper JR, Stern MA, Meyer JH: Comparative efficacy of nadolol and propranolol in the management of migraine. Headache 1987;27:421–426.

38 Havanka-Kanniainen H, Hokkanan E, Myllylä VV: Long acting propranolol in the prophylaxis of migraine. Comparison of daily doses of 80 mg and 160 mg. Headache 1988;28:607–611.

39 Carroll JD, Reidy M, Savundra PA, Cleave N, McAinsh J: Long-acting propranolol in the prophylaxis of migraine: A comparative study of two doses. Cephalalgia 1990;10:101–105.

40 Wörz R, Reinhadt-Benmalek B, Föh M, Grotemeyer KH, Scharafinski HW: Prevention of migraine using bisoprolol. Results of a double-blind study versus metoprolol. Fortschr Med 1992;110:268–272.

41 Grotemeyer KH, Schlake HP, Husstedt IW: Migräneprophylaxe mit Metoprolol und Flunarizin –Eine doppelblind-crossover Studie. Nervenarzt 1988;59:549–552.

42 Ludin HP: Flunarizine and propranolol in the treatment of migraine. Headache 1989;29:218–223.

43 Shimell CJ, Fritz VU, Levien SL: A comparative trial of flunarizine and propranolol in the prevention of migraine. S Afr Med J 1990;77:75–77.

44 Lutschg J, Vassella F: The treatment of juvenile migraine using flunarizine or propranolol. Schweiz Med Wochenschr 1990;120:1731–1736.

45 Sorensen PS, Larsen BH, Rasmussen MJ, Klinge E, Iversen H, Alslev T, Nohr P, Pedersen KK, Schroder P, Lademann A, Olesen J: Flunarizine versus metoprolol in migraine prophylaxis: A double-blind, randomized parallel group study of efficacy and tolerability. Headache 1991;31:650–657.

46 Gawel MJ, Kreeft J, Nelson RF, Simard D, Arnott WS: Comparison of the efficacy and safety of flunarizine to propranolol in the prophylaxis of migraine. Can J Neurol Sci 1992;19:340–345.

47 Verspeelt J, De Locht P, Amery WK: Post-marketing cohort study comparing the safety and efficacy of flunarizine and propranolol in the prophylaxis of migraine. Cephalalgia 1996;16:328–336.

48 Bordini CA, Arruda MA, Ciciarelli MC, Speciali JG: Propranolol vs flunarizine vs flunarizine plus propranolol in migraine without aura prophylaxis. A double-blind trial. Arq Neuropsiquiatr 1997; 55:536–541.

49 Albers GW, Simon LT, Hamik A, Peroutka SJ: Nifedipine versus propranolol for the initial prophylaxis of migraine. Headache 1989;29:214–217.

50 Diener HC, Föh M, Iaccarino C, Wessely P, Isler H, Strenge H, Fischer M, Wedekind W, Taneri Z on behalf of the study group: Cyclandelate in the prophylaxis of migraine: A randomized, parallel, double-blind study in comparison with placebo and propranolol. Cephalalgia 1996;16:441–447.

51 Baldrati A, Cortelli P, Proccaccianti G, Gamberini G, D'Alessandro R, Baruzzi A, Sacquegna T: Propranolol and acetylsalicylic acid in migraine prophylaxis. A double-blind crossover study. Acta Neurol Scand 1983;67:181–186.

52 Grotemeyer KH, Scharafinski HW, Schlake HP, Husstedt IW: Acetylsalicylic acid vs metoprolol in migraine prophylaxis – A double-blind crossover study. Headache 1990;30:639–641

53 Diener HC, Hartung E, Chrubasik J: Acetylsalicylic acid in migraine prophylaxis: A double-blind study in comparison with metoprolol. Cephalalgia 1997;17:434.

54 Kjaersgard Rasmussen MJ, Holt Larsen B, Borg L, Soelberg Sorensen P, Hansen PE: Tolfenamic acid versus propranolol in prophylactic treatment of migraine. Acta Neurol Scand 1994;89:446–450.

55 Kozubski W, Prusinski A: Sodium valproate versus propranolol in the prophylactic treatment of migraine. Neurol Neurochir Pol 1995;29:937–947.

56 Kaniecki RG: A comparison of divalproex with propranolol and placebo for the prophylaxis of migraine without aura. Arch Neurol 1997;54:1141–1145.

Dr. Volker Limmroth, Department of Neurology, University of Essen,
Hufelandstr. 55, D–45122 Essen (Germany)
Tel. +49 201 723 2495, Fax +49 201 723 5901, E-Mail volker.limmroth@t-online.de

Diener HC (ed): Drug Treatment of Migraine and Other Headaches.
Monogr Clin Neurosci. Basel, Karger, 2000, vol 17, pp 269–278

....

Flunarizine for Migraine Prophylaxis

H.C. Diener

Department of Neurology, University Essen, Essen, Germany

Flunarizine has been used for migraine prophylaxis in many countries outside the USA for a long time. The mode of action is unknown, which is true also for most of the other agents used for migraine prophylaxis. Proposed modes of action include antihypoxic properties and the ability to enhance the threshold for cortical spreading depression [1]. The side effect pattern indicates that flunarizine has antidopaminergic [2], antiserotonergic and anti-histaminic [3] action [4]. Pharmacologically, flunarizine is a calcium channel blocker [4]. Originally it was developed for the treatment of dizziness [5]. Later on anti-epileptic properties were detected [6]. This indication was not pursued. This chapter reports most of the published studies performed with flunarizine as migraine prophylaxis starting with open studies, progressing to placebo-controlled trials and finally reporting trials with active comparators. Most studies were performed at times, when standards for the conduct of trials for migraine prophylaxis were not established. This explains in part the variation in outcome.

Open Trials

There were 12 open trials with patient numbers ranging from 20 to 176 (table 1). As could be expected from open trials, flunarizine was effective in all of the studies. Observation periods ranged from 3 to 12 months. All studies had different endpoints, which makes a meta-analytic approach impossible. Martinez-Lage [7] reported a 6-month study in 1,435 patients treated with 10 mg flunarizine at bedtime. 74.4% of the patients were females. After 6 months treatment was terminated, and patients were followed for another 6 months. The evaluation criteria was a rating scale based on frequency, duration,

Table 1. Open studies investigating flunarizine (10 mg dose) in the prophylaxis of migraine ranked according to number of patients recruited

No.	Type of migraine	Follow-up	Primary endpoint	Result for primary endpoint	Comments	Reference
1601	Migraine	8 months	Occurence of extrapyramidal symptoms (EPS) or depression	Two cases of EPS in the flunarizine group, 34 cases of depression with flunarizine and 24 with propranolol	Postmarketing study	[9]
1435	Migraine	6 months	Rating scale: frequency, duration and intensity of attacks	69.5% of patients reported a good or excellent result	Side effects: drowsiness and weight gain	[7]
838	Migraine	8 months	Severity of migraine attacks	Propranolol (n = 763) was somewhat better in reducing the severity of migraine attacks than flunarizine (n = 838)	Postmarketing study	[8]
176	Various types of headache	4 months	25% reduction in frequency, intensity and duration of pain attacks	Symptoms improved in 82% of cases	70 patients had migraine, improvement in 81%	[33]
147	Migraine	5 months	Migraine days/month	50% of patients had at least 50% reduction of migraine days	Reduction of migraine days from 7.8 to 3.6	[34]
137	Migraine	6 months	Number of migraine attacks per month	Baseline = 8.5 3 months = 5.2	Only published as abstract	[35]
120	Migraine with and without aura	3 months	Headache index	60 responders, 50 nonresponders, 10 drop-outs	Headache index not specified	[36]
120	Migraine with and without aura	24 months	Headache index	Responders = 87; responders after 9 months = 10; remaining improved after 24 months on treatment = 18/18	Side effects: drowsiness, weight gain, depression	[37]
108	Migraine with and without aura	3 months	Responders = > 75% reduction in migraine frequency	61 patients were responders	Predictors for responder = familiy history, high pain intensity	[10]

Diener

270

Table 1 (continued)

No.	Type of migraine	Follow-up	Primary endpoint	Result for primary endpoint	Comments	Reference
67	Migraine	12 months	Attack frequency, duration of headache	11 patients attack free, 49 patients improvement	Long-term trial	[38]
64	Migraine with and without aura	3 to 6 months	Efficacy of prophylaxis after discontinuation	16/64 had a long-term benefit after discontinuation	Part of patients used beta-blockers	[39]
40	Migraine	3 months	Side effects, plasma levels of flunarizine	Plasma levels did not correlate with dose (mg/kg), sedation correlates with plasma levels	No efficacy data given	[40]
40	Migraine	4 months	Headache index	31/40 patients had significant improvement	Small numbers	[41]
35	Migraine with and without aura	3 months	Complete elimination of headache	Achieved in 37% of patients	Numbers too small	[42]
25	Migraine with and without aura	6 months	Migraine frequency	Significant reduction	Comparison with nimodipine	[43]
20	Migraine with and without aura	2–6 months	Headache incidence	17/20 reduction in headache incidence	Numbers too small	[44]

intensity and characteristics of the attacks and a checklist of side effects. At the end of the six months a good or excellent result was observed in 69.5% of the patients. This treatment effect outlasted the actual time of drug intake. The most frequent side effects were drowsiness (20.1%) and weight gain (13.6%). The authors claim, that the incidence of these side effects decreased after the first month. This statement is in contrast to studies performed later reporting a continuous weight gain in a certain percentage of patients. It is most likely, that patients with severe side effects dropped out of the study.

Janssen, the producer of flunarizine, initiated a large postmarketing cohort study comparing the safety and efficacy of flunarizine and propranolol in the prophylaxis of migraine [8]. General practitioners in Belgium and the Netherlands recruited patients for whom they would prescribe either flunarizine or propranolol in the normal course of their treatment. Medical events were recorded on follow-up forms for up to 8 months. A total of 1,601 migraine patients were recruited, 838 in the flunarizine cohort and 763 in the propranolol group. Propranolol at a dose between 40 and 120 mg daily was somewhat better than flunarizine in reducing the severity of migraine attacks. The reduction in migraine frequency was comparable. Six percent of the patients receiving flunarizine and 4% of the patients taking propranolol discontinued treatment due to side effects. A total of 58 patients had depressive events, 34 in the flunarizine and 24 in the propranolol cohort. Predictors for a depressive episode were a prior history of depression and a high number of migraine attacks. Although the open design has many shortcomings, the high number of patients compensates for this at least partly. The advantage of this study is, that it mimics the everyday situation in the offices of doctors in private practice.

A second postmarketing study investigated the use of flunarizine in vestibular vertigo and migraine [9]. This study was performed in Germany, Belgium and The Netherlands. Two patients in the migraine population developed extrapyramidal symptoms which were reversible after discontinuation of flunarizine. Patients with migraine were more prone to depression than patients with vertigo, regardless of their treatment.

The study of Lucetti et al. [10] identified a positive family history of migraine and high pain intensity as predictors for a positive response to prophylaxis with flunarizine. D'Amato et al. observed a much higher success rate in patients with migraine with aura compared to migraine without aura [11]

In summary, the open studies indicated, that flunarizine may be effective in the prophylaxis of migraine. Major side effects are drowsiness and weight gain. Some patients may develop depression, in particular when a prior history of depression exists. This, however, also occurs with propranolol. The number of patients with extrapyramidal syndromes due to flunarizine is small.

Placebo-Controlled Studies

Eight studies were performed as placebo-controlled randomized trials (table 2). Four studies had more than 50 patients and reported a significant reduction in migraine frequency with flunarizine both in normal and pediatric migraine [12–15]. In pediatric migraine daily doses of 5 mg were used. Louis et al. [15] reported, that the duration and severity of attacks was not influenced by flunarizine. In summary, the placebo-controlled studies indicate, that flunarizine is superior to placebo in reducing migraine frequency.

Comparative Trials

Three trials compared pizotifen, a 5-HT$_2$-antagonist and flunarizine [16–18]. All studies found no difference between pizotifen and flunarizine in terms of reduction of migraine frequency. Pizotifen and flunarizine caused weight gain and fatigue. Spierings and Messinger [19] summarized six comparative studies comparing 2–3 mg pizotifen with 10 mg flunarizine. Neither a single study nor the pooled data showed a difference between the two drugs. More trials used the more established β-blockers propranolol and metoprolol as comparators (see table 3). Overall there was no significant difference between flunarizine and the β-blockers. Three studies had a good or reasonable study design [20–22]. The study of Ludin [20] found that propranolol furthermore significantly reduced the severity of migraine attacks and the number of analgesics used during the attacks. The largest trial was performed by Sorensen et al. [22]. They found no differences between 200 mg metoprolol and 10 mg flunarizine in terms of efficacy. Both drugs caused day time sedation and flunarizine weight gain. Depression was the most serious side effect occurring in 8% of patients on flunarizine and 3% on metoprolol. Lücking et al. [23] summarized two multicenter double-blind studies comparing propranolol and flunarizine. Eighty-seven patients were recruited in 12 headache centers and 434 patients came from 99 medical practices. There was no difference in terms of number, duration and severity of migraine attacks or analgesic consumption.

Studies comparing flunarizine with valproate [24], citalopram [25], etilefrine pivalate [26], cyclandelate [27] or cinnarizine [28] were too small to allow any conclusions. One study investigated flunarizine and methysergide in 104 patients [29]. Both drugs were equally effective and flunarizine achieved a significant reduction in the intensity of migraine attacks.

Two small studies in pediatric migraine investigated propranolol or acetylsalicyclic acid in comparison to flunarizine [30, 31]. Again all substances were equally effective.

Table 2. Double-blind placebo-controlled studies investigating flunarizine in the prophylaxis of migraine

No.	Type of migraine	Follow-up	Primary endpoint	Result for primary endpoint	Comments	Reference
101	Migraine with and without aura	20 weeks	Migraine frequency	Reduced migraine frequency	Secondary endpoints not significant	[12]
70	Pediatric migraine	8 months, crossover after 3 months	Migraine frequency and duration	Reduction in migraine frequency and duration	Flunarizine dose: 5 mg/day, side effects: sedation, weight gain	[13]
58	Migraine with and without aura	12 weeks	Migraine frequency	Reduced migraine frequency at months 1, 2 and 3	Published only as abstract	[14]
58	Migraine	12 weeks	Migraine frequency	Reduced in 21/29 with flunarizine and 9/29 with placebo	Duration and severity of attacks not influenced	[15]
48	Pediatric migraine	12 weeks	Headache frequency	Headache frequency reduced by 66%	Dose 5 mg/day	[45]
29	Migraine without aura	16 weeks	Frequency of migraine attacks	Significant reduction of migraine frequency	No influence on duration and severity of attacks	[46]
20	Migraine with aura	3–4 months	Migraine index	Migraine index reduced by 82% with flunarizine, increased by 66% with placebo	Few side effects	[47]
17	Migraine with and without aura	12 weeks	Migraine frequency	Reduction of migraine frequency from 3.3 to 1.4/months with flunarizine and 3.8 to 3.2/months with placebo	Side effect: weight gain, small numbers	[48]

Diener

Table 3. Studies with flunarizine (10 mg if not stated differently) and a comparator drug in migraine prophylaxis

No.	Comparative substance; study design	Follow-up	Primary endpoint	Result for primary endpoint	Comments	Reference
27	Pizotifen crossover	2 months	Not defined	No difference between flunarizine and pizotifen	Weight gain more frequent with pizotifen	[49]
35	Pizotifen parallel	4 months	Migraine frequency	Migraine frequency −65% for flunarizine and −45% for pizotifen	Most frequent side effect: weight gain	[16]
42	Pizotifen parallel	3 months	Migraine frequency	No difference between flunarizine and pizotifen	Both substances: weight gain and fatigue	[17]
75	Pizotifen parallel	4 months	Migraine frequency	No difference between pizotifen and flunarizine; flunarizine had effect on migraine severity	Side effects: weight gain similar	[18]
29	Metoprolol 200 mg crossover	2 × 2 months	Migraine frequency	Attack frequency −46% with metoprolol and −43% with flunarizine	Side effects: weight gain with flunarizine	[50]
45	Propranolol 60 mg parallel	120 days	Migraine index plus migraine frequency	Attack frequency on flunarizine 1.2, on propranolol 1.26	15 patients received a combination of both drugs; propranolol dose too low	[51]
58	Propranolol 3 × 60 mg parallel	4 months	Migraine frequency	No difference between propranolol and flunarizine	Side effects flunarizine: weight gain; propranolol: tiredness	[52]
71	Propranolol 3 × 40 mg parallel	4 months	Number of attacks; patient satisfaction	Both drugs resulted in a significant decrease in migraine frequency	Propranolol reduced severity of attacks	[20]
94	Propranolol 2 × 80 mg parallel	4 months	Migraine frequency	Both drugs decreased migraine frequency, flunarizine better in months 1 and 4	No effect on duration and severity of attacks	[21]
149	Metoprolol 200 mg parallel	16 weeks	Number of migraine days/month	Flunarizine −48%, metoprolol −39%, n.s.	Both drugs: daytime sedation, flunarizine: weight gain	[22]

Holroyd et al. published a meta-analysis of clinical trials with flunarizine or propranolol as an abstract [32]. They included data from 31 flunarizine trials and 32 propranol trials with about 3,000 treated patients. The modal propranolol dose was 160 mg/day and the modal dose of fluanrizine 10 mg/day. On average, the trials lasted 16 weeks. The mean improvement in migraine frequency (flunarizine –62%; propranolol –55%) was similar. Propranolol therapy was associated with more drop-outs (18%) compared to flunarizine (13%). The response to flunarizine and propranolol was negatively associated with the chronicity of the migraine disorder.

Finally one study aimed to identify predictive factors for a positive reponse for flunarizine in migraine prophylaxis [10]. Positive factors were a family history of migraine and a high pain intensity. Negative factors were frequent attacks and a history of analgesic abuse.

In summary, the available studies indicate that flunarizine is an effective drug for the prophylaxis of migraine. Most studies performed up to now are either too small or have an inadequate design. The drug deserves to be investigated in trials using a modern design and reasonable number of patients. Typical side effects of flunarizine are weight gain and sedation. The most serious adverse event is major depression. The most widely used dose of flunarizine is 10 mg.

References

1   Wauquier A, Ashton D, Marrannes R: The effects of flunarizine in experimental models related to the pathogenesis of migraine. Cephalalgia 1985;5(suppl 2):119–123.
2   Wöber C, Brücke T, Wöber-Bingöl C, Asenbaum S, Wessely P, Podreka I: Dopamine D2 receptor blockade and antimigraine action of flunarizine. Cephalalgia 1994;14:235–240.
3   Holmes B, Brogden RN, Heel RC, Speight TM, Avery GS: Flunarizine. A review of its pharmacodynamic and pharmakokinetic properties and therapeutic use. Drugs 1984;27:6–44.
4   Amery WK: Flunarizine, a calcium channel blocker: A new prophylactic drug in migraine. Headache 1982;23:70–74.
5   Wouters L, Amery W, Towse G: Flunarizine in the treatment of vertigo. J Laryngol Otol 1983;97: 697–704.
6   Overweg J, Binnie CD, Meijer JWA, Meinardi H, Nuijten STM, Schmaltz S, Wauquier A: Double-blind placebo-controlled trial of flunarizine as add-on therapy in epilepsy. Epilepsia 1984;25:217–222.
7   Martinez-Lage JM: Flunarizine (Sibelium) in the prophylaxis of migraine. An open, long-term, multicenter trial. Cephalalgia 1988;8:15–20.
8   Verspeelt J, De Locht P, Amery WK: Post-marketing cohort study comparing the safety and efficacy of flunarizine and propranolol in the prophylaxis of migraine. Cephalalgia 1996;16:328–336.
9   Verspeelt J, De Locht P, Amery WK: Postmarketing study of the use of flunarizine in vestibular vertigo and in migraine. Eur J Clin Pharmacol 1996;51:15–22.
10 Lucetti C, Nuti A, Pavese N, Gambaccini G, Rossi G, Bonuccelli U: Flunarizine in migraine prophylaxis: Predictive factors for a positive response. Cephalalgia 1998;18:349–352.
11 D'Amato CC, De Marco N, Pizza V: Migraine with and without aura as same or two different disorders: Clinical evidence and response to flunarizine. Headache Quarterly 1996;7:43–47.

12   Diamond S, Freitag FG: A double blind trial of flunarizine in migraine prophylaxis. Headache Quarterly Current Treatment and Research 1993;4:169–172.
13   Sorge F, De Simone R, Marano E, Nolano M, Orefice G, Carrieri P: Flunarizine in prophylaxis of childhood migraine – A double-blind, placebo-controlled, crossover study. Cephalalgia 1988;8:1–6.
14   Baker C: Double-blind evaluation of flunarizine and placebo in the prophylactic treatment of migraine. Headache 1987;27:288.
15   Louis P: A double-blind placebo-controlled prophylactic study of flunarizine (Sibelium®) in migraine. Headache 1981;21:235–239.
16   Rascol A, Montastruc JL, Rascol O: Flunarizine versus pizotifen: A double-blind study in the prophylaxis of migraine. Headache 1996;26:83–85.
17   Wörz R, Drillisch C: Migräne-Prophylaxe durch einen Kalziumeintrittsblocker. Ergebnisse einer Doppelblindstudie Flunarizin vs Pizotifen. Münch Med Wschr 1983;125:711–714.
18   Louis P, Spierings ELH: Comparison of flunarizine (Sibelium®) and pizotifen (Sandomigran®) in migraine treatment: A double-blind study. Cephalalgia 1982;2:197–203.
19   Spierings ELH, Messinger HB: Flunarizine vs. pizotifen in migraine prophylaxis: A review of comparative studies. Cephalalgia 1988;8:27–30.
20   Ludin H-P: Flunarizine and propranolol in the treatment of migraine. Headache 1989;29:218–223.
21   Gawel MJ, Kreeft J, Nelson RF, Simard D, Arnott WS: Comparison of the efficacy and safety of flunarizine to propranolol in the prophylaxis of migraine. Can J Neurol Sci 1992;19:340–345.
22   Sorensen PS, Larsen BH, Rasmussen MJK, Kinge E, Iversen H, Alslev T, Nohr P, Pedersen KK, Schroder P, Lademann A, Olesen J: Flunarizine versus metoprolol in migraine prophylaxis: A double-blind, randomized parallel group study of efficacy and tolerability. Headache 1991;31:650–657.
23   Lücking CH, Oestreich W, Schmidt R, Soyka D: Flunarizine vs. propranolol in the prophylaxis of migraine: Two double-blind comparative studies in more than 400 patients. Cephalalgia 1988;8: 21–26.
24   Mitsikostas DD, Polychronidis I: Valproate versus flunarizine in migraine prophylaxis: A randomized, double-open, clinical trial. Func Neurol 1997;12:267–276.
25   Colucci D'Amato C, Amato D, Alfano V, Giordano E, Marmolo T, Pizza V: Citalopram versus flunarizine in the preventive treatment of migraine. Cephalalgia 1997;17:439.
26   Grotemeyer K-H, Schlake H-P, Husstedt IW: Etilefrine pivalate vs. dihydroergotamin and flunarizine in prophylactic treatment of migraine in patients with low blood pressure – A randomized double-blind-study. Cephalalgia 1989;9:433–434.
27   Nappi G, Sandrini G, Savoini G, Cavallini A, de Rysky C, Micieli G: Comparative efficacy of cyclandelate versus flunarizine in the prophylactic treatment of migraine. Drugs 1987;33:103–109.
28   Drillisch C, Girke W: Ergebnisse der Behandlung von Migräne-Patienten mit Cinnarizin und Flunarizin. MedWelt 1980;51/52:1870–1872.
29   Steardo L, Marano E, Barone P, Denman DW, Monteleone P, Cardone G: Prophylaxis of migraine attacks with a calcium-channel blocker: Flunarizine versus methysergide. J Clin Pharmacol 1986; 26:524–528.
30   Lütschg J, Vassella F: Behandlung der kindlichen Migräne mit Flunarizin bzw. Propranolol. Schweiz Med Wschr 1990;120:1731–1736.
31   Pothmann R: Migräneprophylaxe mit Flunarizin und Azetylsalizylsäure – Eine Doppelblindstudie. Monatsschr Kinderheilkd 1987;135:646–649.
32   Holroyd KA, Penzien DB, Rokicki LA, Cordingley GE: Flunarizine vs propranolol: A meta-analysis of clinical trials. Headache 1992;32:256.
33   Nattero G, Savi L, De Lorenzo C: Flunarizine in the treatment of headache with or without neurological symptoms. Cephalalgia 1985;5(suppl 2):141–143.
34   Gawel M, Kreeft J, Simard D, Nelson R: Flunarizine in the treatment of migraine with and without aura. Can J Neurol Sci 1993;20(suppl 2):S54.
35   Browne K, Shuaib A, Lico S: Migraine prophylaxis with flunarizine: Effectiveness is significantly better at six months compared to three months. Can J Neurol Sci 1993;20(suppl 2):S54.
36   Manzoni GC, Bono G, Sacquegna T, Manna V, Lanfranchi M, Micieli G, Cortelli P, Agnoli A: Flunarizine in common migraine: Italian cooperative trial. I. Short-term results and responders' definition. Cephalalgia 1985;5(suppl 2):149–153.

37 Bono G, Manzoni GC, Martucci N, Baldrati A, Farina S, Cassabgi F, De Carolis P, Nappi G: Flunarizine in common migraine: Italian cooperative trial. II. Long-term follow-up. Cephalalgia 1985;5(suppl 2):155–158.

38 D'Amato C, D'Amato A, Alfano V, Giordani E, Marmo E: Flunarizine in long-term migraine prophylaxis: Clinical evidence. J Med 1990;21:201–207.

39 Wöber C, Wöber-Bingöl C, Koch G, Wessely P: Long-term results of migraine prophylaxis with flunarizine and beta-blockers. Cephalalgia 1991;11:251–256.

40 Albani F, Baldratti A, Cortelli P, Riva R, Baruzzi A: Flunarizine plasma concentrations and side effects in migraine patients. Headache 1990;30:369–370.

41 Micieli G, Sances G, Pacchetti C, Trucco M, Magri M, Piazza D: Flunarizine: A wide spectrum prophylactic for migraine headache. Int J Clin Pharm Res 1984;4:239–245.

42 Balkan S, Aktekin B, Önal Z: Efficacy of flunarizine in the prophylactic treatment of migraine. Gazi Medical Journal 1994;5:81–84.

43 Nuti A, Lucetti C, Pavese N, Dell' Agnello G, Rossi G, Bonuccelli U: Long-term follow-up after flunarizine or nimodipine discontinuation in migraine patients. Cephalalgia 1996;16:337–340.

44 Diamond S, Schenbaum H: Flunarizine, a calcium channel blocker, in the prophylactic treatment of migraine. Headache 1983;23:39–42.

45 Sorge F, Marano E: Flunarizine vs. placebo in childhood migraine. A double-blind study. Cephalalgia 1985;5(suppl 2):145–148.

46 Sorensen PS, Hansen K, Olesen J: A placebo-controlled, double-blind, cross-over trial of flunarizine in common migraine. Cephalalgia 1986;6:7–14.

47 Mentenopoulos G, Manafi T, Logothetis J, Bostantzopoulou S: Flunarizine in the prevention of classical migraine: A placebo-controlled evaluation. Cephalalgia 1985;5(suppl 2):135–140.

48 Frenken CWGM: Flunarizine, a new preventive approach to migraine. Clin Neurol Neurosurg 1984; 86:17–20.

49 Cerbo R, Casacchia M, Formisano R, Feliciani M, Cusimano G, Buzzi MG, Agnoli A: Flunarizine-pizotifen single-dose double-blind cross-over trial in migraine prophylaxis. Cephalalgia 1986;6: 15–18.

50 Grotemeyer K-H, Schlake H-P, Husstedt I-W: Migräneprophylaxe mit Metoprolol und Flunarizin. – Eine doppelblind-cross-over Studie. Nervenarzt 1988;59:549–552.

51 Bordini CA, Arruda MA, Ciciarelli MC, Speciali JG: Propranolol vs. flunarizine vs. flunarizine plus propranolol in migraine without aura prophylaxis. Arquivos de Neru-Psiquiatria 1997;55: 536–541.

52 Shimell CJ, Fritz VU, Levien SL: A comparative trial of flunarizine and propranolol in the prevention of migraine. S Afr Med J 1990;77:7–-78.

Prof. Dr. H.C. Diener, Neurologische Universitäts-Klinik,
Hufelandstrasse 55, D-45122 Essen (Germany)
Tel. +49 201 723 2460, Fax +49 201 723 5901, E-Mail h.diener@uni-essen.de

Diener HC (ed): Drug Treatment of Migraine and Other Headaches.
Monogr Clin Neurosci. Basel, Karger, 2000, vol 17, pp 279–287

....

5-HT Receptor Antagonists in Migraine Prophylaxis

Peer Tfelt-Hansen[a], Pramod R. Saxena[b]

[a] Department of Neurology, Glostrup Hospital, Glostrup, Denmark, and
[b] Department of Pharmacology, Dutch Migraine Research Group, Erasmus University Medical Centre Rotterdam 'EMCR', Rotterdam, The Netherlands

Antiserotonin drugs were the first group of effective agents available for migraine prophylaxis [1, 2]. Originally, these drugs were thought to act via antagonism at serotonin (5-hydroxytryptamine, 5-HT) 'D' receptors [3], which are now classified as $5\text{-}HT_2$ receptors [4]. That this is the case is, however, unlikely (see for extensive discussion [2]). Thus, several selective and potent $5\text{-}HT_2$ receptor antagonists, including ketanserin, ICI 169,369, sergolexole and mianserin, have only minor or no prophylactic effect in migraine [2, 5]. In addition, the antimigraine potency of the antiserotonin drugs does not correlate with their affinity at the $5\text{-}HT_2$ receptor subtypes [6]. For further discussion of possible mechanisms, see the discussions of the individual drugs.

The antiserotonin drugs reviewed in the following will be methysergide, pizotifen and lisuride. For controlled, clinical trials with the other $5\text{-}HT_2$ receptor antagonists ketanserin, ICI 169,369, sergolexole and mianserin, and the ineffective $5\text{-}HT_3$ receptor antagonist tropisetron, see [2].

Methysergide

Methysergide is a semisynthetic compound derived from the ergot alkaloid methylergometrine by adding a methyl group. It was introduced in pharmacotherapy as a specific 5-HT receptor antagonist [1, 7].

During the first years of clinical use of methysergide it became evident that continuous use of the drug for longer periods can induce retroperitoneal, pleural and heart valve fibrosis with an estimated incidence of 1 in 5,000 treated patients [8, 9]. In most cases the fibrotic process regressed after discontinuation of methysergide [9]. The metabolism of methysergide was unchanged in patients who had developed this side effect [10] and its mechanisms remain elusive. This side effect of methysergide limits its clinical use.

Pharmacokinetics

Pharmacokinetic studies in man indicate that methysergide is probably a 'prodrug'; its main metabolite is methylergometrine [11]. After oral administration, the bioavailability of methysergide was about 13%, most likely due to a high degree of first-pass metabolic conversion to methylergometrine [11]. Oral administration of methysergide resulted in an area under the plasma concentration curve (AUC) that was 10 times greater for methylergometrine than for the parent drug. In contrast, after i.v. administration of methysergide the AUC for methysergide and methylergometrine was in the same range. The elimination half-lives of methysergide and methylergometrine were 60 min and 220 min, respectively. Thus, most of orally administered methysergide, synthesized from methylergometrine, is demethylated back to methylergometrine during the first-pass metabolism in the liver.

In contrast to methysergide, methylergometrine has dopaminergic activity [12]. The metabolism of methysergide to methylergometrine probably explains that methysergide has little dopaminergic activity upon parenteral administration [12], but its oral administration can result in a significant decrease in plasma prolactin level [13]. Thus, when the 'pure' 5-HT ligand methysergide is used orally in man, there are serotonergic effects due both to the parent drug and the metabolite methylergometrine (vide infra) as well as some dopaminergic effects due to the metabolite, methylergometrine.

Pharmacological Background

It is well known that methysergide is a potent $5-HT_2$ receptor antagonist, but it does not distinguish between the $5-HT_{2A}$, $5-HT_{2B}$ and $5-HT_{2C}$ subtypes, see [4]. Thus, methysergide antagonises the contractile effects of 5-HT on vascular and non-vascular smooth muscles with a pA_2 of more than 8 [14]. Indeed, in the human isolated temporal artery, which contains predominantly $5-HT_2$ receptors [15], both methysergide and its active metabolite methylergometrine are potent antagonists; the latter compound is some 40 times more active than the parent drug [16]. In addition, methysergide is an agonist at the 'atypical 5-HT' receptor in the carotid vascular bed [17] and selectively decreased carotid blood flow [18] by constricting arteriovenous anastomoses [17]. This atypical 5-HT receptor was later named the $5-HT_1$-like receptor [19]. Although this effect of methysergide is much less marked than that of ergotamine or sumatriptan [20–22], its mediation by novel $5-HT_1$-like receptors provided incentive for the development of sumatriptan, which at the time of its introduction, was regarded as a selective 5-HT$_1$-like receptor agonist [23].

The term '5-HT$_1$-like receptor' is now redundant as the composition of this heterogeneous group has been delineated [24]. This group comprises of the sumatriptan-insensitive 5-HT$_7$ receptor, which mediates tachycardia in cats and vasorelaxation [25–27] as well as sumatriptan-sensitive 5-HT$_{1B}$, 5-HT$_{1D}$ and, in some tissues, even 5-HT$_{1F}$ receptors. Methysergide is a potent antagonist at the 5-HT$_7$ (and 5-HT$_2$) receptor and an agonist at 5-HT$_{1B}$ and, possibly, also 5-HT$_{1D}$ receptors. In vitro functional and radioligand studies confirm that methysergide acts on 5-HT$_{1B}$ receptors. Thus, methysergide contracts canine, bovine and human cerebral arteries [28, 29] and the methysergide-induced contraction of dog isolated saphenous vein is antagonized by the non-selective 5-HT$_1$ and 5-HT$_2$ receptor antagonist methiothepin, but not by the 5-HT$_2$ receptor antagonist ketanserin [23].

The pharmacology of the metabolite, methylergometrine, has been less investigated. However, it is a more potent vasoconstrictor than methysergide both in vivo [30] and in vitro on e.g. canine saphenous vein and human basilar [29] and coronary [31] arteries.

Lastly, chronic but not acute treatment with methysergide has been reported to attenuate dural plasma extravasation following electric stimulation of trigeminal ganglion in the rat [32]. The discrepancy between the effect of acute and chronic treatment with methysergide in this model is most likely due to the presence of methylergometrine during chronic administration of methysergide.

Possible Mechanism of Antimigraine Action

The mechanism of action of methysergide in migraine is not well understood. The efficacy of methysergide has been ascribed to its 5-HT$_2$ receptor antagonist property. This is unlikely since potent 5-HT$_2$ receptor antagonists such as mianserin, sergolexole, ketanserin and ICI 169,369 seem to be without any prophylactic effect in migraine and for cyproheptadine the claimed efficacy [14] has never been confirmed in controlled clinical trials. Therefore, it is highly improbable that 5-HT$_2$ receptor antagonism plays any role in migraine prophylaxis [2, 5]. Inhibition of peptide release from perivascular sensory nerve endings as well as neurogenic inflammation by methysergide, as demonstrated in the rat, has also been invoked as a mechanism of action in migraine [32]. However, as argued elsewhere [33], there is considerable doubt whether inhibition of neurogenic inflammation in experimental animals is connected with antimigraine efficacy, as several such compounds were found clinically ineffective in migraine.

We believe that the vasoconstrictor action of methysergide, and of the metabolite methylergometrine, within the carotid vascular bed [17, 34] is somehow involved in the therapeutic activity. Theoretically, the dopaminergic effect of methylergometrine [12] may also be involved in the prophylactic effect.

Results of Randomized, Controlled, Clinical Trials

Methysergide has been compared with placebo or another drug in nine double-blind randomized clinical trials [35–43]. The daily dosage of methysergide varied from 3 to 6 mg, and in most trials a mixed migraine population (with or without aura) was studied. In two trials methysergide was superior to placebo for either severe headaches [42] or frequency of attacks [39], but in one trial methysergide was not superior to placebo [40]. In four trials [35, 37, 40, 41] methysergide was found comparable to pizotifen. Methysergide was also found comparable to lisuride (25 μg tid) [38], propranolol (40 mg tid) [36] and flunarizine (10 mg daily) [43].

The side effects reported in these trials were dizziness, nausea/vomiting, weight gain, abdominal pain, psychic reactions, and peripheral oedema. Though in some trials only few patients stopped treatment with methysergide because of side effects [36, 37, 40, 41, 43], in others discontinuation of therapy was more frequent: 5% [35], 7% [39], 20% [38] or 26% [42]. The higher drop-out rates of 20% [38] and 26% [42] occurred with a daily dosage of 6 mg methysergide, but apparently this dosage was tolerated in other studies [37, 43]. There was thus no clear-cut dose-response relationship for the side effects of methysergide.

Being the first drug introduced for migraine prophylaxis methysergide has not been evaluated in randomized trials with current methodology [44]. However, taken together, the controlled trials with methysergide show that the drug is efficacious in migraine prophylaxis. The problems with side effects are also demonstrated for this potent drug.

Pizotifen

Pizotifen was introduced in migraine prophylaxis as an antaminic drug based on the idea that not only 5-HT but also other biogenic amines might be involved in migraine [45]. In controlled trials the drug has been more effective than placebo. Its general use is hampered by its main side effects, weight gain and sedation.

Pharmacological Background

Pizotifen is a potent 5-HT_2 receptor antagonist with a pA_2 value of around 9.2 [14, 46]. Pizotifen also has antihistaminic and weak anticholinergic actions and, in some animals, sedative and antidepressant properties [47]. The antidepressant property has been confirmed in man [48]. Furthermore, in both dogs [49] and in man [50], a modest venoconstrictor activity of pizotifen has been demonstrated. It has been suggested that pizotifen should act as a calcium channel blocker [51], but this is unlikely in the concentrations in plasma reached with therapeutic doses in man [49]. In our opinion, the diversity of pharmacological properties of pizotifen precludes a meaningful hypothesis concerning its efficacy in migraine.

Pharmacokinetics

The pharmacokinetics of pizotifen has only been studied with [^{3}H]-labelled drug [52], thus measured concentrations in plasma (total radioactivity) include both parent drug and metabolites. The study indicated maximal therapeutic plasma levels of pizotifen of 9 ng/ml and an extensive metabolism of the drug with less than 1% being excreted unchanged in the urine [52].

Results of Randomized, Controlled, Clinical Trials

In a total of 20 randomized double-blind controlled clinical trials, pizotifen has been compared with placebo in seven trials [53–59] or with other drugs in 13 trials [35, 37, 40, 41, 60–68]. The daily dosage of pizotifen was 1.5 mg to 3 mg.

Pizotifen was superior to placebo for frequency of attacks or headache index in four trials [53, 57, 59, 62] and comparable to placebo for frequency but superior to placebo for severity of headaches in one trial [55]. In two trials with low power to detect a difference, no significant difference was found between pizotifen and placebo [54, 56], and another trial [58] indicated that pizotifen was inferior to placebo, probably due to unsuccessful randomization.

In the comparative trials with methysergide, pizotifen was found to be as efficacious as methysergide [35, 37, 40], and in one trial without any statistics, pizotifen was reported to be superior to methysergide [41]. In four trials pizotifen was found comparable to flunarizine [63–66] and comparable to nimodipine in two trials [67, 68]. Pizotifen was found comparable to prochlor-perazine in one trial [60] and better than [62] or comparable to [61] 1-isopropyl-noradrenochrome-5-monosemicarbazono. In addition, one study indicated that pizotifen 1.5 mg nocte was as effective as 0.5 mg three times daily [69].

The side effects in these controlled trials included drowsiness, increased appetite and weight gain. Thus in one placebo-controlled trial with pizotifen 3 mg per day in 30 patients, the drug induced drowsiness in 15, increased appetite in 12 and weight gain in 24 (>1.5 kg in 21 and >4 kg in three) of the patients; the numbers of patients with these side effects with placebo were 4, 3 and 2, respectively [62]. Drowsiness, however, often diminished with time [62].

In conclusion, the controlled clinical trials demonstrate efficacy of pizotifen in migraine prophylaxis, but side effects, especially weight gain, are frequent and limit the use of the drug.

Lisuride

After its synthesis in 1959, the ergot alkaloid derivative lisuride was first developed as a peripheral 5-HT receptor antagonist, and its similarity to methysergide led to its clinical use in migraine prophylaxis [70]. Later, lisuride's dopaminergic effect was established, and it is now also used in higher doses in the treatment of Parkinson's disease.

Lisuride is a dopamine (D_2) receptor agonist [46], but also has a potent antagonist action at the 5-HT$_2$ [14] as well as 5-HT$_7$ [25]. In addition, lisuride may act as an agonist on CNS 5-HT receptors [70]. The mode of action of lisuride in migraine prophylaxis remains elusive, but the doses used in migraine are probably without any dopaminergic effect [70].

Results of Randomized, Controlled, Clinical Trials

In two double-blind placebo-controlled trials with parallel group design lisuride (0.025 mg tid) was reported to be superior to placebo [71, 72]. In these trials a total of 390 patients were recruited. In both trials [71, 72] patients with up to 21–30 attacks per month were included, making the diagnosis of migraine, which is only defined in one of the trials [72], dubious at least in some patients. In a double-blind trial lisuride (0.025 mg tid) was found comparable with methysergide (2 mg tid) in 253 patients [71]. In this study 11 patients with cluster headache were included and 40% of patients had more than 10 attacks per month making it unlikely that only migraine attacks were treated. In one trial there was no difference between lisuride in doses of 0.025 mg tid and 0.05 mg tid [73].

In conclusion, the controlled clinical trials suggest that lisuride has some efficacy in migraine prophylaxis, but the selection of patients with uncertain diagnosis of migraine for these trials prevents a definitive statement.

References

1   Sicuteri F: Prophylactic and therapeutic properties of 1-methyllysergic acid butanolamide in migraine. Int Arch Allergy 1959;15:300–307.
2   Tfelt-Hansen P, Saxena PR: Antiserotonin drugs in migraine prophylaxis; in Olesen J, Tfelt-Hansen P, Welch KMA (eds): The Headaches, ed 2. New York, Lippincott, Williams & Wilkins (in press).
3   Gaddum JH, Picarelli ZP: Two kinds of tryptamine receptors. Br J Pharmacol 1957;12:323–328.

4   Hoyer D, Clarke DE, Fozard JR, Hartig PR, Martin GR, Mylecharane EJ, Saxena PR, Humphrey PP: International Union of Pharmacology classification of receptors for 5-hydroxytryptamine (serotonin). Pharmacol Rev 1994;46:157–203.

5   Saxena PR, Den Boer MO: Drug therapy of migraine. J Neurol 1991;238(suppl 1):S28–S35.

6   Silberstein SD. Methysergide. Cephalalgia 1998;18:421–435.

7   Fanchamps A, Doepfner W, Weidman H, Cerletti A: Pharmakologische Charakterisierung von Deseril, einem Serotonin-Antagonisten. Schweiz Med Wschr 1960;51:1040–1046.

8   Graham JR, Suby HI, LeCompte PR, Sadowsky NL: Fibrotic disorders associated with methysergide therapy for headache. N Engl J Med 1966;274:360–368.

9   Graham JR: Cardiac and pulmonary fibrosis during methysergide therapy for headache. Am J Med Sci 1967;254:1–12.

10   Bianchine JR, Friedman AP: Metabolism of methysergide and retroperitonal fibrosis. Arch Intern Med 1970;126:252–254.

11   Bredberg U, Eyjolfdottir GS, Paalzow L, Tfelt-Hansen P, Tfelt-HV: Pharmacokinetics of methysergide and its metabolite methylergometrine in man. Eur J Clin Pharmacol 1986;30:75–77.

12   Berde B, Stürmer E: Introduction to the pharmacology of ergot alkaloids and related compounds as a basis of their therapeutic application; in Berde B, Schild HO (eds): Ergot Alkaloids and Related Compounds, Handbook of Experimental Pharmacology. Berlin, Springer-Verlag, 1978, vol 49, pp 1–28.

13   Flückiger E, del Pozo E: Influence on the endocrine system; in Berde B, Schild HO (eds): Ergot Alkaloids and Related Compound, Handbook of Experimental Pharmacology. Berlin, Springer-Verlag, 1978, vol 49, pp 615–690.

14   Mylechrane EJ: 5-HT2 receptor antagonists and migraine therapy. J Neurol 1991;238(suppl 1):S45–S52.

15   Edvinsson L, Jansen I, Olesen J: Characterization of human craniovascular 5-hydroxytryptamine receptors; in Olesen J, Saxena PR (eds): 5-Hydroxytryptamine Mechanisms in Primary Headaches. New York, Ravens Press, 1992, pp 129–136.

16   Tfelt-Hansen P, Jansen I, Edvinsson L: Methylergometrine antagonizes 5-HT in the temporal artery. Eur J Clin Pharmacol 1987;33:77–79.

17   Saxena PR, Verdouw PD: Effects of methysergide and 5-hydroxytryptamine on carotid blood flow distribution in pigs: Further evidence for the presence of atypical 5-HT receptors. Br J Pharmacol 1984;82:817–826.

18   Saxena PR, De Vlaam-Schluter GM: Role of some biogenic substances in migraine and relevant mechanism in antimigraine action of ergotamine-studies in an experimental model for migraine. Headache 1974;13:142–163.

19   Saxena PR, Ferrari MD: From serotonin receptor classification to the antimigraine drug sumatriptan. Cephalalgia 1992;12:187–196.

20   De Vries P, Willems EW, Heiligers JPC, Villalón CM, Saxena PR: Constriction of porcine carotid arteriovenous anastomoses as indicator of antimigraine activity: The role of 5-HT$_{1B/1D}$, as well as unidentified receptors; in Edvinsson L (ed): Migraine & Headache Pathophysiology. London, Martin Dunitz Ltd, 1999, pp 119–132.

21   Den Boer MO, Villalón CM, Heiligers JPC, Humphrey PPA, Saxena PR: Carotid vascular effects of ergotamine and dihydroergotamine in the pig: No exclusive mediation via 5-HT1-like receptors. Br J Pharmacol 1991a;104:183–189.

22   Den Boer MO, Villalón CM, Heiligers JPC, Humphrey PPA, Saxena PR: The role of 5-HT1-like receptors in the reduction of porcine cranial arteriovenous anastomotic shunting by sumatriptan. Br J Pharmacol 1991b;102:323–330.

23   Humphrey PPA, Apperley E, Feniuk W, Perren MJ: A rational approach to identifying a fundamentally new drug for the treatment of migraine; in Saxena PR, Wallis DI, Wouters W, Bevan P (eds): Cardiovascular Pharmacology of 5-Hydroxytryptamine: Prospective Therapeutic Applications. Dordrecht, Kluwer Academic Publishers, 1990, pp 416–431.

24   Saxena PR, De Vries P, Villalón CM: 5-HT$_1$-like receptors: A time to bid goodbye. Trends Pharmacol Sci 1998;19:311–316.

25   De Vries P, Villalón CM, Heiligers JP, Saxena PR. Nature of 5-HT$_1$-like receptors mediating depressor responses in vagosympathectomized rats: Close resemblance to the cloned 5-ht7 receptor. Naunyn Schmiedebergs Arch Pharmacol 1997;356:90–99.

26   Eglen RM, Jasper JR, Chang DA, Martin GR: The 5-HT$_7$ receptor: Orphan found. Trends Pharmacol Sci 1997;18:104–107.

27   Villalón CM, De Vries P, Rabelo G, Centurión D, Sánchez-López A, Saxena PR: Canine external carotid vasoconstriction to methysergide, ergotamine and dihydroergotamine: Role of 5-HT$_{1B/1D}$ receptors and α_2-adrenoceptors. Br J Pharmacol 1998;126:585–594.

28   Müller-Schweinitzer E: Serotonergic receptors in brain vessels; in Owman C, Hardebo JE (eds): Neural Regulation of Brain Circulation. Amsterdam, Elsevier, 1986, pp 219–234.

29   Müller-Schweinitzer E: Ergot alkaloids in migraine: Is the effect via 5-HT receptors? in Olesen J, Saxena PR (eds): 5-Hydroxytryptamine Mechanisms in Primary Headaches. New York, Ravens Press, 1992, pp 297–304.

30   MacLennan SJ, Martin GR: Comparison of the effects of methysergide and methylergometrine with GR43175 on feline carotid blood flow distribution. Br J Pharmacol 1990;99:221P.

31   Maassen Van Den Brink A, Reekers M, Bax WA, Ferrari MD, Saxena PR: Coronary side-effect potential of current and prospective antimigraine drugs. Circulation 1998;98:25–30.

32   Saito K, Markowitz S, Moskowitz MA: Ergot alkaloids block neurogenic extravasation in dura mater: Proposed action in vascular headaches. Ann Neurol 1988;27:732–737.

33   De Vries P, Villalón CM, Saxena PR: Pharmacological aspects of experimental headache models in relation to acute antimigraine therapy. Eur J Pharmacol 1999;375:61–74.

34   Saxena PR: Selective carotid vasoconstriction in carotid vascular bed by methysergide: Possible relevance to its antimigraine effect. Eur J Pharmacol 1974;27:99–105.

35   Andersson PG: BC-105 and deseril in migraine prophylaxis: A double-blind study. Headache 1973; 13:68–73.

36   Behan PO, Reid M: Propranolol in the treatment of migraine. Practitioner 1980;224:201–204.

37   Forssman B, Henriksson K-G, Kihlstrand S: A comparison between BC 105 and methysergide in the prophylaxis of migraine. Acta Neurol Scand 1972;48:204–212.

38   Herrmann WM, Horowski R, Dannehl K, Kramer U, Lurati K: Clinical effectiveness of lisuride hydrogen maleate: A double-blind trial versus methysergide. Headache 1977;17:54–60.

39   Pedersen E, Møller CE: Methysergide in migraine prophylaxis. Clin Pharmacol Ther 1966;7:520–526.

40   Presthus J: BC 105 and methysergide (Deseril) in migraine prophylaxis. Acta Neurol Scand 1971; 47:514–518.

41   Ryan RE: Double-blind crossover comparison of BC-105 methysergide and placebo in the prophylaxis of migraine. Headache 1968;8:118–126.

42   Southwell N, Williams JD, Mackenzie I: Methysergide in the prophylaxis of migraine. Lancet 1964; 1:523–524.

43   Steardo L, Marano E, Barone P, Denman DW, Monteleone P, Cardone G: Prophylaxis of migraine attacks with a calcium-channel blocker: Flunarizine versus methysergide. J Clin Pharmacol 1986; 26:524–528.

44   International Headache Society Committee on Clinical Trials in Migraine: Guidelines for controlled trials of drugs in migraine, ed 1. Cephalalgia 1991;11:1–12.

45   Sicuteri F, Franchi G , del Bianco PL: An antiaminic drug, BC 105, in the prophylaxis of migraine. Int Arch Allergy 1967;31:78–93.

46   Peroutka SJ: Drugs effective in the therapy of migraine; in Hardman JG, Limbird LE, Molinoff PB, Ruddon RW, Gilman AG (eds): Goodman and Gilman's: The Pharmacological Basis of Therapeutics, ed 9. New York, The Macmillan Company, 1996, pp 487–502.

47   Speight TM, Avery GS: Pizotifen (BC-105): A review of its pharmacological properties and its therapeutic efficacy in vascular headaches. Drugs 1972;3:159–203.

48   Standal JE: Pizotifen as an antidepressant. Acta Psychiatr Scand 1977;56:276–279.

49   Müller-Schweinitzer E: Pizotifen, an antimigraine drug with venococonstrictor activity in vivo. J Cardiovasc Pharmacol 1986;8:805–810.

50   Aellig WH: Influence of pizotifen on the vasoconstrictor effect of 5-hydroxytryptamine and noradrenaline in man. Eur J Clin Pharmacol 1983;25:795–762.

51   Peroutka SJ, Banghart SB, Allen GS: Calcium channel antagonism of pizotifen. J Neurol Neurosurg Psychiat 1985;48:381–383.

52   Meier J, Schreier E: Human levels of some anti-migraine drugs. Headache 1976;16:96–104.

53 Arthur GP, Hornabrook RW: The treatment of migraine with BC 105 (pizotifen): A double blind trial. N Z Med J 1971;73:5–9.

54 Carrol JD, Maclay WP: Pizotifen (BC-105) in migraine prophylaxis. Curr Med Res Opin 1975;3: 68–71.

55 Hughes RC, Foster JB: BC 105 in the prophylaxis of migraine. Curr Ther Res 1971;13:63–68.

56 Lance JW, Anthony M: Clinical trial of a new serotonin receptor antagonist, BC 105, in the prevention of migraine. Med J Austral 1968;1:54–55.

57 Lawrence ER, Hossain M, Littlestone W: Sandomigran for migraine prophylaxis: Controlled multi-center trial in general practice. Headache 1977;17:112.

58 Ryan RE: BC-105 a new preparation for the interval treatment of migraine – A double-blind evaluation compared with placebo. Headache 1971;11:6–18.

59 Cleland PG, Barnes D, Elrington GM, Loizou LA, Rawes GD: Studies to assess if pizotifen prophylaxis improves migraine beyond the benefit offered by acute sumatriptan therapy alone. Eur Neurol 1997;38:31–38.

60 Hübbe P: The prophylactic treatment of migraine with an antiserotonin pizotifen (BC 105). Acta Neurol Scand 1973;49:108–114.

61 Kangasneimi P: Placebo, l-isopropylnoradrenochrome-5-monosemicarbazono and pizotifen in migraine prophylaxis. Headache 1979;19:219–222.

62 Osterman PO: A comparison between placebo, pizotifen and 1-isopropyl-3-hydroxy-5-semicarbaz-ono-6-oxo-2,3,5,6-tetrahydroindol (Divascan®) in migraine prophylaxis. Acta Neurol Scand 1977; 56:17–28.

63 Cerbo R, Casacchia M, Formisano R, Feliciani M, Cusimano G, BuzziMG, Agnoli A: Flunarizine-pizotifen single-dose double-blind cross-over trial in migraine prophylaxis. Cephalalgia 1986;6: 15–18.

64 Louis P, Spierings ELH: Comparison of flunarizine and pizotifen in migraine treatment: A double-blind study. Cephalalgia 1982;2:197–203.

65 Rascol A, Montastruc J-L, Rascol O: Flunarizine versus pizotifen: A double-blind study in the prophylaxis of migraine. Headache 1986;26:83–85.

66 Wörz R, Drillisch C: Migräne-Prophylaxe durch einen Kalziumeintrittsblocker. Ergebnisse einer Doppelblindstudie Flunarizin vs. Pizotifen. Münch Med Wschr 1983;125:711–714.

67 Havanka-Kanniainen H, Hokkanen E, Myllylä VV: Efficacy of nimodipine in comparison with pizotifen in the prophylaxis of migraine. Cephalalgia 1987;7:7–13.

68 Micieli G, Trucco M, Agostinis C, Mancuso A, Papalia F, Sinforiani E: Nimodipine vs pizotifen in common migraine: Results of a double-blind cross-over trial. Cephalalgia 1985;5(suppl 3):532–533.

69 Capildeo R, Clifford Rose F: Single-dose pizotifen, 1.5 mg nocte: A new approach in the prophylaxis of migraine. Headache 1982;22:272–275.

70 Horowski R: Some aspects of the dopaminergic action of ergot derivatives and their role in the treatment of migraine. Adv Neurol 1982;33:325–334.

71 Herrmann WM, Kristof M, Sastre y Hernandez M: Preventive treatment of migraine headache with a new isoergonyl derivative. J Int Med Res 1978;6:476–482.

72 Sommerville BW, Herrmann WM: Migraine prophylaxis with lisuride hydrogen maleate – A double-blind study of lisuride versus placebo. Headache 1978;18:75–79.

73 Wilkinson M, Agnoli A, Gerber WD, Grotemeyer KH, Langor HD, Runge I: Multicentre migraine study. Cuvalit® (lisuride 0.025 mg) vs. lisuride 0.05 mg tds. Cephalalgia 1989;9(suppl 10):353–354.

P. Tfelt-Hansen, Department of Neurology, Glostrup Hospital, DK-2600 Glostrup (Denmark)
Tel. +45 43 23 30 50, Fax +45 43 23 39 26, E-Mail tfelt@inet.uni2.dk

Diener HC (ed): Drug Treatment of Migraine and Other Headaches.
Monogr Clin Neurosci. Basel, Karger, 2000, vol 17, pp 288–298

....

Anticonvulsants in Migraine Prophylaxis

Ninan T. Mathew[a], *Steven D. Silberstein*[b]

[a] Houston Headache Clinic, Houston, Tex., USA
[b] Jefferson Headache Center, Thomas Jefferson University, Philadelphia, Pa., USA

In the central nervous system, a balance usually exists between GABAergic inhibition and amino acid-mediated excitation. However, disinhibition due to decreased GABAergic activity may occur in migraineurs, resulting in central neuronal hyperexcitability similar to what occurs in epilepsy. GABA is highly concentrated in the visual cortex and the periaqueductal area of the brainstem, areas intimately connected with migraine pathophysiology. $GABA_A$ receptor subunits are expressed in cerebral blood vessels [1].

Valproate in Migraine Prophylaxis

Valproic acid derivatives, namely sodium valproate and divalproex sodium are migraine preventive drugs. The term valproate will be used in this chapter to include sodium valproate and divalproex sodium. Valproate's central action includes elevation of brain GABA levels, reduction in the firing rates of serotonergic cells in the dorsal raphae nuclei [2] and reduction of central trigeminal activation (as evidenced by reduced C-Fos activation in the trigeminal nucleus caudalis) [3]. Its peripheral effect (outside the brain) includes reduction of experimental neurogenic inflammation in the trigeminal vascular system, which is mediated by $GABA_A$ receptor agonism [4].

Initial Published Open Trials

In 1988, Sorenson conducted an open trial involving 18 patients who received valproate for migraine prophylaxis [5]. Eleven patients became headache-free. Six patients experienced reduction in headache frequency.

In 1991, Viswanathan et al. [6] conducted an open study on 16 patients who had resistant migraine and paroxysmal EEG changes. The patients were treated with sodium valproate, 200 mg three times a day as an add-on medication. After 2 weeks, 12 patients were headache-free and the rest had 50% relief. The drug was continued for 3 months in the totally headache-free patients, while the other four patients increased their dose to 800–1,000 mg a day. Two of these dropped out, and the other two had complete relief.

Moore [7], in 1992, reported a retrospective analysis of 207 patients with refractory headache who were treated with valproate 750–2,000 mg a day. Patients with either migraine (n = 125) or chronic daily headache (CDH) (n = 82) were treated with the drug. Sixty-five percent of patients with migraine without aura and 50% of patients with migraine with aura had a good or excellent response (criteria not defined). Patients with mixed headache had a 52% response, while those with chronic tension-type headache (CTTH) had a 73% response. The average duration of treatment was 246 days.

Controlled Clinical Trails

Hering and Kuritzky [8] subsequently demonstrated superiority of valproate over placebo in a double-blind randomized, crossover study involving 32 patients with migraine. Four patients with migraine with aura and 25 with migraine without aura were included. During the active treatment phase, patients received valproate, 400 mg twice daily, for a period of 8 weeks. Twenty-five of 29 patients (86%) had a positive response. Three patients stopped their participation prematurely (one during active therapy and two while on placebo) and were not included in the final outcome analysis. Valproate reduced migraine attack frequency from 15.6 to 8.8. It also reduced the severity and duration of the attacks. No obvious correlation between valproate and blood levels and clinical response were noted. Valproate was generally well tolerated. One patient discontinued the treatment prematurely during the active phase because of side effects.

Jensen et al. [9] included 43 patients with migraine without aura in a triple-blind, placebo- and dose-controlled crossover study of prophylactic effect of slow release sodium valproate. Thirty-four patients completed the trial. Average number of days with migraine was 3.5 days per 4-week period during treatment with valproate and 6.1 during placebo (p = 0.002). The severity and duration of attacks that did occur were not affected by sodium valproate compared to placebo. Fifty percent were responders; that is, their initial migraine frequency decreased to 50% or less during the valproate phase of the study compared to 18% during the placebo phase. The number of responders increased during the trial to 65 in the last 4 weeks of active treatment. There were no serious side effects that required patients to withdraw from the study. Jensen et al. [9] concluded that sodium valproate is an effective and well-tolerated prophylactic medication for migraine without aura.

Mathew et al. [10] conducted a multicenter, double blind, randomized, placebo- controlled investigation that included a 4-week, single-blind placebo-baseline phase and a 12-week treatment phase (4-week dose adjustment period, 8 week maintenance period). This was the first study using parallel groups. One hundred and seven patients were randomized to divalproex sodium or placebo, with 70 receiving divalproex sodium and 37 receiving placebo. During treatment phase, the mean headache frequency per 4-week period was 3.5 in the divalproex sodium group and 5.7 in the placebo group ($p < 0.001$), compared to 6 and 6.4, respectively during baseline phase. Forty-eight percent of divalproex sodium-treated patients and 14% of patients who received placebo showed a greater than 50% reduction in headache frequency from the baseline phase ($p < 0.001$). Among the migraineurs, divalproex sodium-treated patients used significantly less symptomatic medication and reported significantly less functional restriction on average than the placebo-treated patients. Treatment was stopped in 13% of valproate sodium-treated patients and 5% of placebo-treated patients because of intolerance ($p = NS$). Mathew et al. [10] concluded that divalproex sodium is an effective, well tolerated prophylactic drug for patients with migraine headache.

After the above studies were published, another multicenter, double-blind, placebo-controlled, parallel-group study was done by Klapper et al. [11] The patients were previously untreated or had failed no more than two adequate trials of prophylactic therapy. During the 4-week (single-blind) baseline, all patients received placebo and completed a headache diary. Patients with two or more migraine attacks during the baseline were randomized to divalproex sodium (daily dose of 500, 1,000 or 1,500 mg) or to placebo. The experimental phase (EP) lasted 12 weeks, the first 4 weeks for dose escalation to randomized dose, and the remaining 8 weeks for dose maintenance.

The primary efficacy variable was 4-week migraine frequency during the EP. One hundred and seventy-six patients (44 placebo, 132 divalproex) were randomized. One hundred and seventy-one provided safety data and 137 completed the study. During the EP, after adjustment for differences in baseline migraine attack frequencies, mean reductions in the divalproex sodium groups were 1.7 (500 mg), and 2 (1,000 mg), and 1.7 (1,500 mg) migraine attacks per 4 weeks compared to mean reduction of 0.5 migraine attacks in the placebo group ($p \leq 0.05$ vs. placebo). Forty-four to 45% of divalproex-treated patients (compared to 21% of the patients in the placebo group) achieved more than or equal to 50% reduction in their migraine attack frequencies ($p \leq 0.05$ vs.

placebo). The recommended initial dose of divalproex sodium in migraine prophylaxis is 500 mg a day, although some patients may benefit from higher doses. Adverse events were similar in the divalproex sodium- and placebo-treated groups; however, the incidence rate of nausea, dizziness and tremor was significantly higher in the patients who received 1,500 mg of divalproex sodium than it was in the placebo group. Nausea was also higher in the 500 mg group. Nineteen percent of divalproex sodium-treated patients and 5% of placebo-treated patients stopped treatment prematurely because of medication intolerance (p = 0.03); among the divalproex sodium subgroups, the withdrawal rate was highest in patients receiving 1,500 mg daily dose.

While Hering and Kuritzky [8] suggested that sodium valproate has a positive effect on severity and duration of attacks, study by Jensen et al. [9] and Mathew al. [10] found that the duration and severity of the individual attacks were unchanged during treatment with valproate. Similar findings were reported during prophylactic trials with propranolol [12] and flurinizine [13].

The mean symptomatic medication consumption for the remaining attacks was largely unchanged, while the total symptomatic medication consumed was reduced in the controlled trials. Jensen et al. [9] reported that the number of interictal tension-type headache was unaffected by valproate treatment. This was in contrast to an earlier report from an open trial of valproate in CDH published by Mathew et al. [14] In this prospective series of 30 patients with persistent CDH who were treated openly with divalproex sodium 1,000 to 2,000 mg daily for a period of 3 months, 18 patients experienced significant improvement while taking divalproex, achieving headache-free days and a reduction in the dysfunction days. Nine patients failed to improve significantly and three stopped treatment early because of severe side-effects. Rothrock et al. [15] studied differential responses to divalproex treatment in patients with intractable headache. They consecutively recruited 75 patients with intractable headache syndrome and divided them into three groups based on their clinical headache symptoms. These groups consisted of: (1) frequent migraine (FM); (2) transformed migraine (TM); and (3) tension-type headache (TTH). They treated all 75 patients with divalproex sodium. Thirty-six patients (48%) reported more than a 50% reduction in headache frequency. They noted significantly different treatment response rates in the three groups, with FM patients reporting the highest rate of improvement (11 out of 18 [61%]), TM patients an intermediate rate (22 out of 43 [51%]), and TTH patients the lowest response rate (3 out of 14 [21%]). This data suggests that prophylactic pharmacotherapy with divalproex may be effective in selected patients with intractable headache syndrome and that identification of clinically distinct subtypes may assist in predicting response to treatment.

Comparative Trials with other Substances

No large comparative studies have been done comparing valproate with other migraine prophylactic agents. A small comparative study of divalproex sodium with propranolol and placebo for prophylaxis of migraine without aura was done by Kaniecki [16]. This was a single-investigator, randomized, single-blind, placebo-controlled study with five phases (baseline, week 1 to 4; placebo weeks 5 to 8, first treatment one agent, weeks 9 to 20; wash-out, weeks 21 to 24; and second treatment, crossover to other agent, weeks 25 to 36. Of 37 patients (30 women and 10 men), 32 completed the study. All received placebo, after which half were randomized to divalproex or propranolol and then crossed over after wash-out.

The divalproex sodium and propranolol doses were titrated during the initial 8 weeks of each 12-week treatment cycle. Divalproex, doses were titrated to 1,500 mg per day in 23 patients 2,000 mg per day in two patients, downward in seven patients. The mean valproate dose sodium trough level was 68.5 milligrams per liter. Propranolol was titrated to 180 mg per day and 28 patients, 240 mg per day in one patient, and downward in three patients.

Migraine frequency was reduced in 19% (6/32) of placebo-treated patients, 66% (21/32) of divalproex sodium-treated patients, and 63% (20/32) of propranolol-treated patients. Assessment of migraine days per month revealed significant response to placebo in 22% (7/32) of patients, to divalproex in 66% (21/32), and to propranolol in 69% (22/32). When results were limited to the third month of each active-agent treatment phase, 75% (24/32) of those receiving divalproex and 78% (25/32) of those receiving propranolol had reduced migraine frequency. The study concluded that there is no significant difference between divalproex and propranolol for the prophylaxis of migraine without aura. The longer treatment was continued, the better the result, as evidenced by the third month efficacy.

To date, valproate has not been compared to any other prophylactic agent.

Side Effects

Nausea, vomiting and gastrointestinal distress are the most common side effects of valproate therapy. These are generally self-limited and are slightly less common with divalproex sodium than with sodium valproate. When the therapy is continued, the incidence of gastrointestinal symptoms decreases, particularly after six months.

In an open-label study, Silberstein et al. [17] evaluated the long-term safety of divalproex sodium (Depakote®) in patients who had completed one of two previous double-blind, placebo-controlled studies evaluating the safety and efficacy of divalproex in migraine prophylaxis. Of 163 patients enrolled, 46 had been treated with placebo and 117 had been treated with divalproex. The results, including data from the double-blind study, represented 198 patient-years of divalproex exposure. The average dose was 974 mg/day. Treatment lasted more than 180 days for 71% of patients and more than 360 days for 48% of patients. Improvements in the 4-week change-from baseline migraine headache rates were seen during each of the three- and six-month time intervals considered. Reasons for premature discontinuation (67%) included administrative problems (31%), drug intolerance (21%), and treatment ineffectiveness (15%). The most frequently reported adverse events were nausea (42%), infection (39%), alopecia (31%), tremor (28%), asthenia (25%), dyspepsia (25%), and somnolence (25%). Divalproex was found to be safe prophylactic treatment for migraine headaches, and initial improvements are maintained for periods in excess of 1,080 days. No unexpected adverse events or safety concerns unique to the use of divalproex in the prophylactic treatment of migraine were found.

Valproate has little effect on cognitive functions and it rarely causes sedation. Its hematologic effects are important since valproate may reduce platelet counts. Patients who undergo surgery while on valproate have to be monitored carefully for adverse events that may occur as a result of a lowered platelet count.

On rare occasions, valproate administration is associated with severe adverse reactions, such as hepatitis or pancreatitis. The frequency varies with the number of concomitant medications used, the patient's age, presence of genetic and metabolic disorders and patient's general state of health. These idiosyncratic reactions are unpredictable [18].

The risk of valproate hepatotoxicity is highest in children under the age of 2 years, especially those treated with multiple anti-epileptic drugs, those with metabolic disorders, and those with severe epilepsy accompanied by mental retardation and organic brain disease [19]. The relative risk of valproate for hepatotoxicity is low in migraineurs. Hepatic failure, however, cannot be predicted by laboratory monitoring, since hepatic function tests can be normal until the clinical symptoms are advanced. Some patients progress to fatal hepatotoxicity without ever developing any specific hepatic function abnormalities. Conversely, hepatic function abnormalities and abnormalities of serum ammonia, carnitine, and fibrinogen have been reported without clinical hepatotoxicity. Clinical symptoms, particularly in patients at highest risk, are more reliable indicators of true hepatotoxicity. Vomiting was the most frequently reported initial symptom in fatal cases of hepatotoxicity. Combined symptoms of nausea and vomiting and anorexia occurred in 82% of valproate associated hepatotoxicity cases, whereas lethargy, drowsiness, and coma were described in 40%. In general, fatal hepatotoxicity is extremely rare and has not been reported in any patient undergoing valproate treatment for migraine.

Divalproex sodium is potentially teratogenic and should not be used in pregnant women and women considering pregnancy [20].

Hyperandrogenism, resulting in elevated testosterone levels, ovarian cysts, and obesity, is of particular concern in young women with epilepsy who use valproate [21]. It is uncertain if valproate can cause these symptoms young women with migraine or mania.

Valproate interacts with alcohol, aspirin, chlorpromazine, cimetidine, felbamate, benzodiazepines, erythromycin, phenobarbitone, phenytoin, lamotrigine and rifampin. Because of valproate's interactions with barbiturates, migraine patients who are on valproate should not be given barbiturate-containing combination analgesics for symptomatic headache relief.

Contraindications

Absolute contraindications to valproate are pregnancy and a history of pancreatitis or a hepatic disorder such as chronic hepatitis or cirrhosis of the liver. Other important contraindications are hematological disorders, including thrombocytopenia, pancytopenia and bleeding disorders.

Relative contraindications include those on barbiturates and other drugs listed above.

Practical Advice About Valproate

Silberstein [20] published practical recommendations and clinical guidelines for using valproate in headache prophylaxis. These include the following:

1. Before initiating divalproex sodium, perform a physical examination and take a thorough medical history, with special attention to hepatic, hematologic and bleeding abnormalities. Inform the patient about possible hair loss, weight gain, and teratogenic effects and the signs and symptoms of hepatic and hematologic dysfunction.

Obtain screening baseline laboratory studies to help identify risk factors that could influence drug selection. Suggested studies include: complete blood count, differential, and platelets; prothrombin time and partial thromboplastin time; serum chemistry – glucose, blood urea nitrogen (BUN), electrolytes, calcium, potassium, magnesium, creatinine, urate, cholesterol, bilirubin, alkaline phosphatase, aspartate aminotransferase (AST), alanine aminotransferase (ALT), total protein, and albumin.

2. To minimize gastrointestinal side effects, use the enteric-coated divalproex sodium formulation if available. Begin with a dose of 250 mg at bedtime. If nausea still occurs use the sprinkle formulation (125 mg) and very slowly increase the dose. Slowly increase the dose to 500–750 mg a day (in two to three divided doses) to limit gastrointestinal side effects. Higher doses are needed at times.

3. Obtain follow-up divalproex levels to test for compliance, toxicity, and drug reactions as needed. Rigid adherence to the therapeutic range for epilepsy (50 to 100 µg/ml) is not likely to benefit the patient; trough levels can be pushed to 125 µg/ml.

4. See the patient on a regular basis (every 1 to 2 months) during the first 6 to 9 months of therapy.

5. It is not necessary to monitor blood and urine in otherwise healthy and asymptomatic patients on monotherapy, despite the manufacturer's recommendation that liver function tests be performed at frequent intervals, especially during the first 5 months. Identify patients who belong to one of the high-risk groups at the inception of treatment. Obtain follow-up chemistry, if needed, at most 2 and 6 months following the onset of treatment, particularly in patients on polypharmacy.

6. If mild hepatic transaminase elevation occurs, continue divalproex sodium at the same dose or a lower dose until the enzymes normalize. If the hepatic transaminase elevations are much higher (e.g. 2 to 3 times the upper limit of normal), discontinue valproate, and restart it at a lower dose once the abnormalities have resolved.

7. Avoid divalproex sodium for headache in children under the age of 10 years unless routine treatments have failed, in which case use it as monotherapy. Avoid divalproex sodium in patients with preexistent liver disease. Avoid divalproex sodium for headache in women who are pregnant or attempting to become pregnant.

8. Tremor may occur in 10% of treated patients. If this is bothersome, decrease the dose of divalproex sodium or use propranolol, a β-blocker that is also an effective migraine preventive.

9. Excessive weight gain can occur with an incidence of up to 44%. Advise the patient to exercise regularly and avoid using other medications, such as tricyclic antidepressants that can produce weight gain.

Hair loss occurs with an incidence of 2.6% to 12% [20]. Anecdotally, multivitamins and zinc supplements have been reported to control hair loss. We routinely have our patients take 220 mg a day of zinc (mega zinc) and a multivitamin.

Gabapentin in Migraine Prophylaxis

An initial open-label study of gabapentin in a group of patients with migraine and chronic daily headache of transformed migraine showed substantial reduction in migraine frequency and number of headache days per month [22]. Gabapentin appears to have an antinociceptive (analgesic) effect as well as an anticonvulsant effect. The pharmacologic mechanisms of gabapentin remain unclear at the cellular level and thus may be different for each effect [23]. Gabapentin does not appear to interfere with binding at either the $GABA_A$ or $GABA_B$ receptors, even though GABA is a major inhibitory neurotransmitter. Rather, it seems to enhance GABA synthesis from glutamate by increasing the activity of glutamic acid decarboxylase (GAD), resulting in seizure control [24]. It also appears to bind to gabapentin-binding protein (GBP), a novel, membrane-associated protein in the outer layers of the cerebral cortex, inhibiting monoamine neurotransmitter release, including noradrenaline, dopamine, serotonin, and total cellular calcium content. This may explain its analgesic effect. Another explanation is that by blocking thermal and mechanical hyperalgesia when administered intrathecally, gabapentin may be operating at the spinal cord level by altering N-methyl-D-aspartate (NMDA) responses. It has not been found to activate opiate receptors.

Recently, the Mathew et al. [25] trial compared gabapentin with placebo in migraineurs (with or without aura) in a randomized, double-blind, placebo-controlled multicenter trial [25]. After screening and a 4-week single-blind, placebo-baseline period, 145 patients were randomized to 12 weeks of treatment with gabapentin (n=99) or matching placebo (n=46). The 12-week treatment period consisted of a 4-week titration (gabapentin 300 mg/day to 2,400 mg/day) and an 8-week stable dosing phase. Of the 99 patients randomized to receive gabapentin, 76.2% titrated to 2,400 mg/day and the remaining patients to 1,800 mg/day. The majority of patients were white (91.7%) and female (80.7%) with a mean age of 40 years. Both groups were evenly matched for age, sex, race, weight and height.

The mean 4-week migraine headache rate at the end of the 12-week treatment phase was 2.9 for the gabapentin patients and 3.4 for the placebo-treated patients, compared with 4.5 and 4.2, respectively, during the single-blind baseline period. In addition, 36.4% of patients receiving gabapentin and 13.9% receiving placebo demonstrated a 50% or greater reduction in a 4-week migraine headache rate.

Thirty-five patients (24.1%) discontinued the study, primarily due to adverse events (n=20, 13.8%). Of this group, 13% were gabapentin-treated patients, who reported somnolence and dizziness, and 7% were placebo-treated patients. The study concluded that gabapentin is generally well tolerated and an effective prophylactic agent for patients with migraine headaches.

Advantages of Gabapentin Over Valproate
- Absence of disturbing adverse events such as weight gain, tremor, hair loss.
- Absence of concern about liver toxicity.
- Overall, better tolerated.

Place of Anticonvulsants in Migraine Prophylaxis

While β-blockers remain the first-line drug, valproate or gabapentin may be considered first line under many circumstances. When β-blockers are contraindicated in conditions like asthma, congestive cardiac failure, low blood pressure, orthostatic hypotension, and cardiac conduction defects, valproate or gabapentin would become the first-line drug. Beta-blockers are known to produce depression in some patients; therefore, they can be replaced by valproate or gabapentin. Patients with migraine who are on immunotherapy for allergy treatment should not be taking β-blockers concomitantly and therefore may be switched to these agents. Beta-blockers are known to reduce exercise tolerance in those who exercise regularly. Gabapentin and divalproex sodium have no effect on exercise tolerance.

Valproate is the only approved drug for migraine without any direct cardiovascular effects. Gabapentin also does not exhibit any cardiovascular effects. Valproate is now approved for three different indications, which include epilepsy, migraine, and mania. When there is comorbid epilepsy and migraine or epilepsy and bipolar illness, valproate may be considered as a first-line drug. Similar beneficial effects are expected with gabapentin when the above disorders coexist.

References

1   Limmorth V, Lee WS, Cutrer FM, Waeber C, Moskowitz MA: Meningeal GABA$_A$ receptors located outside the blood-brain barrier mediate sodium valproate blockade of neurogenic and substance P-induced inflammation. Possible mechanism in migraine. Cephalalgia 1995;13:102.
2   Nishikawa T, Scatton B: Inhibitory influence of GABA on central serotoninergic transmission. Raphi nuclei as the neuroanatomical side of GABAergic inhibition of cerebral serotoninergic neurons. Brain Res 1985;1:331–391.
3   Cutrer FM, Limmroth V, Ayata G, Moskowitz MA: Valproate reduces C-Fos expression in trigeminal nucleus caudalis (TNC) after noxious meningeal stimulation. Cephalalgia 1995;15(suppl 14):96.
4   Cutrer FM, Moskowitz MA: Actions of valproate and neurosteroids in a model of trigeminal pain. Headache 1996;36:285.
5   Sorensen KV: Valproate: a new drug in migraine prophylaxis. Acta Neurol Scand 1988;78:346–348.
6   Viswanathan KN, Sundraram N, Rajendran C, Manohar DS, Balaraman VT: Sodium valproate in therapy of intractable headache with EEG changes. Cephalalgia 1991;11:282–283.

7   Moore KL: Valproate in the treatment of refractory recurrent headaches: A retrospective analysis of 207 patients. Headache Qu 1992;3:323–325.

8   Hering R, Kuritzky A: Sodium valproate in the prophylaxis treatment of migraine: A double-blind study versus placebo. Cephalalgia 1992;12:81–84.

9   Jensen R, Brink T, Olesen J: Sodium valproate has a prophylactic effect in migraine without aura: A triple-blind, placebo-controlled crossover study. Neurology 1994;44:647–651.

10 Mathew NT, Saper J, Silberstein S, Rankin L, Markley H, Solomon S, Rapoport AM, Silber CJ, Deaton RL: Migraine prophylaxis with divalproex. Arch Neurol 1995;52:281–286.

11 Klapper J: Divalproex sodium in migraine prophylaxis: A dose-controlled study. Cephalalgia 1997; 17:103–108.

12 Ramadan NM, Schultz LL, Gilkay SJ: Migraine prophylactic drugs: Proof of efficacy, utilization, and cost. Cephalalgia 1997;17:73–80.

13 Lucetti C, Nuti A, Pavese N, Gambaccini G, Rossi G, Bonucelli U: Flunarizine in migraine prophylaxis: Prediction factors for a positive response. Cephalalgia 1998;16:349–352.

14 Mathew NT, Ali S: Valproate in the treatment of persistent chronic daily headache. An open label study. Headache 1982;31:71–74.

15 Rothrock JF, Kelly NM, Brody ML, Golbeck A: A differential response to treatment with divalproex sodium in patients with intractable headache. Cephalalgia 1994;14:241–244.

16 Kaniecki RG: A comparative study of propanolol and divalproex sodium in the prophylaxis of migraine. Arch Neurol 1997;54:1141–1144.

17 Silberstein SD: Safety of divalproex sodium in migraine prophylaxis – An open label long-term study. Headache 1999 (in press).

18 Pellock JM, Willmore LJ: A rational guide to routine blood monitoring in patients receiving antiepileptic drugs. Neurology 1991;41:961–964.

19 Driefuss FE, Santilli N, Langer DH, Sweeney KP, Moline KA, Menander KB: Valproic acid hepatic fatalities: A retrospective review. Neurology 1987;37:379–385.

20 Silberstein SD: Divalproex sodium in headache: Literature review and clinical guidelines. Headache 1996;36:547–555.

21 Vainionpaa LK, Rattya J, Knip M, Tapanainen JS, Pakarinen AJ, Lanning P, Tekay A, Myllyla VV, Isojarvi JI: Valproate-induced hyperandrogenism during pubertal maturation in girls with epilepsy. Ann Neurol 1999;45:444–450.

22 Mathew NT: Gabapentin in migraine prophylaxis. Cephalalgia 1996;16:357.

23 Taylor CP, Gee NS, Su Tz, Kocsis JD, Welty DF, Brown JP, Dooley DJ, Boden P, Singh L: A summary of mechanistic hypotheses of gabapentin pharmacology. Epilepsy Res 1998;29:233–249.

24 Petroff OA, Rothman DL, Behar KL, Lamoureux D, Mattson RH: The effect of gabapentin on brain GABA in patients with epilepsy. Ann Neurol 1996;39:95–99.

25 Mathew NT, Magnus-Miller L, Saper J, Poddinck P, Klapper J, Tepper S, Stacey B, Rapoport A, Ranadan N: Efficacy and safety of gabapentin (Neurontin) in migraine prophylaxis. Cephalalgia 1999;19:380.

Ninan T. Mathew, MD, Houston Headache Clinic,
1213 Hermann Drive, Suite 350, Houston, TX 77004 (USA)
Tel. +1 713 528 1916, Fax +1 713 526 6369, E-Mail ntmathew@houstonheadacheclinic.com

Diener HC (ed): Drug Treatment of Migraine and Other Headaches.
Monogr Clin Neurosci. Basel, Karger, 2000, vol 17, pp 299–306

....

Migraine Prophylaxis – Other Drugs

Volker Pfaffenrath[a], Jean Schoenen[b], Peer Tfelt-Hansen[c]

[a] Neurological Praxis, München, Germany, and
[b] University Department of Neurology, C.H.R. de la Citadelle, Liege, Belgium, and
[c] Department of Neurology, Glostrup Hospital, Glostrup, Denmark

In the treatment of the acute migraine attack some very successful substances have been developed. Nonetheless, there is still a need for migraine prophylactics which combine high efficacy with few side effects. Drugs with established efficacy in migraine prophylaxis and details of their therapeutic use have been presented in previous chapters. Other drugs with dubious or possible effects and either anecdotal or scientific evidence are widely and traditionally used. In the following, only agents which have been scientifically assessed in the last two decades are dealt with:

- Magnesium
- Riboflavin
- Feverfew
- Clonidine
- Amantadine
- Antidepressants

Magnesium

For many years a migraine prophylactic effect has been attributed to magnesium. This, however, has never been proved in a controlled study, with the exception of a small trial with magnesium for menstrual migraine [1]. Previous investigations have not convincingly been able to show where magnesium interacts in the pathophysiology of migraine and whether those findings were not merely coincidental.

Recent studies have generated interesting hypotheses. In vivo phosphorus-magnetic resonance spectroscopy showed a reduced brain tissue magnesium without a pH shift during a migraine attack. Furthermore, it was found that erythrocyte magnesium was low in patients with interictal migraine without aura between attacks [1–3]. Reduced magnesium levels were seen in serum and cerebrospinal fluid (CSF) during, as well as between, migraine attacks. Also, reduced magnesium levels were found in the serum and saliva of migraine patients with and without aura compared to healthy controls, and the magnesium levels dropped further during the migraine attacks [2, 3]. More recently, Mauskop et al. [2] emphasized the importance of serum ionized magnesium measurements in determining the magnesium state in migraine. Animal experiments have demonstrated a relationship between magnesium deficiency and cortical spreading depression (CSD) [2, 3]. Reduced magnesium levels increase the sensitivity of N-methyl-D-aspartate (NMDA) [2, 3]. Despite the above-mentioned laboratory evidence supporting an association between migraine and magnesium deficiency, the role of magnesium supplementation in the prevention of migraine has rarely been examined.

Two double-blind, placebo-controlled trials have demonstrated contradictory therapeutic efficacy of magnesium in migraine prophylaxis:

In the first study, 10 mmol magnesium twice daily were evaluated in a 12-week treatment phase after a 4-week baseline period [1]. With a calculated total sample size of 150 patients, an interim analysis with 69 patients was performed. With regard to the number of migraine days, migraine attacks, tolerability and safety, there was no benefit with magnesium compared to placebo.

In the second study, a placebo-controlled trial with 81 patients [3], the prophylactic effect of 24 mmol oral magnesium daily for 12 weeks after a prospective baseline period of four weeks was examined. In weeks 9–12 the attack frequency was reduced by 41.6% in the magnesium group and by 15.8% in the placebo group compared to baseline. The therapeutic effect was already statistically significant at weeks 5–8. The number of migraine days was significantly less in the verum group but the protocol-correct collective analysis showed the difference to be of no statistical significance. There was no significant correlation between the magnesium verum levels prior to therapy and the reduction of frequency. Magnesium concentrations were not measured during the study.

The positive effect of 360 mg magnesium daily in a select placebo-controlled sample of 24 women with menstrual migraine [4] is uncertain (small number of patients, efficacy measured by a 'total pain index'), as are results in uncontrolled studies with parenteral magnesium for acute migraine and cluster headache attacks [2].

The side effects of high-dose (20–24 mmol) oral magnesium include diarrhoea and gastric complaints which are usually mild and tolerable.

In conclusion, these studies are currently not sufficient in assessing the role of oral magnesium in migraine prophylaxis despite its favourable side effect profile and interactions in the pathophysiology of migraine.

Riboflavin (Vitamin B2)

A reduction of mitochondrial phosphorylation potential in the brain has been reported between attacks in migraine with and without aura [5]. In a recent study published in abstract form, reduced plasma riboflavin levels were detected in a subgroup of children with transformed migraine [6]. Riboflavin has the potential of increasing mitochondrial energy efficiency and has been used with some clinical benefit in mitochondriopathies.

In a preliminary open pilot study [7] 49 migraine patients were treated with a single 400 mg dose of riboflavin for at least three months. Twenty-three patients received in addition 75 mg aspirin. Efficacy was assessed after at least 3–5 months of treatment and expressed as change of 'migraine severity', i.e. the arithmetic mean between a subjective disease severity score given on a 10-point scale and the monthly number of migraine days between the month prior to treatment and the last month of therapy. Mean global improvement after therapy was 68.2% with no difference between the two groups. No drug-related side effects were reported.

The results of this open study must be interpreted with caution and for this reason a randomized clinical trial was performed, in which 400 mg riboflavin was compared to placebo in 55 patients over a period of three months [8]. Using an intent-to-treat analysis, riboflavin was superior to placebo in reducing attack frequency (59% vs. 15%) and headache days. The therapeutic gain of riboflavin over placebo for reduction of attacks by at least 50% ('responders') was 37% and close to that calculated from studies of other established prophylactics: 42% for beta blockers and flunarizine or 37% for valproate [8]. The effect of riboflavin begins after one month and is maximal after three months of treatment. There were no side effects except in one patient who dropped out because of diarrhoea.

This is up to now the only controlled study of riboflavin. The dosage of 400 mg was chosen because comparable high doses were previously used in the treatment of mitochondropathies and because of the lack of toxicity.

Recommendations for the use of riboflavin cannot be made before additional dose-finding studies are available, even though it seems to have a very positive efficacy/side effect profile compared to other unconventional prophylactic therapies in migraine.

Feverfew

Feverfew (*Tanacetum parthenium*) is a long used herbal treatment [9] for fever, women's ailments and inflammations. During the last few decades the plant has been increasingly applied as a herbal therapy for migraine prophylaxis. Its role is based on its inhibitory effects on platelet aggregation and release of serotonin from blood platelets and leukocytes [9]. Furthermore, feverfew seems to exert inhibiting effects on prostaglandin biosynthesis. A definite link between the pathophysiology of migraine and feverfew has, however, not yet been established. In a systematic review Vogler et al. [9] deals with all of the five currently available randomized controlled trials. While the studies with the lowest and highest scientific score showed no benefit, three trials with a dosage range from 50–100 mg, including 67% of the total studied population, were in favour of feverfew. The sample size of all five studies ranged from 17 to 72 patients, the main outcome measures differed substantially. In the reviewed trials adverse events were mild and reversible, the most frequently reported being mouth ulceration and gastrointestinal symptoms. Oral medication is relatively safe, but further data on long-term use are necessary.

The clinical effectiveness of feverfew for migraine prevention has not been established beyond reasonable doubt, and the possible active ingredients have not been determined [10]. More clinical trials are needed, both on a larger scale and reported in a uniform manner to enable statistical assessment of trial results [10].

Clonidine

The antihypertensive agent clonidine is a centrally acting selective alpha 2-adrenoceptor agonist. It has vasoconstrictor activity in vascular smooth muscle. It was found to reduce the responsiveness of the cat femoral artery bed to vasoconstrictor and vasodilator substances such as noradrenaline, adrenaline and angiotensin [11]. Such vascular reactions were then believed to cause the aura and headache phases of a migraine with aura attack, and it seemed that clonidine might block them. A Danish double-blind crossover trial with 21 patients found clonidine to be no better than placebo. This result was supported by a further Danish crossover study with 49 patients. Some later crossover trials have compared clonidine with pizotifen, propranolol and metoprolol and showed clonidine to be either equally effective or inferior [11]. All in all, the methodology used in these studies is questionable or peculiar.

Clonidine seems unlikely to be effective in migraine prophylaxis.

Amantadine

In the course of a study with Levodopa on Parkinson patients, four patients described a favourable effect of amantadine on their frequent headaches [12]. In a subsequent double-blind crossover study vs. placebo, 14 patients with frequent attacks were given 100 mg amantadine orally twice a day. The duration of attacks and its severity were recorded and showed no difference between the two groups.

Amantadine is unlikely to be an effective prophylactic drug in migraine.

Antidepressants

Antidepressants of the major categories – tri- and tetracyclics, serotonin re-uptake inhibitors and monoamine oxidase inhibitors – have demonstrated effects mostly in the treatment of chronic tension-type headache. Of these agents, however, only amitriptyline has shown efficacy in migraine prevention. Clinical trials have clearly demonstrated that its anti-migraine effect occurs independently of its antidepressive activity. In four placebo-controlled randomized clinical trials, doses of 10 to 150 mg amitriptyline daily were found to be superior to placebo [10]. It should be stressed that there is not a single trial performed according to IHS criteria and IHS guidelines confirming the effectivity of tricyclics in migraine.

The effective dosage varies considerably among subjects and should be commenced with 10 mg at night and can be increased weekly up to an average dose of 50 mg. Some patients with sleep disorder or depression require doses of 100 to 150 mg. Common side effects are weight gain, drowsiness, dry mouth, blurred vision and urinary retention [13]. The addition of amitriptyline to propranolol does not improve the results in migraine headache, however, the combination is superior to either preparation in the management of headaches which combine the features of migraine and tension headache [14].

The tricyclic antidepressants imipramine and clonipramine are both inactive in migraine. Similarly, the atypical antidepressant mianserin appears to have no prophylactic effect in migraine [15] despite a study in which 30 mg mianserin was superior to placebo both in frequency and severity of attacks. With altogether 34 patients completing the study the results are to be interpreted with caution [16].

Since monoamine oxidase inhibitors (MAOIs) were thought to maintain or increase serotonine levels in migraine, they seemed to be a logical form of treatment [15]. Modulation of central nervous system monoaminergic neurotransmission is more likely to be responsible for the effect of phenelzine in migraine [15]. There are no controlled trials for MAOIs such as phenelzine (15 mg t.i.d.). This form of treatment should be reserved for patients resistant to other drugs and they should be provided with a notice specifying the foods and drugs to be avoided. Naratriptan (2.5 mg) and zolmitriptan (5 mg or less) are safe to use with MAO-A inhibitors while sumatriptan and rizatriptan should be avoided. The MAO-B inhibitor selegeline is not helpful in the management of migraine [17].

The specific serotonin re-uptake inhibitors (SSRIs) are not as effective in treatment as the tricyclic antidepressive amitriptyline, especially in pure migraine without concomitant depression or tension-type headache. The combination of the two is to be avoided because of the serotonin syndrome (agitation, myoclonus and other movement disorders) [18]. The SSRI are notable for their benign side effect profile as they are associated with fewer anticholinergic and cardiovascular side effects than the tricyclics. Fluoxetine specifically blocks serotonin re-uptake. A small placebo controlled trial (n = 36) with doses from 20–40 mg showed a significant improvement in the verum group [19]. A larger trial involving 58 migraine patients given 20 mg daily [20] did not demonstrate any improvement compared to placebo. In a study with S-fluoxetin, the long-acting enantiomer of fluoxetine, in a dosage of 40 mg at night, 33 patients out of 65 provided a complete data set. There was a significant decrease of attacks in month 2 and month 4. As it was a phase II study and the number of patients was relatively small results should be interpreted conservatively [21]. The same holds true for a small trial with fluvoxamine (50 mg) vs. amitriptyline (25 mg) without placebo control [22].

Conclusion

The goals of the preventive therapy of migraine are to decrease the frequency, intensity and duration of attacks as well as to reduce disability and improve functional ability. Medication for prophylactic treatment should be selected on the basis of relative drug efficacy, side effect profile, related indications (e.g. epilepsy, depression, hypertension, sleep disorders), contraindications, ease of use and potential for inter-drug interactions.

Of the drugs reviewed are:

- Of no efficacy:
  clonidine, amantadine, clomipramine, trimipramine, mianserin, SSRIs

- Of potential yet to be confirmed efficacy:
  riboflavin, magnesium, feverfew

- Of efficacy in migraine with concomitant tension-type headache, depression or for treatment resistant cases:
  amitriptyline (and probably other tricyclics).

References

1   Pfaffenrath V, Wessely P, Meyer C, Isler HR, Evers S, Grotemeyer KH, Taneri Z, Soyka D, Göbel H, Fischer M: Magnesium in the prophylaxis of migraine – A double-blind placebo-controlled study. Cephalalgia 1996;16:436–440.
2   Mauskop A, Altura BM: Magnesium for migraine – rationale for use and therapeutic potential. CNS Drugs 1998;3:185–190.
3   Peikert A, Wilimzig C, Köhne-Wolland R: Prophylaxis of migraine with oral magnesium: Results from a prospective, multi-center, placebo-controlled and double-blind randomized study. Cephalalgia 1996;16:257–263.
4   Facchinetti F, Sances G, Borella P, Genazzani AR, Nappi G: Magnesium prophylaxis of menstrual migraine: Effects on intracellular magnesium. Headache 1991;31:298–301.
5   Montagna P: High-dose riboflavin as a prophylactic treatment. Cephalalgia 1994;14:317.
6   Hershey AD, Powers SW, Bentti A-L, de Grauw TJ: Chronic daily headaches (CDH) in children: Characteristics and treatment response. Headache 1999;39:358.
7   Schoenen J, Lenaerts M, Bastings E: High dose riboflavin as a prophylactic treatment of migraine: Results of an open pilot study. Cephalalgia 1994;14:328–329.
8   Schoenen J, Jacquy J, Lenaerts M: Effectiveness of high-dose riboflavin in migraine prophylaxis – A randomized controlled trial. Neurology 1998;50:466–470.
9   Vogler BK, Pittler MH, Ernst E: Feverfew as a preventive treatment for migraine: A systematic review. Cephalalgia 1998;18:704–708.
10 Mylecharane EJ, Tfelt-Hansen P: Nonsteroidal antiinflammatory and miscellaneous drugs in migraine prophylaxis; in Olesen J, Tfelt-Hansen P, Welch KMA (eds): The Headaches. New York, Lippincott, Williams & Wilkins, 2000 (in press).
11 Clonidine in migraine prophylaxis – Now obsolete. Drug Ther Bull 1990;28:79–80.
12 Baxter RCH, Marsden CD, Parkes JD, Zilkha KJ: Amantadine in migraine. Lancet 1972; August 26:429.
13 Rapaport AM: Pharmacological prevention of migraine. Clinical Neurosci 1998;5:55–59.
14 Mathew NT, Stubits E, Nigam M: Transformation of migraine into daily headache: Analysis of factors. Headache 1982;22:66–68.
15 Mylecharane EJ, Tfelt-Hansen P: Miscellaneous drugs; in Olesen J, Tfelt-Hansen P, Welch KMA (eds): The Headaches. New York, Raven Press, 1993, pp 397–402
16 Monro P, Swade C, Coppen A: Mianserin in the prophylaxis of migraine: A double-blind study. Acta Psychiatr Scand 1985;72:96–103.

17 Kuritzky A, Zoldan Y, Melamed E: Selegeline, a MAO B inhibitor, is not effective in the prophylaxis of migraine without aura – An open study. Headache 1992;32:416.

18 Mathew NT, Tiejen GE, Lucker C: Serotonin syndrome complicating migraine pharmacotherapy. Cephalalgia 1996;16:323–327.

19 Adly C, Straumanis J, Chesson A: Fluoxetine prophylaxis in migraine. Headache 1992;32:101–104.

20 Saper JR, Silberstein SD, Lake AE, Winters ME: Double-blind trial of fluoxetine: Chronic daily headache and migraine. Headache 1994;34:497–502.

21 Steiner TJ, Ahmed F, Findley LJ, MacGregor EA, Wilkinson M: S-fluoxetine in the prophylaxis of migraine: A phase II double-blind randomized placebo-controlled study. Cephalalgia 1998;18: 283–286.

22 Bank J: A comparative study of amitriptyline and fluvoxamine in migraine prophylaxis. Headache 1994;34:476–478.

Pfaffenrath Volker, MD, Neurologist, Leopoldstr. 59/II, D-80802 München (Germany)
Tel. +49 89 334003, Fax +49 89 332942, E-Mail vpfa@aol.com

Diener HC (ed): Drug Treatment of Migraine and Other Headaches.
Monogr Clin Neurosci. Basel, Karger, 2000, vol 17, pp 307–312

....

Priority of Drugs and Treatment Regimens

Timothy J. Steiner

Imperial College School of Medicine, London, UK

Introduction

The formal evidence-base for all prophylactic antimigraine drugs is not good by current clinical trials standards, though adequate for most agents in use. They are generally old, which has allowed the accumulation of vast informal evidence based on experience in clinical use. It is this informal evidence which justifies their continued use, and it is from this, mainly, that priorities are determined.

Indications for Prophylaxis

When indicated, prophylactic therapy is used *in addition to*, not instead of, acute therapy. The intention in prescribing prophylactic medication is to reduce the number of attacks in circumstances when best acute therapy has failed to bring symptoms adequately under control. Therefore, the threshold for prophylaxis is not necessarily defined in terms only of attack frequency, although this is clearly an important factor. Over frequent use of acute therapy is also a criterion for migraine prophylaxis, but with the proviso that prophylactic drugs are inappropriate and will be ineffective for medication misuse headache.

The ultimate judge of when prophylaxis is needed ought, usually, to be the patient, who nonetheless is not in a position to exercise this choice unless the offer is made. The prescriber therefore remains in control, but of course must exercise this dutifully.

Priority of Drugs

There are no sound criteria based on efficacy for preferring one prophylactic drug to another. Side effects vary between them and, to a large extent, drive drug selection which is made in the light of comorbidity and contraindications (including risks in pregnancy).

One major factor likely to detract from the efficacy of all prophylactic drugs is poor compliance [1, 2]. No matter how intelligently prescribed, a drug not taken does not work well. There is evidence, sufficient that it should be considered when selecting treatment for prophylaxis, that once-daily dosing is preferable [2].

First-Line Prophylactic Drugs
The choice, usually, is between β-adrenergic blockers without partial agonism, sodium valproate, pizotifen and amitriptyline. Specifically for menstrually-related migraine, there are other options that may be worth considering.

There is at least some evidence of efficacy for most β-blockers that lack partial agonist activity. Adequate clinical trials evidence supports the use of propranolol, metoprolol and atenolol [3], but it is difficult to take a view on their comparative efficacy. Cardioselectivity and hydrophilicity both tend to improve side effect profile, and this suggests grounds for preferring one drug to another, as does dosing simplicity. On all counts, propranolol, effective in the range 40–240 mg or more daily, is at a disadvantage compared with *atenolol* or *metoprolol*, 100–200 mg daily, and atenolol is more cardioselective and more hydrophilic than metoprolol.

Nonetheless, *propranolol* has best evidence of safety during pregnancy and lactation [4]. Fortunately, most women with migraine improve during pregnancy but, if not and prophylaxis is necessary, this is the drug of choice. Women should be counselled with regard to the relative risks and benefits.

Lethargy, impaired sleep quality and reduced exercise tolerance may prevent use of β-blockers or lead to a preference for alternatives. Important relative contraindications to β-blockers are asthma, which is becoming very common; depression, which is prevalent in people with migraine; and diabetes. Cardioselective β-blockers can often be used successfully in mild asthma but clearly require care. Heart failure, 2nd or 3rd degree AV block and peripheral vascular disease are absolute contraindications to use of β-blockers for migraine; whilst these are uncommon amongst migraine patients it would be most unfortunate to overlook them.

Clear clinical trials evidence of efficacy supports the use of *sodium valproate* [5], or the 1:1 molar ratio combination of sodium valproate and valproic acid (*divalproex*). The trials do not well-establish the therapeutic dose range which, in practice, is 0.5–2.0 g daily. Valproate is well-tolerated. Nausea, asthenia and drowsiness were most frequent in trials [6], but weight gain and the possibility of transient hair loss are the side effects that most concern patients; both are reversible if they occur. This drug is not safe during pregnancy nor, therefore, when there is any likelihood that pregnancy may occur. Hepatic dysfunction also contraindicates use absolutely; liver function should be assessed before start of treatment. Nevertheless, hepatotoxicity is idiosyncratic and rare, and liver function tests are not predictive and therefore not worth monitoring [7].

Pizotifen, 1.5 mg daily, is widely used but, in fact, clinical trials evidence of efficacy is limited. There is no evidence of greater efficacy from higher doses. Whilst the formal evidence is poor indeed that a single daily dose is as effective as three of 0.5 mg, long-standing clinical practice has shown preference for the former regimen. It probably produces fewer side effects and is better for compliance. Pizotifen is a sedative and should be taken at bedtime. It enhances appetite, with a degree of weight gain that many sufferers, the majority of whom are women, will not accept; obesity should firmly rule out its use.

Clinical trials evidence of efficacy is equally limited for *amitriptyline*, but nonetheless it is often recommended as first-line prophylactic if migraine coexists with troublesome tension-type headache or is associated with depression or disturbed sleep. It may be used concomitantly with a β-blocker (see below). Unless the choice of this drug is explained to patients who do not consider themselves depressed, they may well reject it (and the doctor). The dose is difficult, particularly as side effects are common. A reasonable regimen is to start with 10–25 mg at night, increased in 25-mg increments as quickly as possible until there is efficacy or unremitting and unacceptable side effects, or 150 mg is reached. Usual side effects are sedation and dry mouth, sometimes constipation, and urinary retention occasionally troubles men. Use for migraine should be avoided with epilepsy or glaucoma. Amitriptyline is not generally recommended for children.

Second-Line Prophylactic Drugs

On rather doubtful evidence but perhaps on the basis of clinical experience, *methysergide*, 1–2 mg three times daily, is sometimes considered to be the most effective prophylactic. It is held in reserve because of its association with retroperitoneal and pleural fibrosis. The drug does not have this side effect in courses of less than 6 months (see *Duration of use* below), but abdominal discomfort, leg cramps and weight gain may be troublesome. Repeat prescribing without review is clearly unwise. Pregnancy or likelihood of it, and breastfeeding, and any evidence of cardiac or vascular disease, are absolute contraindications to methysergide.

Flunarizine is not available everywhere, but popular where it is and supported by adequate evidence of efficacy in migraine prophylaxis [8]. It may have particular value in patients with prolonged aura, or hemiparetic migraine [9]. Depression, an occasional side effect of flunarizine [8], is potentially serious in migraine which has established comorbidity with this illness.

A β-*blocker* and *amitriptyline* may be used together. Although no trial has evaluated the combination, synergistic effect is claimed for it. It appears logical if there may be a depressive trait.

Desipramine, nortriptyline and *protriptyline* are less sedative alternatives to amitriptyline, but there is no formal evidence of efficacy of these or other tricyclics.

Prophylaxis for Menstrually-Related Migraine

The effect of hormones on migraine is common, and greater for migraine without aura [10]. Empirical evidence implicates oestrogen withdrawal as a trigger for migraine in some women [11]. Correct diagnosis of menstrual migraine, a rare condition defined as attacks of migraine without aura that occur regularly on day 1 ± 2 of menstruation and at no other time [12], is essential for successful hormonal management. The diagnosis is clinical and confirmed by diary cards maintained over at least three months. Depending on need for contraception, several options can be tried in whatever order seems appropriate.

Mefenamic acid, 500 mg three to four times daily, may be given from the onset of menstruation until the last day of bleeding. This non-hormonal prophylactic option does not depend on regular menstruation. It may reasonably be tried as first-line in migraine associated with menorrhagia and/or dysmenorrhoea.

Transdermal oestrogen, 50–100 µg daily, is used from 3 days before the onset of menses for 7 days. Alternatively, *oestradiol gel*, 1.5 mg in 2.5 g daily, applied over the same period, produces higher, more stable levels of oestrogen. Clearly these regimens depend for success on predictable periods. Hormones used intermittently for menstrual migraine are supplements: no progestogens are necessary in a woman with an intact uterus who is menstruating regularly.

Combined oral contraceptives (COCs) and *injectable depot progestogens* inhibit the ovarian cycle, if that is the cause of problems. Migraine then occurring in the pill-free interval with COCs, more common with high-progestogen contraceptives [13], can often be resolved or reduced in frequency by changing to a more oestrogen-dominant pill or reduced by using them for three cycles consecutively. Oral contraceptives sometimes exacerbate migraine and should be changed or discontinued if they do. They should be stopped forthwith, and are contraindicated, if exacerbation includes the development of focal neurological signs.

Other Drugs, with Limited Efficacy

Other calcium channel antagonists are of uncertain value. *Verapamil* 120–240 mg modified release twice daily, is well-tolerated although headache is sometimes a side effect. Clinical trials evidence of efficacy is very limited.

Selective serotonin reuptake inhibitors are second-line to tricyclics. *Fluoxetine*, 20 mg on alternate days to 40 mg once daily, is best studied but evidence from clinical trials of efficacy against migraine is inconclusive. Against depression, its value in higher doses is well-established.

Drugs to Avoid in Prophylactic Intervention

Clonidine is ineffective against migraine. There is insufficient evidence to justify the use of anti-epileptic drugs other than valproate or valproic acid.

Treatment Regimens

Specific recommendations have been made, where appropriate, for each drug. There are some general points of importance.

Duration of Use

Migraine is very much prone to cyclical variation. Prophylactic treatment in most cases is required only for periods of exacerbation. Therefore, the issue will arise of how long to continue prophylactic drugs that are effective. Whilst there is no basis for firm or invariable rules, uninterrupted use over a year or longer is rarely appropriate. A reasonable empirical approach is to withdraw after 4–6 months of benefit to establish continued need. Depending on dose, β-blockers and methysergide may need to be withdrawn slowly; most patients, rightly or wrongly fearing rebound, prefer this anyway.

It may be more difficult to judge when prophylactic drugs that are apparently *not* effective should be discontinued. Reacting too soon risks prematurely labelling patients as non-responders, eventually, perhaps, to every drug. Again, no evidence-based guide exists for what should be the minimum period. Patients may well decide for themselves, but should be discouraged from pre-empting a considered evaluation. Since efficacy may develop slowly, 3–4 weeks may be a minimum once the right dose has been achieved. This is what makes use of drugs with a wide therapeutic dose range, such as propranolol, so difficult. Three cycles is a reasonable minimum in the case of specific therapy for menstrually-related migraine.

Multiple Therapy

Beta-blockers are sometimes used with amitriptyline (see above). This and other combinations are used purely empirically, since none have been formally evaluated. As in all therapeutic areas, drug combinations risk a higher incidence of side effects and the possibility of interaction arises.

If Prophylaxis Fails

Reasons for failure of a range of prophylactics include wrong diagnosis and poor compliance. Both should be reviewed, though the latter is difficult to check unless electronic monitoring devices are used [2]. If they are, it may be found that whilst overall consumption is close to expected, concordance with the dosing schedule is *very* poor, especially with multiple daily doses. Detailed and repeated explanations do not always resolve this problem, and a decision may have to be taken to abandon what is futile.

Other medication, particularly symptomatic therapy, should also be reviewed. Medication misuse will render prophylaxis ineffective, and indeed it is a contraindication to the use of prophylactics. If prophylaxis still fails to have measurable benefit, discontinue it.

References

1   Steiner TJ, Catarci T, Hering R, Whitmarsh T, Coutourier EGM: If migraine prophylaxis does not work, think about compliance. Cephalalgia 1994;14:463–464.
2   Mulleners WM, Whitmarsh TE, Steiner TJ: Noncompliance may render migraine prophylaxis useless, but once-daily regimens are better. Cephalalgia 1998;18:52–56.
3   Ramadan NM, Schultz LL, Gilkey SJ: Migraine prophylactic drugs: Proof of efficacy, utilization and cost. Cephalalgia 1997;17:73–80.
4   Hopkinson HE: Treatment of cardiovascular diseases; in Rubin P (ed): Prescribing in pregnancy. London, BMJ Publishing Group, 1995, p 98.
5   Rothrock JF: Clinical studies of valproate for migraine prophylaxis. Cephalalgia 1997;17:81–83.
6   Steiner TJ, Tfelt-Hansen P: Anti-epileptic drugs in migraine prophylaxis; in Olesen J, Tfelt-Hansen P, Welch KMA (eds): The Headaches, ed 2. Philadelphia, Lippincott-Raven (in press).
7   Silberstein SD, Wilmore LJ: Divalproex sodium: Migraine treatment and monitoring. Headache 1996;36:239–242.
8   Diener H-C: Flunarizine. This volume, p 269.
9   Lance JW: Indication for drug therapy. This volume, p 250.
10   Rasmussen BK, Olesen J: Migraine with aura and migraine without aura: An epidemiological study. Cephalalgia 1992;12:221–228.
11   Somerville BW: Estrogen withdrawal migraine. Neurology 1975;25:239–250.
12   MacGregor EA: Menstruation, sex hormones and headache. Neurol Clin 1997;15:125–141.
13   Whitty CWM, Hockaday JM, Whitty MM: The effect of oral contraceptives on migraine. Lancet 1966;i:856–859.

Dr. T.J. Steiner, Division of Neuroscience and Psychological Medicine, Imperial College School of Medicine, Charing Cross Campus, St. Dunstan's Road, London W6 8RP (UK)
Tel. +44 181 846 1191, Fax +44 181 741 7808, E-Mail t.steiner@ic.ac.uk

Drug-Treatment of Other Headaches

Diener HC (ed): Drug Treatment of Migraine and Other Headaches.
Monogr Clin Neurosci. Basel, Karger, 2000, vol 17, pp 314–321

....

Tension-Type Headache

Jean Schoenen

Departments of Neurology and Neuroanatomy, University of Liège, Belgium

Various treatment modalities are used in tension headache (TH). Only some of them have been proven effective in good quality controlled clinical trials. Designing and performing such trials is more difficult in TH than in migraine for various reasons. TH has a highly variable attack and disease cause; the headache is lower in intensity and aggravating factors such as those listed under the fourth digit code may play a confounding role. Most patient with episodic tension headache (ETH) treat themselves with over-the-counter drugs without meeting a physician [1]. At the other end of the spectrum chronic tension headache (CTH) is much more difficult to treat than migraine, because of the lower intensity of the pain and possibly because of other physiological and psychological factors. The placebo effect may be superior in TH, exceeding 30% in many studies [2].

Guidelines for clinical drug trials in TH were recently proposed by a subcommittee of the International Headache Society (IHS) [3]. This can be recommended to the reader as a standard against which he can compare the scientific value of treatment trials published in the literature.

As for migraine, therapies for TH can be schematically subdivided in acute, mainly pharmacologic treatment of the individual headache attack and prophylactic, pharmacologic or non-pharmacologic, treatments which may prevent the headache in the long term.

Acute Pharmacotherapy

Many controlled studies of simple analgesics and non-steroidal anti-inflammatory drugs (NSAIDs) have been performed in tension-type headache, using the headache attack as a model for acute pain. Several among them

Table 1. Recent trials of acute pharmacotherapy in episodic TTH

Study objective	Design	Results	Authors
Ibuprofen vs. paracetamol	RCT, parallel • ibuprofen 400 mg • paracetamol 1,000 mg • placebo	ibu > para > plac	Schachtel et al. 1996 [4]
Ketoprofen vs. ibuprofen vs. naproxen	RCT, parallel • ketoprofen 25 mg • ketoprofen 12.5 mg • ibuprofen 200 mg • naproxen 275 mg	equal efficacy	Lange & Lentz 1995 [6]
Ketoprofen vs. ibuprofen	RCT, parallel, home-monitored (electr. diary) • ketoprofen 50 mg • ketoprofen 25 mg • ibuprofen 200 mg • placebo	keto50 = keto25 > ibu200 > plac	Vangerven et al. 1996 [7]
Ketoprofen vs. paracetamol	RCT, crossover • ketoprofen 50 mg • ketoprofen 25 mg • paracetamol 500 mg • paracetamol 1,000 mg • placebo	keto50 > plac keto50 > para plac < keto25 = para < keto50	Dahlöf & Jacobs 1996 [8]
Ketoprofen vs. paracetamol	RCT, parallel • ketoprofen 25 mg • paracetamol 1,000 mg • placebo	keto25 = para > plac	Steiner & Lange 1998 [9]
Ketoprofen vs. ES Tylenol®	RCT, parallel • ketoprofen 25 mg • ketoprofen 12.5 mg • ES Tylenol® 1,000 mg • placebo	keto25 > keto12.5 = ES Tyl = plac	Mehlisch et al. 1997 [10]

fulfill the standards recommended for drug trials in tension-type headache (TTH) by the International Headache Society [3]. From these studies, one may conclude that NSAIDs are the drugs of first choice. The following is a review of recent randomized controlled trials comparing various NSAIDs and simple analgesics. Although differences between drugs may be small or variable, a hierarchical classification of compounds emerges when efficacy data are considered (table 1, fig. 1).

Table 1 (continued)

Study objective	Design	Results	Authors
Naproxen sodium vs. ibuprofen	RCT, parallel • naproxen 220 mg • ibuprofen 200 mg	napro = ibu	Autret et al. 1997 [21]
Caffeine as adjuvant	RCT, crossover (6 studies) 1) para 1,000 + caf 130 2) para + asp 500 + caf 130 3) paracetamol 1,000 mg 4) placebo	1 = 2 > 3 > 4	Migliardi et al. 1994 [14]
Caffeine as adjuvant	RCT, parallel 1) ibu 400 + caf 200 2) ibu 400 3) caf 200 4) placebo	1 > 2 > 3 = 4	Diamond et al. 1997 [15]
Ketoralac vs. meperidine + promethazine	RCT, parallel 1) ketoralac 60 mg IM 2) meperidine 50 mg + promethazine 25 mg IM 3) normal saline IM	1 > 3 (at 30&60 min) 1 = 3 (from 2 h on) 2 < / = 3	Harden et al. 1998 [11]

RCT = Randomised controlled trial.

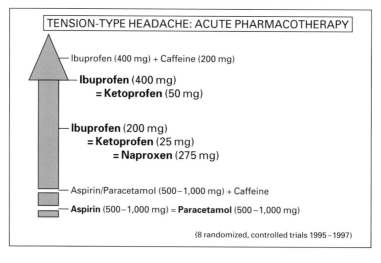

Fig. 1. Tension-type headache: acute pharmacotherapy: compounds of increasing efficacy are listed in the direction of the arrow.

Aspirin (500 mg or 1,000 mg) is more effective for the relief of acute TTH than placebo; its efficacy is comparable to that of paracetamol (500 mg or 1,000 mg). Paracetamol may be the most frequently used OTC drug for TH in certain countries [1], although in most trials the simple analgesics were found inferior to the classical antirheumatic NSAIDs.

Ibuprofen 400 (or 800) mg is significantly more effective than placebo or paracetamol 1,000 mg [4]. Even at a low dose of 200 mg ibuprofen is superior to aspirin 500 mg [5]. Five comparative trials of ketoprofen have been published in recent years [6–10]. They indicate that ketoprofen 50 mg is more effective than ibuprofen 200 mg or paracetamol 1,000 mg whereas ketoprofen 25 mg is not clearly superior to the latter. The efficacy of ketoprofen 12.5 mg did not significantly exceed that of placebo in one study, nor did extra-strength Tylenol®. Naproxen 550 mg provided superior analgesia compared with paracetamol or placebo, while the 220 mg dose was equally effective as ibuprofen 200 mg. Other NSAIDs such as ketoralac, diclofenac or indomethacin are also effective, but less well studied.

The therapeutic efficacy of NSAIDs in TTH, though undisputable, has to be put in perspective. For instance, the low proportion of patients becoming pain-free 2 h after dosing in most trials underscores the relative insufficiency of these drugs: 32% for ketoprofen 50 mg, 28% for the 25 mg dose; 17–22% for paracetamol 1,000 mg; 17% for placebo. Ketorolac 60 mg IM was superior to normal saline only up to 1 h after dosing and in the same study a combination of meperidine 50 mg and promethazine 25 mg IM was equal to placebo at any time-point [11]. There is thus clearly room for better acute treatments of TTH and a need for prophylactic therapy for frequent TTH attacks.

At present time, ibuprofen (400–800 mg) can probably be considered the first choice for acute TTH, followed by naproxen sodium (275–550 mg) because of the all-over better gastrointestinal tolerability. Several surveys have indeed shown that ibuprofen is associated with the lowest risk of gastrointestinal bleeding or perforation (odds ratio: 2.9) while ketoprofen carries a much higher risk (odds ratio: 23.7), naproxen occupying an intermediate position (odds ratio: 9.1) [12–13]. It remains to be determined whether the newer COX-2 inhibitors, assumed to have a lower gastrointestinal toxicity, are also effective as analgesics in TTH.

In some patients, combination of analgesics with caffeine, sedatives or tranquilizers may be more effective than simple analgesics or NSAIDs, but in many cases this impression comes from too low a dosage of the latter. It has been proven nonetheless in controlled trials that the adjunction of caffeine (130 or 200 mg) significantly increases the efficacy of simple analgesics [14] and of ibuprofen [15] (see table 1). Whenever possible, combination analgesics for TTH should be avoided because of the risk of dependency, abuse and chronification of the headache.

Topical applications on the forehead of Tiger balm [16] and peppermint oil [17] were also found superior to placebo in TTH treatment and they were not significantly different from paracetamol.

There is at present no scientific basis for the use of muscle relaxants in the treatment of TH.

Prophylactic Pharmacotherapy

The tricyclic antidepressants are the most widely used first-line therapeutic agents for CTH. Surprisingly, few controlled studies have been performed and not all of them have found an efficacy superior to placebo (table 2). The drawbacks of these studies are small patient numbers, inadequate efficacy parameters or short duration. Only a few of them can be considered adequate according to the 1995 IHS guidelines.

One major problem that arises with trials showing statistical differences between placebo and tricyclics is to evaluate whether the observed effect is clinically relevant. In one study for instance a reduction in average daily headache duration was selected as the primary efficacy parameter. Amitriptyline reduced daily headache duration from 11.1 h per day to 7.9 h per day by an average of 3.2 h. This effect was significantly different from placebo, but the clinical significance of such a reduction is questionable.

Nonetheless, in clinical practice the tricyclic antidepressants remain the most useful prophylactic drugs for CTH or frequent ETH. In a recent open-label study [18], amitriptyline 25 mg/day was found effective in non-depressed patients suffering from CTH, but not in those having ETH. Amitriptyline is the most frequently used drug. Clomipramine may be slightly superior, but has more side effects. Other antidepressants, such as doxepin, maprotiline or mianserin can be used as a second choice.

The initial dosage of tricyclics should be low: 10–25 mg of amitriptyline or clomipramine at bed-time. Many patients will be satisfied by such a low dose. The average dose of amitriptyline in CTH, however, is 75–100 mg per day. If a patient does not sufficiently improve on this dose, a trial of higher doses of amitriptyline or clomipramine is warranted. If the headache is improved by at least 80% after 4 months, it is reasonable to attempt discontinuation of the medication. Decrease the daily dose by 20–25% every 2–3 days may avoid rebound headache.

The mechanism of action of antidepressants in CTH remain to be determined. Their effect on the headache may be partly independent from their antidepressant effect. Tricyclics have a variety of pharmacological activities. Serotonin increase by inhibition of its re-uptake, endorphin release or inhibi-

Table 2. Controlled studies on prophylactic pharmacotherapy for TH

Drugs tested	No. of subjects	Results	Significance	Ref.
Amitriptyline (75 mg/d) Placebo	27	> 50% improved 56% 11%	$p < 0.01$	[22]
Placebo Amitriptyline 10 mg (up to 6/day) Amitriptyline 25 mg (up to 6/day)	29 28 28	Improvement in headache intensity 33% 54% 38%	$p < 0.05$	[23]
Doxepin Placebo	23	Headache days decreased 15% by doxepin compared to placebo	$p < 0.05$	[24]
Maprotiline (75 mg/day) Placebo	30	Headache intensity diminished by 25% and headache-free days increased by 40% on Maprotiline	$p < 0.001$	[25]
Placebo Clomipramine Mianserine	36 28 28	% intensity improvement (day 43) 49% 57% 54%	Non-significant	[26]
Placebo Amitriptyline (50–75 mg/day) Amitriptylinoxide (60–90 mg/day)	64 67 66	50% reduction in duration × frequency and in intensity 21.9% 22.4% 30.3%	Non-significant	[27]
Placebo Amitriptyline (75 mg/day)	29 24	Change in mean daily duration –0.28 h –3.2 h	$p \le 0.001$	[28]

tion of NMDA receptors which play a role in pain transmission may all be relevant for the pathophysiology of TH.

The recent generation of antidepressants blocking selectively the re-uptake of serotonin (e.g. fluoxetine) have as yet not been proven to be effective in TH prophylaxis. In clinical practice, they seem less efficient than the tricyclics, but they may be useful in subgroups of patients.

Botulinum toxin injections in head or neck muscles were found ineffective in one open study [19], but helpful in another study of four patients [20].

References

1   Forward SP, McGrath PJ, MacKinnon D, Brown TL, Swann J, Currie EL: Medication patterns of recurrent headache sufferers: A community study. Cephalalgia 1998;18:146–151.

2   Couch JR, Micieli G: Tension-type headache, cluster headache, and miscellaneous headaches: Prophylactic pharmacotherapy; in Olesen J, Tfelt-Hansen P, Welch KMA (eds): The Headaches. New York, Raven Press, 1993, pp 537–542.

3   International Headache Society Committee on Clinical Trials: Guidelines for trials of drug treatments in tension-type headache, ed 1. Cephalalgia 1995;15:165–179.

4   Schachtel BP, Furey SA, Thoden WR: Nonprescription ibuprofen and acetaminophen in the treatment of tension-type headache. J Clin Pharmacol 1996;36:1120–1125.

5   Nebe J, Heier M, Diener HC: Low-dose ibuprofen in self-medication of mild to moderate headache: A comparison with acetylsalicylic acid and placebo. Cephalalgia 1995;15:531.

6   Lange R, Lentz R: Comparison ketoprofen, ibuprofen and naproxen sodium in the treatment of tension-type headache. Drugs Exp Clin Res 1995;21:89–96.

7   Vangerven JMA, Schoemaker RC, Jacobs LD, Reints A, Ouwerslootvandermeij MJ, Hoedemaker HGJ, Cohen AF: Self-medication of a single headache episode with ketoprofen, ibuprofen or placebo, home-monitored with an electronic patient diary. Br J Clin Pharmacol 1996;42:475–481.

8   Dahlöf CGH, Jacobs LD, Ketoprofen, paracetamol and placebo in the treatment of episodic tension-type headache. Cephalalgia 1996;16:117–123.

9   Steiner TJ, Lange R: Ketoprofen (25 mg) in the symptomatic treatment of episodic tension-type headache: Double-blind placebo-controlled comparison with acetaminophen (1,000 mg). Cephalalgia 1998;18:38–43.

10 Mehlisch DR, Weaver M, Fladung B: Ketoprofen 12.5 and 25 mg, extra strength Tylenol® 1000 mg and placebo for the treatment of patients with episodic tension-type headache. Cephalalgia 1997;17:274.

11 Harden RN, Rogers D, Fink K, Gracely RH: Controlled trial of ketorolac in tension-type headache. Neurology 1998;50:507–509.

12 Langman MJS, Weil J, Wainwright P, Lawson DH, Rawlins MD, Logan RFA, Murphy M, Vessey MP, Colin-Jones DG: Risks of bleeding peptic ulcer associated with individual non-steroidal anti-inflammatory drugs. Lancet 1994;343:1075–1078.

13 Garcia Rodriguez LA, Jick H: Risk of upper gastrointestinal bleeding and perforation associated with individual non-steroidal anti-inflammatory drugs. Lancet 1994;343:769–772.

14 Migliardi JR, Armellino JJ, Friedman M, Gillings DB, Beaver WT: Caffeine as an analgesic adjuvant in tension headache. Clin Pharmacol Ther 1994;56:576–586.

15 Diamond S, Freitag FG, Balm TK, Berry DA: The use of a combination agent of ibuprofen and caffeine in the treatment of episodic tension-type headache. Cephalalgia 1997;17:446.

16 Schattner P, Randerson D: Tiger Balm as a treatment of tension headache. A clinical trial in general practice. Aust Fam Physician 1996;25:216.

17 Göbel H, Heinze A, Dworschak M, Stolze H, Lurch A: Oleum menthae piperitae significantly reduces the symptoms of tension-type headache and its efficacy does not differ from that of acetaminophen. Cephalalgia 1997;17:446.

18 Cerbo R, Barbanti P, Fabbrini G, Pascali MP, Catarci T: Amitriptyline is effective in chronic but not in episodic tension-type headache: Pathogenetic implications. Headache 1998;38:453–457.

19 Zwart JA, Bovim G, Sand T, Sjaastad O: Tension headache: Botulinum toxin paralysis of temporal muscles. Headache 1994;34:458–462.

20 Wheeler A: Botulinum toxin A, adjunctive therapy for refractory headaches associated with pericranial muscle tension. Headache 1998;38:468–471.

21 Autret A, Unger Ph, EURAXI group, Lesaichot JL: Naproxen sodium versus ibuprofen in episodic tension headache. Cephalalgia 1997;17:446.

22 Lance JW, Curran DA: Treatment of chronic tension headache. Lancet 1964;1:1236–1239.

23 Diamond S, Baltes BJ: Chronic tension headache treated with amitriptyline: A double blind study. Headache 1971;11:110–116.

24 Morland TJ, Storli OV, Mogstad TE: Doxepin in the prophylactic treatment of mixed 'vascular' and tension headache. Headache 1979;19:382–383.

25 Fogelholm R, Murros K: Maprotiline in chronic tension headache: A double-blind cross-over study. Headache 1985;25:273–275.

26 Langemark M, Loldrup D, Bech P, Olesen J: Clomipramine and mianserin in the treatment of chronic tension headache. A double-blind, controlled study. Headache 1990;30:118–121.

27 Pfaffenrath V, Hummelsberger J, Pöllmann W, Kaube H, Rath M: MMPI personality profiles in patients with primary headache syndromes. Cephalalgia 1991;11:215–228.

28 Göbel H, Hamouz V, Hansen C, Heininger K, Hirsch S, Lindner V, Soyka D: Effect of amitriptyline prophylaxis on headache symptoms and neurophysiological parameters in tension-type headache; in Olesen J, Schoenen J (eds): Tension-Type Headache: Classification, Mechanisms and Treatment. New York, Raven Press, 1993, pp 275–280.

Prof. J. Schoenen, University Department of Neurology,
CHR Citadelle, Bld. du 12ème de Ligne 1, B-4000 Liège (Belgium)
Tel. +32 4 225 61 11, Fax +32 4 225 64 51, E-Mail schoenen.j@village.uunet.be

Diener HC (ed): Drug Treatment of Migraine and Other Headaches.
Monogr Clin Neurosci. Basel, Karger, 2000, vol 17, pp 322–328

....

Drug Treatment of Cluster Headache

Karl Ekbom[a]*, Jan Erik Hardebo*[b]

[a] Department of Neurology, Huddinge University Hospital, Huddinge, Sweden, and
[b] Department of Neurology, University Hospital, Lund, Sweden

Pain in cluster headache is so intense that over-the-counter medications are ineffective. Furthermore, oral preparations are too slowly absorbed to cure pain within reasonable time. Combinations with codeine at a high dose are often used by the undiagnosed patient, but usually only reduces pain. Besides, such medication may lead to drug-induced headache, and should therefore be avoided. The peak of pain arises within a few minutes, which demands a parenteral or pulmonary drug administration in order to become successful. Today most attacks can be effectively and rapidly aborted by sumatriptan injections or inhalation of oxygen. In severe and chronic cases with a frequency of attacks exceeding two per day reasonably effective prophylactic treatments are available. Evaluation of treatment should consider that cluster headache occurs in periods ('clusters') that are separated by sudden, spontaneous remission periods lasting for months or years. The course of disease is therefore not seldom unpredictable. Dosage of drugs and the administration mode should be individualized and adapted to the rhythm of the attacks. Patients should be encouraged to keep a headache diary and be followed on frequent visits. General advice about triggers such as alcoholic beverages, nitroglycerin and horizontal body position may be given. As with migraine, treatment can be divided into 1) acute symptomatic treatment of individual attacks and 2) prophylactic treatment.

Acute Symptomatic Treatment

Triptans
Sumatriptan is now regarded as the most effective acute treatment of cluster headache. A randomized, double-blind, placebo-controlled, crossover study was

conducted in 39 evaluable patients [1]. Patients were given one dose of suma-triptan 6 mg s.c. to treat one attack and one dose of placebo to treat another, the order being randomized. Seventy-four percent of sumatriptan-treated attacks responded by 15 min, as compared to 26% of placebo-treated attacks. Thirty-six percent of the patients given sumatriptan were pain-free already within 10 min, as compared to 3% of those given placebo. Another randomized, double-blind, placebo-controlled crossover study [2] showed that sumatriptan injection 12 mg was not more effective than sumatriptan injection 6 mg in alleviating cluster headache attacks, but was associated with a higher incidence of adverse events than the 6 mg dose. Long-term results in open clinical trials [3, 4] have shown very good effects. There has been no evidence of tachyphylaxis and suma-triptan has generally been very well tolerated. Side effects and contraindications are described in chapter by Diener, Sumatriptan–Therapy.

Several patients report that pain relief starts as early as 2–5 min after injection [4–6] and the great majority of patients become nearly or completely pain-free within 10–15 min. Sufferers from chronic cluster headache are less responsive [4]. This clinical effect parallels the peak plasma concentration, and occurs considerably faster than in migraine therapy. As suggested by the manufacturer, the autoinjector should be pressed to the skin of the lateral aspect of the mid-thigh area. Particularly in the male patients, such injections are liable to deposit intramuscularly because of a thin subcutaneous tissue depth at this location [7]. In males, therefore, injections should be preferentially made in the gluteal area or an abdominal skin fold.

The nasal spray formulation of sumatriptan has also been tested in an open study in cluster headache [6]. The highest dose commercially available, 20 mg, applied in the nostril on the painful or pain-free side, had a considerably weaker effect on pain than injections. In addition, the onset of effect was slow. At 15 min about half of the patients had not started feeling any relief of pain.

Zolmitriptan, in a placebo-controlled study [8], provides a meaningful pain relief after oral administration of 5 or 10 mg in the majority of patients with episodic, but not in chronic cluster headache. The effect is, however, not significant until 30 min after intake.

Oxygen

Inhalation of 100% oxygen, usually at 6–7 l/min, is long known to be effective and rapid in relieving pain during attacks in the majority (50–80%) of sufferers [9, 10]. The best responders are patients under the age of 50 with episodic cluster headache. An arterial constrictory effect has been suggested as mechanism. The pain declines after 5–15 min of continuous breathing through a loosely applied facial mask. Oxygen should be discontinued if no effect occurs after 15–20 min. Oxygen causes no side effects. Oxygen can be given parallel to prophylactic treatment, but a draw-back of oxygen inhalation treatment is that the patient must have continuous access to the oxygen supply, which in some instances may be impractical. Oxygen tanks should be placed both at home and in the work place. Its use is surrounded by precautions from fire authorities, and this type of treatment is sometimes inconvenient since it cannot be carried around, as for a tablet or an autoinjector. Further, it forces the patient to sit still during treatment, a behavior that usually is incompatible with the intense pain. Only about 1/3 of the patients who accept oxygen continue its use [10].

As a consequence, hyperbaric oxygen (2.5 ATA) has been tested as a prophylactic treatment [11]. Some studies have indicated an effect lasting from a few days to one month, whereas a recent, double-blind placebo-controlled crossover study on episodic and chronic cluster headache showed no significant effect [12].

Ergotamine, Dihydroergotamine

Oral or rectal administration of ergotamine tartrate is of limited value in the treatment of acute attacks. Ergotamine inhalation may give some relief, but there are practical problems with inhaling ergotamine. Ergotamine inhalators are no longer available in many countries. Dihydroergotamine administered by a nasal spray (1 mg) has been compared with placebo in a limited number of patients [13]. There was no difference in the duration of the attacks, but a significantly better effect on the intensity of individual attacks. It was suggested that the investigation should be repeated using a higher dosage. Dihydroergotamine given intravenously or intramuscularly is used in some quarters and has been claimed to be an excellent method of aborting attacks.

Local Anesthetics

Anesthetics, applied deep in the nostril on the painful side, have been tried in attempts to block pain close to its anticipated origin (deep behind the eye). In earlier trials *cocaine* was used, but has won no widespread acceptance because of its addictive potential. *Lidocaine* is preferred today [14, 15]. Lidocaine 20–60 mg given as nasal drops or spray, results in mild to moderate relief within 1–10 min in the majority of patients, but only single patients obtain full pain relief. Accordingly, lidocaine may be useful in the short-term for a limited number of cluster headache sufferers, perhaps as an adjunct to other treatments. *Capsaicin* desensitizes pain neurons by depleting substance P. Daily application of 0.025% capsaicin cream for one week in the nostril on the painful side has been shown to reduce attack frequency and intensity [16]. It may be tried in selected cases.

Prophylactic Treatment

The main aim of treatment is usually to prevent the attacks. *Ergotamine tartrate* given 1/2–1 h before an expected attack has been the standard therapy for many years. Most commonly, this alleviates or entirely eliminates the attack. The daily dose of ergotamine is generally 3 to 4 mg. However, other drugs are now generally preferred.

Calcium-Channel Blockers

By unknown mechanisms calcium-channel blockers are effective as prophylactic treatment of episodic and chronic cluster headache. *Verapamil* is today the most widely used agent; it has a high efficacy in many patients and gives few side effects, also in the high doses that are sometimes needed. Constipation, postural hypotension, water retention and fatigue are the most common side effects. Around 2/3 of the patients improve more than 50% at daily doses of 240–480 mg or higher; severe chronic cases may need from 720 mg up to around 1,200 mg per day [17, 18]. It may be combined with lithium in chronic cases.

Lithium

Lithium is effective against episodic, and notably chronic cluster headache [18–21]. Most patients are improved within a few days of treatment and are also helped by treatment during several years. Others, however, seem to develop drug tolerance. Lithium is effective at rather low serum concentrations, between 0.3 and 0.8 μmol/l, and most patients will benefit from a daily dose of 600–900 mg of lithium carbonate. Side effects are tremor, polyuria, and diarrhea. Renal and thyroid functions should be checked before and during treatment, and the serum levels determined at regular intervals. Lithium affects internal biological rhythms but the exact mechanism of its action in cluster headache is unknown.

Corticosteroids

The corticosteroids prednisone and dexamethasone are effective and rapid-acting prophylactic drugs in the treatment of episodic and also, but to a much lesser extent, chronic cluster headache. The mechanism of action is uncertain. *Prednisone* 40–60 (–80) mg daily or *dexamethasone* 8 mg daily or *methylprednisolone* 500–1,000 mg i.v. usually eliminates or strongly reduces the number of attacks within 1–2 days [22, 23]. Since side effects of steroids increase with long-term use, these agents are utilized only to induce remission in severe cases with attacks of high frequency and intensity. Usually, the headache returns when the dose of prednisone or dexamethasone is reduced below 25 mg and 4 mg per day, respectively. Treatment should be finished within about 3 weeks. This short-term treatment may guide the patient through the mid-part of a severe cluster period, while waiting for it to decline or other drugs to reach effective doses.

Serotonin Inhibitors

Serotonin antagonists have been used for many years as prophylactics against cluster headache. Many investigators have shown that *methysergide* in a daily dose of 3–6 mg is effective in about 70% of cases [24]. Treatment should be interrupted every four months for a two-week interval, to minimize the risk of fibrotic complications. Other side effects are nausea, dizziness, epigastric pain, leg cramps. It has been suggested that the metabolite, methylergometrine, is the active agent. Another serotonin antagonist, *pizotifen* (not available in the United States), may be tried in those cluster headache patients, who do not respond to conventional treatment. There is one single-blind trial of pizotifen in cluster headache with positive results [25]. The dose is normally between 2 to 3 mg per day. Side effects are sedation, increase of appetite and weight gain.

Other Treatments

A recent therapeutic approach is resetting of internal pacemakers by shifting sleep-wake cycles and/or exposure to bright light. Other medications that have been tried recently are sodium valproate, melatonin, somatostatin, tizanidine or clonidine transdermally. The results are mostly based upon single reports on rather small patient series.

To summarize, cluster headache is one of the most severe pain conditions known to mankind. The suffering of the patient is enormous, which places special demands on the treating physician as regards his/her empathy and understanding of the patient's whole situation. Prioritization of drugs for the prevention of cluster headache is shown in the following, which is a summary of a recent consensus discussion at the Ninth International Headache Research Seminar in Copenhagen on November 20–22, 1998 [26]. It also accords well with the treatment recommendations given by Ekbom and Solomon [27].

Prophylactic Treatment of Episodic Cluster Headache
a) Single drug:
1. Verapamil
2. Prednisone
3. Ergotamine tartrate
4. Methysergide
5. Lithium carbonate
6. Pizotifen.

b) Combination of drugs:
1. Verapamil + prednisone
2. Verapamil + ergotamine
3. Verapamil + lithium.

Prophylactic Treatment of Chronic Cluster Headache
a) Single drug:
1. Verapamil
2. Lithium carbonate
3. Methysergide
4. Pizotifen.
b) Combination of drugs:
1. Verapamil + lithium
2. Verapamil + ergotamine
3. Verapamil + ergotamine + lithium.

References

1   The Sumatriptan Cluster Headache Study Group: Treatment of acute cluster headache with suma-triptan. N Engl J Med 1991;325:322–326.
2   Ekbom K, Monstad I, Prusinski A, Cole J, Pilgrim AJ, Noronha D: Subcutaneous sumatriptan in the acute treatment of cluster headache: A dose comparison study. Acta Neurol Scand 1993;88:63–69.
3   Ekbom K, Krabbe A, Micieli G, Prusinski A, Cole JA, Pilgrim A, Noronha D for the Sumatriptan Cluster Headache Long-Term Study Group: Cluster headache attacks treated for up to three months with subcutaneous sumatriptan (6 mg). Cephalalgia 1995;15:230–236.
4   Göbel H, Lindner V, Heinze A, Ribbat M, Deuschl G: Acute therapy for cluster headache with sumatriptan: Findings of a one-year long-term study. Neurology 1998;51:908–911.
5   Hardebo JE: Subcutaneous sumatriptan in cluster headache: A time study of the effect on pain and autonomic symptoms. Headache 1993;33:18–21.
6   Hardebo JE, Dahlöf C: Sumatriptan nasal spray (20 mg/dose) in the acute treatment of cluster headache. Cephalalgia 1998;18:487–489.
7   Frid A, Hardebo JE: The thigh may not be suitable as an injection site for patients self-injecting sumatriptan. Neurology 1997;49:559–561.
8   Bahra A, Gawel M, Hardebo JE, Millson D, Breen SA, Goadsby PJ: Oral zolmitriptan is effective in the acute treatment of cluster headache. Neurology (in press).
9   Kudrow L: Response of cluster headache attacks to oxygen inhalation. Headache 1981;21:1–4.
10 Gallagher RM, Mueller L, Ciervo CA: Analgesic use in cluster headache. Headache 1996;36:105–107.
11 Di Sabato F, Fusco BM, Pelaia P, Giacovazzo M: Hyperbaric oxygen therapy in cluster headache. Pain 1993;52:243–245.
12 Nilsson-Remahl AIM, Ansjön R, Lind F, Waldenlind E: No prophylactic effect of hyperbaric oxygen during active cluster headache: A double-blind placebo-controlled cross-over study. Cephalalgia 1997;17:456.
13 Andersson PG, Jespersen LT: Dihydroergotamine nasal spray in the treatment of attacks of cluster headache. Cephalalgia 1986;6:51–54.
14 Hardebo JE, Elner A: Nerves and vessels in the pterygopalatine fossa and symptoms of cluster headache. Headache 1987;27:528–532.

15   Robbins L: Intranasal lidocaine for cluster headache. Headache 1995;35:83–84.
16   Marks DR, Rapoport A, Padla D, Weeks R, Rosum R, Sheftell F, Arrowsmith F: A double-blind placebo-controlled trial of intranasal capsaicin for cluster headache. Cephalalgia 1993;13:114–116.
17   Gabai IJ, Spierings ELH: Prophylactic treatment of cluster headache with verapamil. Headache 1989;29:167–168.
18   Bussone G, Leone M, Peccarisi C, Micieli G, Granella F, Magri M, Manzoni GC, Nappi G: Double blind comparison of lithium and verapamil in cluster headache prophylaxis. Headache 1990;30: 411–417.
19   Ekbom K: Litium vid kroniska symtom av cluster headache. Opusc Med 1974;19:148–156.
20   Kudrow L: Comparative results of prednisone, methysergide, and lithium therapy in cluster headache; in Greene R (ed): Current Concepts of Migraine Research. New York, Raven Press, 1978, pp 159–163.
21   Manzoni GC, Bono G, Lanfranchi M, Micieli G, Terzano MG, Nappi G: Lithium carbonate in cluster headache: Assessment of its short- and long-term therapeutic efficacy. Cephalalgia 1983;3: 109–114.
22   Anthony M, Daher BN: Mechanism of action of steroids in cluster headache; in Clifford Rose F (ed): New Advances in Headache Research: 2. London, Smith-Gordon, 1992, pp 271–274.
23   Cianchetti C, Zuddas A, Marchei F: High dose intravenous methylprednisolone in cluster headache. J Neurol Neurosurg Psychiat 1998;64:418.
24   Curran DA, Hinterberger H, Lance JW: Methysergide. Res Clin Stud Headache 1967;1:74–122.
25   Ekbom K: Prophylactic treatment of cluster headache with a new serotonin antagonist, BC 105. Acta Neurol Scand 1969;45:601–610.
26   Olesen J, Goadsby P: Cluster headache and related conditions. Ninth International Headache Research Seminar, Copenhagen, November 20–22, 1998.
27   Ekbom K, Solomon S: Management of cluster headache; in Olesen J, Tfelt-Hansen P, Welch KMA (eds): The Headaches, ed 2. New York, Lippincott-Raven (in press).

Karl Ekbom, MD, PhD, Department of Neurology, Huddinge University Hospital,
SE-141 86 Huddinge (Sweden)
Tel. +46 8 585 82655, Fax +46 8 774 4822

Diener HC (ed): Drug Treatment of Migraine and Other Headaches.
Monogr Clin Neurosci. Basel, Karger, 2000, vol 17, pp 329–336

....
Post-Traumatic Headache

Matthias Keidel

Department of Neurology, University of Essen, Essen, Germany

Headache which occurs as the result of a head trauma (HT) or whiplash injury (WI) is known as post-traumatic headache. Also included here are localized headaches with scalp or cranial vault injuries and symptomatic headaches with trauma related intracranial, epidural, subdural, subarachnoid and intracerebral haemorrhage or raised intracranial pressure. The post-traumatic headache shows a manifold clinical picture (tension-type headache, migraine headache, cluster headache, cervicogenic headache), although the post-traumatic tension-type headache is the most common [1–3]. This has to be distinguished from the well-known primary idiopathic headache form as a secondary headache. An acute post-traumatic headache (onset <14 days, end <8 weeks after the trauma) is differentiated from a chronic post-traumatic headache (onset <14 days, duration >8 weeks) [4]. For a clear-cut classification there must be the temporal relationship of the post-traumatic headache to a head injury or a whiplash injury with a description of amnesia or loss of consciousness present in head trauma. In addition to this, according to the classification criteria of the IHS (International Headache Society) abnormalities should be expected in the clinical neurological examination as well as in the radiological, neurophysiological or neuropsychological investigations [4].

Epidemiology

Approximately 90% of minor head injuries are followed by a post-traumatic headache. Headache following minor head injuries is more common and protracted than the headache following severe head injuries. The incidence and severity of the post-traumatic headache does not correlate with the length of the traumatic loss of conciousness or the cerebral lesions observed on CT or MRI.

The incidence following 'minor' whiplash injury (grade I or II) is also about 90%. In half of the patients with a whiplash injury the post-traumatic headache is associated with a feeling of heaviness of the head. The incidence of post-traumatic headache following head trauma or whiplash injury is observed in the following decreasing order: tension-type headache 90%, cervicogenic headache 8%, migraine 2.5% [2, 3, 5]. The exact incidence of cluster headache is not known. Anecdotally described are the post-traumatic occurrence of a basilar migraine or a post-traumatic headache associated with sexual activity [1].

History and Clinical Findings

Different from the primary, idiopathic headache, the post-traumatic headache (with or without accompanying neck symptoms) is the cardinal symptom found in the manifold symptomatology of the post-traumatic syndrome. In addition to the pain syndrome this is characterized in the acute phase (i) by a vegetative syndrome (e.g. non-systematic vertigo, nausea/vomiting, orthostatic dysregulation, thermodysregulation), (ii) by a neurasthenic-depressive syndrome (e.g. subjectively impaired cognitive performance with eventual neuropsychological deficits, depressive mood, nervousness, irritability) and (iii) by a 'sensory' syndrome with mainly oversensitivity to light and noise [6, 7].

The generally seen post-traumatic headache of the *tension-type* (90%) is characterized by a holocephalic localization (67%), or else distributed in a band, helmet or cap-like form. It has a dull-pressing or dragging character (77%). It is seldom experienced as episodic, usually as continuous, fluctuating in intensity with an increase in pain during the evening [6, 8, 9].

The post-traumatic *cervicogenic headache* (8% following an acute whiplash injury of the cervical spine) is clinically characterized by a strongly unilateral nuchal pain without side change and with limited cervical spine mobility. The pain has a dragging character and radiates from occipital to frontotemporal without accompanying brachialgia. The pain can be triggered by turning the head, by defined positioning of the head or pressure on the occipital nerve entry points. The diagnosis can be confirmed by relief from pain after local anaesthetic infiltration of the tender greater occipital nerve entry point or C2 root [10].

Post-traumatic *migraine-like* headache is mainly experienced as a pulsating, hemicranial and side-changing head pain. Accompanying vegetative complaints like nausea, vomiting, dizziness or photo- and/or phonophobia are common. An aura with neurological sensations and/or deficits is possible. Usually the trauma acts as the trigger for an accumulation of attacks, it is not however considered as the cause of migraine.

The post-traumatic *cluster-type* headache cannot be clinically distinguished from the primary cluster headache. The clinical picture is characterized by unilateral, periorbital and frontotemporal pressing or throbbing head or facial pain, accompanied by local autonomic signs like ptosis, miosis, enophthalmus, lacrimation, rhinorrhea and conjunctival injection.

Clinically important, as it is often not recognized as a post-traumatic tension-type headache, is a persistent *drug-induced headache* which has developed after whiplash injury or head trauma due to prolonged or inadequate intake of analgesics.

Differential Diagnosis

The following symptomatologies can cause problems in the differential diagnosis of post-traumatic headache: (i) unilateral nuchal pain as part of a vertebral dissection, (ii) unilateral neck and facial pain as part of a traumatic carotid artery dissection, (iii) local circumscript headache as part of an isolated head contusion, (iv) half-sided or mainly one-sided headache in intracranial bleeding (e.g. epi- or subdural, subarachnoid or intracerebral haemorrhage) and (v) holocephalic headache with vegetative signs as part of raised intracranial pressure.

Course

Following minor head injury, within the first month 90% of patients suffer from a post-traumatic headache, after one year 35%, after two years 22% and after three years still 20%. Over 80% of patients with post-traumatic headache after HT are free of headache after 6 months. 10–15% develop a chronic 'post-concussion' syndrome including headache. Prognostically unfavourable factors for the development of a chronic post-traumatic syndrome following HT are: female gender, age >40 years, high self-expectations, pending litigation, lower educational standard, lower intellectual and socio-economic level, chronic alcohol abuse, positive history of repeated HT and previous headache as well as polytraumatization.

Patients with chronic post-traumatic syndrome after head injury with post-traumatic headache suffer from depressive mood, show raised levels of anxiety and have accumulated (secondary) social problems [8, 11].

The post-traumatic headache after minor whiplash injury generally resolves within 3 months with an average duration of the post-traumatic headache of three weeks. Longer post-traumatic headache duration is found in patients with: initially severe headache, marked limitation of passive cervical spine mobility, an initially poor general well-being, depressive mood and the presence of numerous somatic-vegetative complaints, increased age, a previous history of head injury, a positive headache history, abnormal cervical spine X-ray findings (fracture, luxation, kink formation) and with neurological abnormalities [6].

Treatment

The treatment possibilities of the different types of post-traumatic headache are summarized below [2–4]. Recommendations of the general management of the post-traumatic syndrome are given in addition to the specific strategies of drug therapy of the distinct post-traumatic headache types. Most recommendations are based on experience and not on randomized controlled trials.

Drug Treatment

The acute and prophylactic drug treatment is listed for the acute and chronic post-traumatic tension type headache, the post-traumatic migraine-type headache, the post-traumatic cluster-type headache and the drug-induced persistent headache.

Acute Post-Traumatic Tension-Type Headache

Before onset of drug treatment a secondary, symptomatic headache e.g. due to fracture or intracranial (e.g. subdural, subarachnoidal or intracerebral) bleeding should not be overseen. Because of the danger of inducing a rebleeding it has to be taken care that ASS is only prescribed after exclusion of any intracranial haemorrhage. Analgetic combination preparations should not be prescribed, because of the high probability of developing drug-induced headache, which is often misclassified as a post-traumatic headache by the patient. The danger of an analgesic-induced persistent headache increases with a drug intake >4 weeks. This has to be prevented by a controlled and short-lasting prescription of analgetics and by narrow timed re-examinations of the patient (table 1).

Table 1. Drug treatment of acute post-traumatic tension type headache

Analgesics/Anti-inflammatories	
Acetylsalicylic acid (ASS)	500–1,000 mg daily, max. 1,500 mg daily
Alternatives	
Paracetamol	500–1,000 mg daily, max. 1,500 mg daily
Ibuprofen	400–600 mg daily
Naproxen	500–1,000 mg daily

Adapted from the recommendations of the German Migraine and Headache Society [2, 5].

Table 2. Drug treatment of chronic post-traumatic tension type headache

Antidepressants	(daily doses)
Amitriptyline: evening dose of	25–100 mg or 25–0–75 mg
Alternative: Amitryptiline-N-oxide	30–90 mg
2nd choice: doxepine	50–100 mg, max. 150 mg
2nd choice: imipramine	75–100 mg, max. 150 mg
MAO blockers: Tranylcypromine	20–40 mg

Adapted from the recommendations of the German Migraine and Headache Society [2–5].

Chronic Post-Traumatic Tension-Type Headache

If post-traumatic tension-type headache lasts longer than 8 weeks and becomes chronic according to the definition of the IHS, the prescription of tricyclic anti-depressants should be considered.

The specialist, who performs the treatment, should be aware, (i) of a slow increase of dosage; (ii) of a sufficient dosage, (iii) of a sufficiently long intake (treatment success can only be evaluated after 8 weeks of intake) and (iv) of the contraindications (among others prostatism, glaucoma). An ECG should be done before treatment with tricyclic thymoleptics. MAO blockers should be given only in refractory cases and fully controlled (table 2).

Table 3. Drug treatment of post-traumatic migraine-type headache

Treatment of attacks	
Antiemetic: Metoclopramide	10–20 mg p.o.
Alternative: Domperidone	10–20 mg p.o.
Analgesics: ASS	1,000 mg as effervescent tablet (20 min after antiemetic)
Alternatives:	
Paracetamol	1,000 mg supp.
Ibuprofen	600 mg dissolved
Prophylactic treatment	
Beta blockers: Metoprolol	up to 200 mg daily
Alternative: Propranolol	up to max. 240 mg daily

For further details see migraine chapters.

Post-Traumatic Migraine-Type Headache

The treatment of the post-traumatic migraine-type headache is based on the therapeutic standards of the idiopathic migraine (for further treatment recommendations see the migraine chapters in this volume) (table 3).

Post-Traumatic Cluster-Type Headache

The drug treatment of post-traumatic cluster-type headache is summarized in table 4.

Drug-Induced Persistent Headache

The drug-induced persistent headache is treated by discontinuing analgesic, anti-inflammatory, relaxant or ergotamine preparation and by tailing off of barbiturates or benzodiazepines. A too sudden discontinuation of benzodiazepines may provoke cerebral fits! Antiemetics can be prescribed if necessary. For tiding over the initial headache exacerbation naproxen 2×500 mg daily can be given. For an eventual introduction of a prophylaxis for an underlying tension-type headache it is referred to the relevant chapter in this volume.

Table 4. Recommendations of acute treatment of post-traumatic cluster attacks and of prophylaxis of post-traumatic cluster-type headache

---

Attack treatment
  Inhalation of 100% oxygen (7l/min) over 15 min and/or
  Nasal instillation of 4% lignocaine and/or
  DHE (1–2 mg) s.c. or
  Sumatriptan (6 mg) s.c.

Prophylaxis
  Verapamil increasing dosages up to 3×80 mg daily
  Alternative: lithium 600–900 mg daily (plasma levels of max. 0.9 mmol/l)
  Alternative: 'breakthrough attempt' with steroids: prednisone 60 mg for 3
    days; gradual tailing of over 14 days

Non-Drug Treatment

The general (drug-free) management of the post-traumatic headache together with neck pain in the context of a cervicocephalic pain syndrome following head trauma with accompanying cervical spine distortion or following whiplash injury includes:

(i) immobilization of the cervical spine by means of a cervical collar as short as possible (if any); (ii) supplementary physical therapy only in the acute phase with dry heat (infrared light, warm air, heat pillows), with moist heat (fango (volcanic mud) packs) or better with cold packs; (iii) physiotherapy with e.g. passive and active movement of the cervical spine, isometric tension, complex movements and postural strengthening; (iv) manual treatment attempts for releasing vertebral segmental blockade; (v) general physical health recommendations (sport, avoidance of alcohol, nicotine or caffeine, vegetative stabilization with e.g. hot and cold showers, brush massage, regular lifestyle); (vi) learning of automobilization of the cervical spine and of muscle relaxation techniques of the shoulder-neck musculature (according to Jacobson), possibly in combination with EMG biofeedback techniques; (vii) in cases of chronification concomitant psychotherapy-based (among others) on concepts of cognitive coping strategies for pain and stress; (viii) course-dependent approach of an interdisciplinary and multi-modal regime of therapy; (ix) empathetic guidance of the patient; (x) explanation of the good prognosis in general; (xi) narrow timed re-examinations of the patient in the acute phase and (xii) fast solving of accident-related medico-legal problems.

The Following Procedures Should be Avoided

(i) Cervical support longer than a few days (avoidance of immobilization-related hypotrophy of the neck musculature); (ii) late start of physiotherapy; (iii) manual traction of the cervical spine or manual-medical treatment (cave: vertebral dissection); (iv) longer bedrest (danger of chronification of the post-traumatic syndrome including post-traumatic headache).

Nonbeneficial and Unnecessary Therapies

These include massage of the stretched musculature, reflex zone massages, local invasive anaesthetic measures like infiltration or neural therapy, acupuncture, acupressure, fresh cells or ozone therapy, local nuchal unguent treatment, systemic treatment with steroids and antihistamines or the use of neuroleptics, ergotamine preparations or opioids in the post-traumatic headache treatment.

References

1   Keidel M, Diener HC: Der posttraumatische Kopfschmerz. Nervenarzt 1997;68:769–777.
2   Keidel M, Ramadan N: Acute posttraumatic headache; in Olesen J, Welch KMA, Tfelt-Hansen P (eds): The Headaches, ed 2. Philadelphia, Lippincott-Raven Publishers, 1999 (in press).
3   Ramadan N, Keidel M: Chronic posttraumatic headache; in Olesen J, Welch KMA, Tfelt-Hansen P (eds): The Headaches, ed 2. Philadelphia, Lippincott-Raven Publishers, 1999 (in press).
4   Headache Classification Committee of the International Headache Society: Classification and diagnostic criteria for headache disorders, cranial neuralgias and facial pain. Cephalalgia 1988;8(suppl 7): 1–96.
5   Keidel M, Neu IS, Langohr HD, Göbel H: Therapie des posttraumatischen Kopfschmerzes nach Schädel-Hirn-Trauma und HWS-Distorsion. Empfehlungen der Deutschen Migräne- und Kopfschmerzgesellschaft. Schmerz 1995;12:350–367.
6   Keidel M, Pearce JMS: Whiplash injury; in Brandt Th, Dichgans J, Diener HC, Caplan LR, Kennard Ch (eds): Neurological Disorders: Course and Treatment. San Diego, Academic Press, 1996, pp 65–76.
7   Narayan RK, Wilberger JE, Povlishock JT (eds): Neurotrauma. New York, McGraw-Hill, 1996, pp 119–135.
8   Keidel M, Miller JD: Head trauma; in Brandt Th, Caplan LR, Dichgans J, Diener HC, Kennard Ch (eds): Neurological Disorders: Course and Treatment. San Diego, Academic Press, 1996, pp 531–544.
9   Kügelgen B (ed): Neuroorthopädie VI. Berlin/Heidelberg/New York, Springer, 1995, pp 73–113.
10   Pöllmann W, Keidel M, Pfaffenrath V: Headache and the cervical spine: A critical review. Cephalalgia 1997;17:801–816.
11   Haas DC: Chronic post-traumatic headaches classified and compared with natural headaches. Cephalalgia 1996;16:486–493.

PD Dr. Matthias Keidel, University of Essen, Department of Neurology,
Hufelandstrasse 55, D–45122 Essen (Germany)
Tel. +49 201 723 2364, Fax +49 201 723 5919, E-Mail keidel@uni-essen.de

Diener HC (ed): Drug Treatment of Migraine and Other Headaches.
Monogr Clin Neurosci. Basel, Karger, 2000, vol 17, pp 337–346

....

Paroxysmal Hemicranias

Holger Kaube

Department of Neurology, University Hospital of Essen, Essen, Germany, and
Institute of Neurology, London, UK

A common feature of all paroxysmal headaches is the short duration of
the headache attacks. In contrast to migraine and tension-type headache,
attacks may only last for seconds to minutes. In this chapter the focus will lie
on the more common hemicranial manifestations as a subset of paroxysmal
headaches. In sequence of prevalence the following headache syndromes and
their treatments will be discussed in detail: trigeminal neuralgia, idiopathic
stabbing headache, episodic and chronic paroxysmal hemicrania, hemicrania
continua, SUNCT-syndrome (short lasting neuralgia with conjunctival injection and tearing) and cluster-tic syndrome. For cluster headache see chapter
by Ekbom and Hardebo. Paroxysmal hemicranias present a very heterogenous
group with regard to epidemiology, aetiology, pathophysiology, associated
symptoms and responsiveness to treatment. Principally, as is true for all headache syndromes the diagnosis of paroxysmal hemicranias is entirely based on
the headache history with regard to frequency and duration of attacks, severity,
associated symptoms and again responsiveness to treatment (for summary see
table 1). Additional diagnostic certainty may be derived from clinical signs
and further investigations. For review see [1].

Diagnostic Features of Paroxysmal Hemicranias

Characteristics of Pain. Most paroxysmal hemicranias are side constant
unilateral and the pain maximum is concentrated in a particular region of the
headache. In cluster headache, chronic and episodic paroxysmal hemicrania,
hemicrania continua and SUNCT the typical localization is retro-ocular, orbital or temporal. In rare cases occipital and extracranial manifestations have
been described [2]. In trigeminal neuralgia the stabbing/shooting and electrify-

Table 1. Differential diagnosis of paroxysmal hemicranias

Headache	Sex (m:f)	Pain: type	Pain: severity	Site	Attack: duration	Attack: freq.	Auton. signs	Indo- meth.	Alcohol- sensitive
CH	9:1	boring	very severe	orbital temporal	15–180 min	1–8/day	+	−	+
CPH	1:3	throbbing/ boring	very severe	orbital temporal	2–45 min	1–40/day	+	+	+
EPH	1:1	throbbing	very severe	orbital temporal	1–30 min	3–30/day	+	+	+
SUNCT	8:1	stabbing	mod. to severe	orbital temporal	5–250 sec	1/day to 30/h	+	−	+
ISH	f>m	stabbing	severe	any part	<1 sec	few to many/day	−	+	−
TN	f>m	stabbing	very severe	V2/V3>V1	<1 sec	few to many/day	−	−	−
HC	1:1.8	steady	mod. to severe	unilateral	cont.	5–12/day	+	+	−

CH = Cluster headache; CPH = chronic paroxysmal hemicrania; EPH = episodic paroxysmal hemicrania; ISH = idiopathic stabbing headache; TN = trigeminal neuralgia; HC = hemicrania continua. Adapted from Goadsby and Lipton, 1997 [1].

ing pain usually projects to the maxillary and mandibular less often the ophthalmic territory of the trigeminal nerve. Idiopathic stabbing headaches occur at any cranial localization and frequently change sites [3]. The most severe headache intensities occur in cluster headache, chronic and episodic paroxysmal hemicrania, and trigeminal neuralgia. In descending order idiopathic stabbing headaches, hemicrania continua and SUNCT-syndrome only reach severe to moderate severity. A very distinctive and diagnostically valuable feature is the headache duration and frequency: idiopathic stabbing headaches and trigeminal neuralgia attacks last for subseconds to seconds and occur 1–100 times daily. SUNCT attacks vary between 5 seconds to 5 minutes 1–30 times daily. Longer attack durations between a few min to 45 min up to 30 times daily are typical for chronic and episodic paroxysmal hemicrania [1]. Not truly paroxysmal is hemicrania continua – the headache is permanent but may undulate in severity over hours [4].

Autonomic Symptoms. Similar to cluster headache chronic and episodic paroxysmal hemicrania, hemicrania continua and SUNCT-syndrome are typically accompanied by one or several of the following autonomic signs: conjunctival injection, lacrimation, nasal congestion, rhinorrhea, ptosis or eyelid oedema. In contrast, classic trigeminal neuralgia and idiopathic stabbing headaches [3] have no clinically apparent autonomic dysfunction.

Precipitating Factors. Trigeminal neuralgia attacks are typically elicited by touch or brush in the affected trigeminal territory, chewing, drinking or eating. Consumption of alcohol may precipitate cluster headache attacks, chronic and episodic paroxysmal hemicrania and SUNCT-syndrome [1]. In many cases SUNCT attacks follow movement of the neck or touch and manipulations in the face or even extracranially similar to trigeminal neuralgia [2].

As a rare exception, cluster-tic syndrome is described as a cluster headache with autonomic signs triggerable in the same way as trigeminal neuralgia [5, 6].

In some of the paroxysmal hemicranias indomethacin is the only prophylactic treatment available. Although some exceptions have been published, as a rule of thumb and as an additional diagnostic feature, a positive treatment response to indomethacin can be expected in chronic and episodic paroxysmal hemicrania, hemicrania continua and idiopathic stabbing headaches [3, 7].

Further Diagnostic Investigations

Most paroxysmal hemicranias described, mainly occur as primary headache syndromes, i.e. no underlying structural, metabolic, inflammatory or infectious causes for the headache can be found. However, there are some important exceptions. In most cases of trigeminal neuralgia a microvascular compression syndrome between the trigeminal nerve root and cerebellar arteries or veins is the aetiopathogenetic cause of the disease. Bilateral occurrence and manifestations in the young must raise suspicion of inflammatory lesion, multiple sclerosis, tumors or vascular malformations and necessitate further investigations including cranial MR and lumbar puncture. The same is true for all patients with paroxysmal hemicranias and pathological neurological findings. Also patients who only respond to unusually high doses of indomethacin or with diminishing response after initially successful treatment warrant further diagnostic work-up [1]. Therefore, a typical positive response to a recommended treatment does not exclude the possibility of a potentially dangerous secondary headache syndrome.

Treatment

Trigeminal neuralgia (TN): Pharmacological Treatment
Since the 1960s the pharmacological treatment of TN has been the domain of classic anticonvulsants [8]. Drug of first choice is carbamazepine (CBZ), followed by phenytoin (PHT) [9]. New studies, partly uncontrolled and with smaller numbers, also show efficacy of gabapentine [10–14], lamotrigine [15, 16] and oxcarbazepine [17]. However, the results of larger trials must be awaited before general recommendations can be made. For therapeutic regimens and dosage see table 2.

Table 2. Treatment of trigeminal neuralgia: medication

- First choice
  Carbamazepine
  Increasing doses, towards 200 mg three times daily (rapid saturation only in in-patients) up to a maximum of 6×200 mg orally or toxic symptoms (>15 μg/ml). Initial pain relief 80–90%; after 6 months 25–50%.
  Side effects: dizziness, ataxia, nausea, diplopia, exanthema, idiosyncratic reactions e.g. leucopaenia, thrombocytopaenia, hepatic dysfunction, atrioventricular block.
  Contraindications: Pregnancy, lactation, hepatic damage.
  Carbamazepine is a potent enzyme inducer and interacts with oral contraceptives, steroids, anticoagulants. Drugs e.g. cimetidine, danazol, erythromycin, verapimil, etc. inhibit its metabolism with resultant neurotoxicity.

- Second choice
  Phenytoin
  Initial oral administration 3×100 mg/day up to a maximum 5×100 mg or toxic symptoms. Pain relief after 2 weeks 50–70%; after 6 months approximately 25%.
  Side effects: Anorexia, dyspepsia, nausea, vomiting, ataxia, drowsiness, gum hypertrophy, hirsutism, megaloblastic anaemia, hepatotoxicity.
  Contraindications: Pregnancy, lactation, hepatic damage.
  Phenytoin is a potent enzyme inducer and interacts with other anti-epileptic drugs, anti-coagulants, steroids, cyclosporin, oral contraceptives.

- Third choice
  Baclofen
  Initial oral administration 4×10 mg up to a maximum 4×20 mg/day possibly combined with carbamazepine or phenytoin.
  Side effects: Nausea, vomiting, hypotension, constipation, headache, dizziness, infrequently psychosis and seizures.
  Contraindications: Gastrointestinal ulcer, liver damage, epilepsy, recent stroke, psychiatric disorder.

- Fourth choice
  Pimozide 4–12 mg/day
  Side effects: Cholinergic e.g. fatigue, dizziness, hypersalivation, bradycardia, hypotension, increased GIT motility and akinesia and delayed akinesia.

Adapted from Brandt et al. 1996 [41].

The initial response rate after CBZ and PHT is usually excellent with 70–90%, but may drop to 25% during the course of treatment over weeks or months In the case of intolerable side effects with CBZ and PHT alternative but less effective substances are the GABA-agonist baclofen (BAC) [18, 19] and the neuroleptic pimozide [20]. Also, combinations of BAC with CBZ or

Table 3. Treatment of trigeminal neuralgia: surgery

- First choice
  Microvascular decompression (Gardner-Jannetta)
  Satisfactory success of approx. 80% (relapse rate of approx. 20% within 2 years) involves
    some risk, particularly among elderly patients (>70 years) and patients in poor state
    of health and should only be done by surgeons experienced in the technique.

- Second choice (first choice for elderpatients and patients with trigeminal neuralgia of
    the ophthalmic division)
  Percutaneous thermocoagulation (Sweet)
  Satisfactory success sometimes only after repetition of up to 80% (relapse rate of approx.
    20% within years) minimum strain involved in operation, possible even for elderly
    patients in a poor state of health.
  Percutaneous microcompression (even simpler operation) or percutaneous postganglionic
    glycerine instillation.

- Step 3. Last resorts in the case of anaesthesia dolorosa
  Stimulation therapy via implanted electrodes of the gasserian ganglion or in the brain
    stem

Adapted from Brandt et al. 1996 [41].

PHT and CBZ and PHT have been suggested. Other neuroleptics such as haloperidol and tricyclic antidepressants are not effective in TN.

Although, the analgesic effect of anticonvulsants correlates with plasma levels [21] the therapeutic regimen is not governed by plasma level measurements but dosage depends on the clinical response. In order to avoid unnecessary transient side effects that may lead to premature disrupture of treatment, dosages should generally be increased slowly. Once an effective dose has been reached, slow-release formulations should be preferred. Before pharmacological treatment is abandoned in favour of surgical interventions, a trial attempt with gabapentin, lamotrigine or oxcarbazepine may seem worthwhile considering the possibly more favourable spectra of side effects.

Surgical Treatment

If pharmacological treatment does not allow satisfactory control of TN two surgical interventions have been shown to be most successful. For a short overview see table 3. In younger patients with normal operative risks microvascular decompression of the trigeminal root according to Janetta is the treatment of first choice . The trigeminal root is identified after suboccipital

---

craniotomy and a small sponge inserted between the nerve and aberrant or elongated arteries. Compressing veins are coagulated. The initial response rate is 80% [22]. Long-term follow-up studies report remission rates between 70–80% [22]. In cases of relapse decompressive surgery can be repeated. Perioperative mortality is between 0.22% and 1.5%. Postoperative morbidity can be severe including cerebellar oedema, subdural and epidural haematoma. Permanent cranial nerve lesions occur in up to 5%.

For patients with increased operative risks thermocoagulation of the trigeminal ganglion according to Sweet has proven particularly suitable [23, 24]. Under short anaesthesia a thermo-controlled radiofrequency electrode is inserted through the foramen ovale. Careful monitoring of the coagulation temperature allows preferential destruction of nociceptive fibres and minimal loss of normal aesthesia to touch in the corresponding skin area. The operative mortality and morbidity (<4%) is lower than after open surgery for decompressive interventions. However, the recurrence rate after 5 years varies between 21% and 100% depending on the initial extent of the postoperative sensory deficit, indicating regeneration of trigeminal fibres [25].

Other percutanous interventions are the postganglionic glycerol instillation [26] and microcompression of the Gasserian ganglion [27]. Both methods show similar results to thermocoagulation but are not used as widely.

A rare (<4%) but awesome sequelae after all surgical lesions is anaesthesia dolorosa as neuropathic pain syndrome after deafferentiation. Because of its central nature anaesthesia dolorosa does not respond to further surgical interventions and may not respond satisfactorily to classical treatment of neuropathic pain such as oral slow-release opioids and tricyclic antidepressants. As ultima ratio electrode implants in the region of the central grey have been used [28].

Since 1991 the use of the gamma knife has also been advocated for the treatment of TN [29]. The most recent 2-year follow-up study reports on a 70% remission rate [30], however numbers are still too small to make general recommendations. The possible long-term sequelae of the radiation are not yet known.

Treatment of Rare Paroxysmal Hemicranias

Indomethacin responsive headache syndromes: Idiopathic stabbing headache, chronic and episodic paroxysmal hemicrania and hemicrania continua.

Idiopathic stabbing headache (ISH) occurs in all ages and predominantly in females and patients with other primary headache syndromes. Despite the severe intensity of the headache, most patients only experience a few of the very short-lasting stabs (≤1 second) per day or week and do not contact a

Table 4. Treatment of idiopathic stabbing headache (ISH), chronic and episodic paroxysmal hemicrania (CPH, EPH) and hemicrania continua

---

Indomethacin
- For a short indomethacin test, 50 mg once or twice daily can be administered intramuscularly.
- Indomethacin 25–50 mg 2–3 times daily orally or as suppositories.
- If necessary increase dose up to 250 mg/day within the first week.
- After effective dose is reached: successive reduction to determine minimal daily dose.
- Alternative oral and rectal administration to minimize gastric and rectal mucosal irritation.
- Consider additional medication with H2-blockers or proton pump inhibitors.
- Side effects: gastrointestinal disorders with pain, occult haemorrhage, ulcers, allergic reactions, suppression of haematopoiesis, impairment of renal and hepatic function, sodium and water retention; long-term use can induce continuous headaches
- Contraindications: gastric and intestinal ulcers, proctitis, pregnancy and lactation, clotting disorders

---

physician or require daily medication for prevention, but may only require reassurance about the benign nature of the symptoms. Obviously, attack treatment is not possible because of the short duration. In cases with high attack frequency and interference with daily activities symptomatic treatment with indomethacin may be commenced (see table 4 for details) [3].

In chronic paroxysmal hemicrania (CPH) and episodic paroxysmal hemicrania (EPH) the painful attacks of high severity with durations of up to 45 min and pronounced autonomic symptoms occur many times a day, disrupting normal life. Treatment of first choice is indomethacin (IND) (see table 4 for details) [1, 31]. Usually after discontinuation of treatment with indomethacin the symptoms reappear. As a diagnostic measure and initiation of therapy an intramascular injection of IND has been suggested [7]. If treatment with IND is ineffective other treatments with NSAIDS such as naproxen [32] and acetylsalicylic have been suggested [33, 34] based on small numbers of treated cases. Also in case studies, verapamil [35, 36] and acetazolamide [37] have shown some beneficial effects in CPH. Because of the relatively short duration of the attacks a report on effective treatment with oral sumatriptan does not seem convincing [38]. Recently reevaluation of the effect of oxygen as in cluster headache [1] was suggested.

In contrast to the paroxysmal hemicranial headaches, hemicrania continua (HC) shows continuous unilateral pain which usually does not reach intolerable intensity with occasional superimposed exacerbations. Only during the more intensive pain phases autonomic signs coexist. Except for very few cases HC is reliably responsive to treatment with IND (see table 4 for details). Patients who do not respond to IND can be treated with slow-release opioids.

Indomethacin Non-Responsive Headache Syndromes: SUNCT and Cluster-tic Syndrome (CLT)

In SUNCT and cluster-tic syndrome the autonomic features of cluster headache and triggering by touch or manipulation of cranial and extracranials site of trigeminal neuralgia are combined. However, in SUNCT the attacks are usually considerably shorter (5–250 sec) than in cluster headache and cluster-tic syndrome. Both syndromes do not respond to indomethacin. Otherwise, the pharmacological responsiveness differs considerably. Whereas, in cases of CLS successful individual treatments of the cluster and trigeminal neuralgia component were reported [39], most patients with SUNCT seem to be refractory to any pharmacological intervention. Irreproducible or questionable partial relief was seen after oral sumatriptan and valproate [40]. After verapamil SUNCT worsened in some cases [40]. Ineffective treatments in SUNCT included: NSAIDS (aspirin, naproxen, indomethacin, ibuprofen), ergotamine, dihydroergotamine, subcutaneous sumatriptan, prednisone, methysergide, lithium, propranolol, tricyclic antidepressants, carbamazepine, intravenous lignocaine, and local infiltrations of the greater occipital nerve [40].

References

1   Goadsby PJ, Lipton RB: A review of paroxysmal hemicranias, SUNCT syndrome and other short-lasting headaches with autonomic feature, including new cases. Brain 1997;120:193–209.
2   Pareja JA, Sjaastad O: SUNCT syndrome. A clinical review. Headache 1997;37:195–202.
3   Pareja JA, Ruiz J, de Isla C, al-Sabbah H, Espejo J: Idiopathic stabbing headache (jabs and jolts syndrome). Cephalalgia 1996;16:93–96.
4   Sjaastad O, Spierings EL: 'Hemicrania continua': Another headache absolutely responsive to indomethacin. Cephalalgia 1984;4:65–70.
5   Watson P, Evans R: Cluster-tic syndrome. Headache 1985;25:123–126.
6   Klimek A: Cluster-tic syndrome. Cephalalgia 1987;7:161–162.
7   Antonaci F, Pareja JA, Caminero AB, Sjaastad O: Chronic paroxysmal hemicrania and hemicrania continua. Parenteral indomethacin: The 'indotest'. Headache 1998;38:122–128.
8   Blom S: Trigeminal neuralgia: Its treatment with a new anticonvulsant drug. Lancet 1962;1:839–840.
9   McQuay H, Carroll D, Jadad AR, Wiffen P, Moore A: Anticonvulsant drugs for management of pain: a systematic review. Br Med J 1995;311:1047–1052.
10 Sist T, Filadora V, Miner M, Lema M: Gabapentin for idiopathic trigeminal neuralgia: Report of two cases. Neurology 1997;48:1467.
11 Merren MD: Gabapentin for treatment of pain and tremor: A large case series. South Med J 1998;91:739–744.
12 Khan OA: Gabapentin relieves trigeminal neuralgia in multiple sclerosis patients. Neurology 1998;51:611–614.

13 Attal N, Brasseur L, Parker F, Chauvin M, Bouhassira D: Effects of gabapentin on the different components of peripheral and central neuropathic pain syndromes: A pilot study. Eur Neurol 1998; 40:191–200.

14 Solaro C, Lunardi GL, Capello E, Inglese M, Messmer Uccelli M, Uccelli A, Mancardi GL: An open-label trial of gabapentin treatment of paroxysmal symptoms in multiple sclerosis patients. Neurology 1998;51:609–611.

15 Lunardi G, Leandri M, Albano C, Cultrera S, Fracassi M, Rubino V, Favale E: Clinical effectiveness of lamotrigine and plasma levels in essential and symptomatic trigeminal neuralgia. Neurology 1997;48:1714–1717.

16 Zakrzewska JM, Chaudhry Z, Nurmikko TJ, Patton DW, Mullens EL: Lamotrigine (lamictal) in refractory trigeminal neuralgia: Results from a double-blind placebo controlled crossover trial. Pain 1997;73:223–230.

17 Grant SM, Faulds D: Oxcarbazepine. A review of its pharmacology and therapeutic potential in epilepsy, trigeminal neuralgia and affective disorders. Drugs 1992;43:873–888.

18 Fromm GH, Terrence CF, Chattha AS: Baclofen in the treatment of trigeminal neuralgia: Double-blind study and long-term follow-up. Ann Neurol 1984;15:240–244.

19 Fromm GH, Shibuya T, Nakata M, Terrence CF: Effects of D-baclofen and L-baclofen on the trigeminal nucleus. Neuropharmacology 1990;29:249–254.

20 Lechin F, van der Dijs B, Lechin ME, Amat J, Lechin AE, Cabrera A, Gomez F, Acosta E, Arocha L, Villa S, et al: Pimozide therapy for trigeminal neuralgia. Arch Neurol 1989;46:960–963.

21 Tomson T, Tybring G, Bertilsson L, Ekbom K, Rane A: Carbamazepine therapy in trigeminal neuralgia: Clinical effects in relation to plasma concentration. Arch Neurol 1980;37:699–703.

22 Jannetta PJ: Microsurgical management of trigeminal neuralgia. Arch Neurol 1985;42:800.

23 Sweet WH, Wepsic JG: Controlled thermocoagulation of trigeminal ganglion and rootlets for differential destruction of pain fibers. 1. Trigeminal neuralgia. J Neurosurg 1974;40:143–156.

24 Sweet WH: The treatment of trigeminal neuralgia (tic douloureux). N Engl J Med 1986;315:174–177.

25 Latchaw JP, Hardy RW, Forsythe SB, Cook AF: Trigeminal neuralgia treated by radiofrequency coagulation. J Neurosurgery 1983;59:479–484.

26 Hakanson S: Trigeminal neuralgia treated by the injection of glycerol into the trigeminal cistern. Neurosurgery 1981;9:638–646.

27 Meglio M, Cioni B: Percutaneous procedures for trigeminal neuralgia: Microcompression versus radiofrequency thermocoagulation. Personal experience. Pain 1989;38:9–16.

28 Nittner K: Possibilities of neurological pain relief. Fortschr Neurol Psychiatr Grenzgeb 1980;48: 571–602.

29 Lindquist C, Kihlstrom L, Hellstrand E: Functional neurosurgery – A future for the gamma knife? Stereotact Funct Neurosurg 1991;57:72–81.

30 Pollock BE, Gorman DA, Schomberg PJ, Kline RW: The Mayo Clinic gamma knife experience: Indications and initial results. Mayo Clin Proc 1999;74:5–13.

31 Sjaastad O, Apfelbaum R, Caskey W, Christoffersen B, Diamond S, Graham J, Green M, Horven I, Lund-Roland L, Medina J, Rogado S, Stein H: Chronic paroxysmal hemicrania (CPH). The clinical manifestations. A review. Ups J Med Sci 1980;31(suppl):27–33.

32 Hannerz J, Ericson K, Bergstrand G: Chronic paroxysmal hemicrania: Orbital phlebography and steroid treatment. A case report. Cephalalgia 1987;7:189–192.

33 Kudrow DB, Kudrow L: Successful aspirin prophylaxis in a child with chronic paroxysmal hemicrania. Headache 1989;29:280–281.

34 Evers S, Husstedt IW: Alternatives in drug treatment of chronic paroxysmal hemicrania. Headache 1996;36:429–432.

35 Shabbir N, McAbee G: Adolescent chronic paroxysmal hemicrania responsive to verapamil monotherapy. Headache 1994;34:209–210.

36 Schlake HP, Bottger IG, Grotemeyer KH, Husstedt IW, Schober O: Single photon emission computed tomography (SPECT) with 99mTc-HMPAO (hexamethyl propylenamino oxime) in chronic paroxysmal hemicrania – A case report. Cephalalgia 1990;10:311–315.

37 Warner JS, Wamil AW, McLean MJ: Acetazolamide for the treatment of chronic paroxysmal hemicrania. Headache 1994;34:597–599.

38   Hannerz J, Jogestrand T: Intracranial hypertension and sumatriptan efficacy in a case of chronic paroxysmal hemicrania which became bilateral. (The mechanism of indomethacin in CPH.) Headache 1993;33:320–323.

39   Pascual J, Berciano J: Relief of cluster-tic syndrome by the combination of lithium and carbamazepine. Cephalalgia 1993;13:205–206.

40   Pareja JA, Kruszewski P, Sjaastad O: SUNCT syndrome: Trials of drugs and anesthetic blockades. Headache 1995;35:138–142.

41   Brandt T, Illingworth RD, Peatfield RC: Trigeminal and glossopharyngeal neuralgia; in Brandt T, Caplan LR, Dichgans J, Diener HC (eds): Neurological Disorders. Course and Treatment. San Diego, Academic Press, 1996, p 51.

Dr. Holger Kaube, Clinical Neurology, Institute of Neurology,
Queen Square, London WC1N 3BG (UK)
Tel. +44 171 837 3611, Fax +44 171 813 0349, E-Mail holgerk@ion.ucl.ac.uk

Diener HC (ed): Drug Treatment of Migraine and Other Headaches.
Monogr Clin Neurosci. Basel, Karger, 2000, vol 17, pp 347–356

....

Drug-Induced Headache

Hans Christoph Diener[a], *Ninan T. Mathew*[b]

[a] Department of Neurology, University of Essen, Essen, Germany, and
[b] Houston Headache Clinic, Houston, Tex., USA

Inappropriate use of headache medication may contribute to the development of chronic daily headache which is refractory to most treatments. Physicians experienced in the treatment of migraine and other headaches are well aware that the daily intake of antipyretic or anti-inflammatory analgesics, ergotamine, DHE, 'triptans' and opioids may result in chronic daily headache. Conversely, if a patient complains of chronic daily headache and takes pain medication every day, this headache is most likely to be caused and sustained by the medication and will vanish or improve with abstinence.

It should be noted that almost no experimental work has been done in this field, and the following is based mainly on clinical series describing patients presenting at headache clinics with this problem, with subsequent treatment and follow-up.

Epidemiology

Prevalence and incidence rates of chronic drug-induced headache are not available. Most headache centers report that between 5 and 10% of the patients they see fulfill the criteria of drug-induced headache [1–6]. Micieli et al. [7] observed an incidence of 4.3% in 3,000 consecutive headache patients. In a population-based study, Castillo et al. [8] reported 18.4% of chronic tension-type headache and 40% of transformed migraine patients overused medications. Since headache centers and clinics see a negative selection of headache sufferers, the true prevalence is estimated to be 0.5–1% of patients with migraine and 0.3–0.5% of patients with chronic tension headache. Higher numbers are seen in patients who have a combination of both migraine and tension-type headache. Patients with cluster headache rarely develop drug-induced headache. A survey in family doctors showed, that drug-induced headache was the third most common cause of headache [9]. Taken together, these studies indicate that drug-induced headache is a major health problem. This is also true if one considers the side effects of chronic intake of analgesics, ergotamine and triptans.

Pathophysiology

Most headache experts agree that patients with migraine and tension-type headache have a higher potential for drug-induced headache. Relapses of migraine occur in migraineurs who have been placed on analgesics for other ailments [10]. The association between analgesic overuse and headache has been studied in conditions other than primary headache disorders. Chronic overuse of analgesics does not cause increased headache in nonmigraineurs. For example, a group of arthritis patients who were consuming fairly large amounts of analgesics regularly for arthritis did not show increased incidence of headache [11]. There are no major differences in the abilities of the various types of analgesics used in the treatment of chronic headache to produce analgesic rebound headache [12]. The conclusion drawn from various clinical observations and studies is that analgesic rebound headache may be restricted to those who are already headache sufferers. The basis for this could either be genetic or the fact that migraine pain is more severe than joint pain. Different mechanisms probably contribute to the transition from the original headache to drug-induced headache. Psychological factors include the reinforcing properties of pain relief by drug consumption, a very powerful component of positive conditioning. Many patients report taking migraine drugs prophylactically because they are worrying about missing work (or, inevitably, the job) or missing an important social event (dinner, theater, etc.). More importantly, patients often fear an imminent headache and take analgesics or specific migraine drugs prophylactically. They are often instructed by the physicians or by the instructions supplied with the medication to take the migraine drug as early as possible at the start of either the aura or the headache phase of a migraine attack.

Withdrawal headache is an additional factor. Whenever the patient tries to stop or reduce the medication, he experiences a worsening of the preexisting headache. Barbiturates are contained in drugs for the treatment of tension-type headache and have a high potency for addiction and cause headache. The psychotropic side effects of analgesic or migraine drugs such as sedation or mild euphoria and their stimulating action may lead to drug dependency.

Barbiturates, codeine, other opioids and caffeine are the most likely substances to have this effect. Caffeine increases vigilance, relieves fatigue, and improves performance and mood. The typical symptoms of caffeine withdrawal such as irritability, nervousness, restlessness and especially 'caffeine withddrawal headache' [13–15], which may last for several days, encourage the patients to continue their abuse. Despite the fact that caffeine may enhance the analgesic action of acetylsalicylic acid and acetaminophen [16, 17], it should be removed from analgesics. Similarly, caffeine and meprobamat, the main metabolite of carisoprodol, should be removed from ergotamine-containing formulations.

There are reports on physical dependence on codeine and other opioids in headache patients [18, 19]. There are no studies that have investigated the effects of codeine intake over periods as long as 10 years as many headache patients have done. It should be remembered that up to 10% of codeine is metabolized to morphine [20].

Ergotamine and DHE may certainly lead to physical dependency [21]. Many patients who feel a migraine attack may take ergotamine as prophylactic treatment. Professional women are particularly likely to do this, e.g. teachers [22]. The withdrawal headache confirms the patient's belief that she or he is better off with than without the drugs. The reason for the physical dependency on ergotamine remains obscure. Verhoeff et al. [23] observed no upregulation of D2-receptors in the brain of patients with ergotamine abuse. Ergotamine abusers react similarly to other migraine patients to the vasoconstrictor effect of ergotamine [24]. In one study the tyramine-induced mydriasis after ergotamine administration was increased during abuse but not after withdrawal of ergot-amine, indicating a central inhibition of pupillary sympathetic activity during abuse [25]. Thus a possible CNS effect of ergotamine can be observed after chronic use but not after a single dose of the drug. Other studies investigating the effect of chronic use of ergotamine on the CNS regulation of the autonomic nervous system are needed.

Clinical Features

For the purpose of this chapter, a meta-analysis was performed summarizing 29 studies comprising a total of 2,612 patients with chronic drug-induced headache [1–5, 10, 22, 26–31]. Sixty-five percent of the patients reported migraine as primary headache, 27% of patients reported tension-type headache, and 8% of patients reported mixed or other headaches (e.g. cluster headache). Women were more prone to drug-induced headache than men (3.5:1; 1,533 women, 442 men). This ratio is slightly higher than could be expected from the gender differences in frequency of migraine. The mean duration of primary headache was 20.4 years. The mean admitted time of frequent drug intake was 10.3 years in one study [26], and the mean duration of daily headache was 5.9 years.

The drugs leading to chronic drug-induced headache vary considerably in the different series depending probably on both selection of patients (e.g. 'pure' ergotamine abusers being reported) [1, 2, 27, 30, 32–37], and cultural factors. Probably, potentially each component contained in analgesics or drugs for the treatment of migraine attacks can induce headache. This is also true for acetylsalicylic acid and paracetamol [29, 38, 39]. It is, however, difficult to identify a single substance as 90% of patients take more than one compound at a time. Four studies [4, 7, 40, 41] investigated the frequency of the chemical compounds of drugs used. Combination analgesic containing butalbital (short-acting barbiturate), caffeine, aspirin with or without codeine was the leading candidate for drug-induced headache in one study [41]. Sumatriptan can also lead to drug-induced headache. This was first observed in patients who abused ergotamine [42, 43]. Later de novo cases were reported [44–46]. Recently, patients who developed drug-induced headache from naratriptan and zolmi-triptan were reported [47]. Due to the delay between frequent intake of triptans and the development of drug-induced headache, it is likely, that similar cases will be observed in future with zolmitriptan, naratriptan and rizatriptan. The risk appears to be particularly high in headache patients with a former history of misuse of analgesics and/or ergotamine.

Results from headache diaries show that the number of tablets or supposi-tories taken per day averages 4.9 (range 0.25–25). Patients take on average 2.5–5.8 different pharmacological components simultaneously (range 1–14).

In our experience, patients with migraine as the primary headache report two different kinds of headaches:

- A constant, diffuse, dull headache without associated symptoms.
- Often patients who take ergotamine or a triptan daily also experience a throbbing, pulsating headache in the early morning, sometimes combined with nausea. The headache disappears between 30 and 60 min after the intake of ergotamine or a triptan. This headache is probably a minor withdrawal headache.

- In addition to the diffuse, daily headache, patients may still experience migraine attacks with intensified unilateral headaches and associated symp-toms. Patients with chronic tension-type headache or post-traumatic headache as the primary headache are most often not able to discriminate the character-istics of their primary headache and chronic drug-induced headache.

- The withdrawal headache experienced after stopping of medication resembles a severe and prolonged migraine attack in patients with migraine as primary headache.

The psychological examination reveals a high prevalence of depression, as it is observed in many patients with chronic pain [41, 48].

Recognizing Drug-Induced Headache

Several clinical characteristics are helpful in identifying the occurence of analgesic rebound headache in patients with primary headache disorders [41]. The following are the clinical features of drug-induced headache:

The headaches are refractory, daily, or nearly daily.

The headaches occur in a patient with primary headache disorders who uses immediate relief medications very frequently, often in excessive quantities.

The headache itself varies in its severity, type and location from time to time.

The slightest physical or intellectual effort may bring on headache. In other words, the threshold for head pain appears to be low.

Headaches are accompanied by asthenia, nausea and other gastrointestinal symptoms, restlessness, anxiety, irritability, memory problems, and difficulty in intellectual concentration and depression. Those consuming large quantities of ergot derivatives may exhibit cold extremities, tachycardia, paresthesias, diminished pulse, hypertension, lightheadedness, muscle pain of the extremities, weakness of the legs and depression.

There is a drug-dependent rhythmicity of headaches. Predictable early morning (2:00 a.m. to 5:00 a.m.) headaches are frequent, particularly in patients who use large quantities of analgesic, sedative, caffeine or ergotamine combinations. Barbiturate-containing analgesics, such as butalbital with caffeine and aspirin (Fiorinal) or with caffeine and acetaminophen (Esgic), suppress rapid eye movement (REM) sleep, which is followed by REM rebound and results in awaking with severe headache.

There is evidence of tolerance to analgesics over time, with patients needing progressively larger doses.

Withdrawal symptoms are observed when patients are taken off pain medications abruptly.

Spontaneous improvement of headache occurs on discontinuing the medications. Concomitant prophylactic medications are relatively ineffective while the patients are consuming excess amounts of immediate relief medications.

Prognosis

The success rate of withdrawal therapy within a time window of 1–6 months is 72.4% (17 studies, N = 1,101 patients). Success is defined as no headache at all or an improvement of more than 50% in terms of headache days. Three studies had a longer observation period between 9 and 35 months [4, 26, 37]. The success rates in these studies were 60, 70 and 73%, respectively. A 5-year follow-up study found a relapse rate of 40% [49]. Whereas Baumgartner et al. [4] could not identify prognostic factors that predicted a favorable outcome, Diener et al. [26] reported, that migraine patients responded better than patients with tension-type headache or patients with both. Regular intake of ergotamine for less than 10 years was also a positive prognostic factor.

Management

A careful history is necessary in evaluating chronic headache patients. It is very common that these patients take several different substances daily despite the fact that the effect is negligible. The mechanism behind this behavior is merely an attempt to avoid a disabling withdrawal headache. The present and prior use of prescription drugs, nonprescription compounds and caffeine intake should be recorded. Many patients also abuse other substances, such as tranquilizers, opioids, decongestants, and laxatives [50–52]. In addition, it is often helpful to let the patient keep a diagnostic headache diary for 1 month in order to actually register headache pattern and drug use [53]. History and examination should also search for possible complications of regular drug intake, e.g. recurrent gastric ulcers, anemia and ergotism (for details, see above). A good indicator is the number of physicians consulted by the patient and the number of previous unsuccessful therapies. Thus in one study [26] the headache patients had consulted an average of 5.5 physicians who had pre-scribed 8.6 different therapies.

Abrupt drug withdrawal seems to be the first treatment of choice for drug-induced headache. There are, however, no prospective and randomized trials comparing continuation of drug intake and drug withdrawal. A survey of 22 studies dealing with therapy of drug-induced headache shows that most centers used drug withdrawal as the primary therapy (see [54]). Clinical experience indicates that medical and behavioral headache treatment fails, as long as the patient continues to take symptomatic drugs daily. The typical withdrawal symptoms last for 2–10 days (average 3.5 days) and include withdrawal headache, nausea, vomiting, arterial hypotension, tachycardia, sleep disturbances, restlessness, anxiety and nervousness. Seizures or hallucinations were only rarely observed even in patients abusing barbiturate-containing migraine drugs. Drug withdrawal is performed differently. Most authors prefer inpatient programs. Hering and Steiner [29] abruptly withdrew the offending drugs on an outpatient basis by adequate explanation of the disorder, regular follow-up, and amitriptyline (10 mg at night) and naproxen (500 mg) for relief of headache symptoms. A consensus paper by the German Migraine Society [55] recommends outpatient withdrawal for patients who do not take barbiturates or tranquilizers with their analgesics and are highly motivated. Inpatient treatment should be performed in patients who take tranquilizers, codeine, or barbiturates who failed to withdraw the drugs as outpatients or who have a high depression score.

Treatment

Treatment recommendations for the acute phase of drug withdrawal vary considerably between the 22 studies mentioned above. They include fluid replacement, analgesics, tranquilizers, neuroleptics, amitriptyline, valproate, intravenous DHE, oxygen and electrical stimulation (see also [56]). Valproate has been shown to have beneficial effects in the prophylactic treatment of chronic daily headache complicated by excessive analgesic intake [57]. A double-blind study showed a single subcutaneous dose of sumatriptan to be better than placebo in the treatment of ergotamine withdrawal headache but the headache reappeared within 12 h [58]. An open randomized study indicated that naproxen was better than symptomatic treatment with antiemetics and analgesics [59]. Further double-blind controlled trials are needed. In contrast, Dichgans et al. [22] favored giving no replacement therapy at all during the first days of withdrawal, with the intention of reversing the conditioning response learned before. In this way, patients experience headache improvement without taking any medication.

If more than three migraine attacks per month continue after withdrawal, medical and behavioral prophylaxis should be initiated. The clinical experience shows that many patients respond to prophylactic treatment, e.g. with beta-blockers or flunarizine, after drug withdrawal despite the fact that these drugs seemingly had been unsuccessful before. Ergotamine, triptans and possibly analgesics counteract the action of prophylactic therapy and will not improve drug-induced headache. The same phenomenon can be observed for the action of amitriptyline [52] and behavioral therapy [59] in patients with tension-type headache.

Prevention

The most important preventive measure is proper instruction and an appropriate surveillance of patients. The migraine patients at risk often have a mixture of migraine and tension-type headaches and should be instructed carefully to use specific antimigraine drugs only for migraine attacks. This point was already stressed in 1951 by Peters and Horton concerning ergotamine abuse, i.e. complications can be avoided if enough time is taken for proper instruction of the patient, so that he or she can distinguish between vasodilating and nondilating headache [35].

Restricting the dose of ergotamine per attack (4 mg ergotamine), per week (no more than twice per week) and per month (no more than 20 mg ergotamine) is also helpful in avoiding dependency. In a similar way, the number of doses of triptans should be limited per attack and per month. Migraine drugs that contain barbiturates, codeine, or tranquilizers as well as mixed analgesics should be avoided. Probably an early start of migraine prophylaxis, either by medical or behavioral treatment, can be a preventive measure to avoid drug-induced headache.

References

1   Ala-Hurula V, Myllylae V, Hokkanen E: Ergotamine abuse: Results of ergotamine discontinuation, with special reference to the plasma concentrations. Cephalalgia 1982;2:189–195.
2   Andersson PG: Ergotamine headache. Headache 1975;15:118–121.
3   Andersson PG: Ergotism – The clinical picture; in Diener HC, Wilkinson M (eds): Drug-Induced Headache. New York, Heidelberg, Springer, 1988, pp 16–19.
4   Baumgartner C, Wessely P, Bingöl C, Maly J, Holzner F: Long term prognosis of analgesic withdrawal in patients with drug-induced headaches. Headache 1989;29:510–514.
5   Granella F, Farina S, Malferrari GC: Drug abuse in chronic headache; a clinico-epidemiologic study. Cephalalgia 1987;7:15–19.
6   Medina JL, Diamond S: Drug dependency in patients with chronic headaches. Headache 1977;17:12–14.
7   Micieli G, Manzoni GC, Granella F, Martignoni E, Malferrari G, Nappi G: Clinical and epidemiological observations on drug abuse in headache patients; in Diener HC, Wilkinson M (eds): Drug-Induced Headache. Berlin, Heidelberg, New York, Springer, 1988, pp 20–28.
8   Castillo J, Guitera V, Munoz P, Pascual J: Prevalence and diagnostic distribution of chronic daily headache in the general population. Cephalalgia 1997;17:283.
9   Rapoport A, Stang P, Gutterman DL, Cady R, Markley H, Weeks R, Sairs J, Fox AW: Analgesic rebound headache in clinical practice: Data from a physician survey. Headache 1996;36:19–19.
10 Isler H: Migraine treatment as a cause of chronic migraine; in Rose CF (ed): Advances in Migraine Research. New York, Raven Press, 1982, pp 159–164.
11 Lance E, Parkes C, Wilkinson M: Does analgesic abuse cause headaches de novo? Headache 1988;28:61.
12 Bowlder I, Kikan J, Gansslen-Blumberg S: The association between analgesic abuse and headache-coincidental or cause? Headache 1988;28:494.
13 Abbott PJ: Caffeine: A toxicological overview. Med J Austral 1986;145:518–521.
14 Silverman K, Evans SM, Strain EC, Griffiths RR: Withdrawal syndrome after the double-blind cessation of caffeine consumption. N Engl J Med 1992;327:1109–1114.
15 van Dusseldorp M, Katan MB: Headache caused by caffeine withdrawal among moderate coffee drinkers switched from ordinary to decaffeinated coffee: A 12-week double-blind trial. Br Med J 1990;300:1558–1559.
16 Laska EM, Sunshine A, Mueller F, Elvers WB, Siegel C, Rubin A: Caffeine as an analgesic adjuvant. JAMA 1984;251:1711–1718.

17   Lipton RB, Stewart WF, Ryan RE, Saper J, Silberstein S, Sheftell F: Efficacy and safety of acetamin-
      ophen, aspirin and caffeine in alleviating migraine headache pain – Three double-blind, randomized,
      placebo-controlled trials. Arch Neurol 1998;55:210–217.

18   Fisher MA, Glass S: Butorphanol (Stadol): A study in problems of current drug information and
      control. Neurology 1997;48:1156–1160.

19   Ziegler DK: Opiate and opioid use in patients with refractory headache. Cephalalgia 1994;14:
      5–10.

20   Meadows B: Codeine combinations in clinical practice. Curr Ther Res 1984;35:501–510.

21   Saper JR, Jones JM: Ergotamine tartrate dependency: Features and possible mechanisms. Clin
      Neuropharmacol 1986;9:244–256.

22   Dichgans J, Diener HC, Gerber WD, Verspohl EJ, Kukiolka H, Kluck M: Analgetika-induzierter
      Dauerkopfschmerz. Dtsch med Wschr 1984;109:369–373.

23   Verhoeff NPLG, Visser WH, Ferrari MD, Saxena PR, van Royen EA: Dopamine D2 receptor imaging
      with 123-I-iodobenzamide SPECT in migraine patients abusing ergotamine: Does ergotamine cross
      the blood brain barrier? Cephalalgia 1993;13:325–329.

24   Tfelt-Hansen P, Olesen J: Arterial response to ergotamine tartrate in abusing and non-abusing
      migraine patients. Acta Pharmacol Toxicol 1989;48:69–72.

25   Fanciullacci M, Alessandri M, Pietrini U, Briccolani-Bandini E, Beatrice S: Long-term ergotamine
      abuse: Effect on adrenergically induced mydriasis. Clin Pharmacol Ther 1992;51:302–307.

26   Diener HC, Dichgans J, Scholz E, Geiselhart S, Gerber WD, Bille A: Analgesic-induced chronic
      headache: Long-term results of withdrawal therapy. J Neurol 1989;236:9–14.

27   Dige-Petersen H, Lassen NA, Noer J, Toennesen KH, Olesen J: Subclinical ergotism. Lancet 1977;
      i:65–66.

28   Henry P, Dartigues JF, Benetier MP, Lucas J, Duplan B, Jogeix M, Orgogozo JM: Ergotamine-
      and analgesic-induced headaches. Controlled study of the use of electrical stimulation by high
      frequency current; in Clifford Rose F (ed): Migraine. Proceedings of the 5th International Migraine
      Symposium, London, 1984. Basel, Karger, 1985, pp 197–205.

29   Hering R, Steiner TJ: Abrupt outpatient withdrawal of medication in analgesic-abusing migraineurs.
      Lancet 1991;337:1442–1443.

30   Horton BT, Peters GA: Clinical manifestations of excessive use of ergotamine preparations and
      management of withdrawal effect: Report of 52 cases. Headache 1963;3:214–226.

31   Osborne MMJ, Austin RCT, Dawson KJ, Lange DL: Is there a problem with long-term use of
      sumatriptan in acute migraine? Br Med J 1994;8:308.

32   Hokkanen E, Waltimo O, Kallanranta T: Toxic effects of ergotamine used for migraine. Headache
      1978;18:95–98.

33   Lippman C: Characteristic headache resulting from prolonged use of ergot derivates. J Nerv Ment
      Dis 1955;121:270–273.

34   Lucas RN, Falkowski W: Ergotamine and methysergide abuse in patients with migraine. Br J
      Psychiat 1973;122:199–203.

35   Peters GA, Horton BT: Headache: With special reference to the excessive use of ergotamine prepara-
      tions and withdrawal effects. Proceed Staff Meet Mayo Clin 1951;26:153–161.

36   Rowsell AR, Neylan C, Wilkinson M: Ergotamine induced headaches in migrainous patients.
      Headache 1973;13:65–67.

37   Tfelt-Hansen P, Krabbe AA: Ergotamine abuse: Do patients benefit from withdrawal? Cephalalgia
      1981;1:29–32.

38   MacGregor EA, Vorah C, Wilkinson M: Analgesic use: A study of treatments used by patients for
      migraine prior to attending the City of London migraine clinic. Headache 1990;30:571–574.

39   Rapoport A, Weeks R, Sheftell F: Analgesic rebound headache: Theoretical and practical implica-
      tions; in Olesen J, Tfelt-Hansen P, Jensen K (eds): Proceedings 2nd International Headache Congress,
      Copenhagen. Kopenhagen 1985, pp 448–449.

40   Diener HC, Bühler K, Dichgans J, Geiselhart S, Gerber WD, Scholz E: Analgetikainduzierter
      Dauerkopfschmerz. Existiert eine kritische Dosis? Arzneimitteltherapie 1988;6:156–164.

41   Mathew NT, Kurman R, Perez F: Drug induced refractory headache – Clinical features and
      management. Headache 1990;30:634–638.

42   Catarci T, Fiacco F, Argentino C, Sette G, Cerbo R: Ergotamine-induced headache can be sustained by sumatriptan daily intake. Cephalalgia 1994;14:374–375.
43   Kaube H, May A, Diener HC, Pfaffenrath V: Sumatriptan misuse in daily chronic headache. Br Med J 1994;308:1573.
44   Gaist D, Hallas J, Sindrup SH, Gram LF: Is overuse of sumatriptan a problem? A population-based study. Eur J Clin Pharmacol 1996;3:161–165.
45   Gaist D, Tsiropoulus I, Sindrup SH, Hallas J, Rasmussen BK, Kragstrup J: Inappropriate use of sumatriptan: Population-based register and interview study. Br Med J 1998;316:1352–1353.
46   Pini LA, Trenti T: Case report: Does chronic use of sumatriptan induce dependence? Headache 1994;34:600–601.
47   Limmroth V, Kazarawa S, Fritsche G, Diener HC: Headache after frequent use of new 5-HT agonists zolmitriptan and naratriptan. Lancet 1999;353:378.
48   Saper JR: Daily chronic headache. Neurologic Clinics 1990;8:891–901.
49   Schnider P, Aull S, Baumgartner C, Merterer A, Wöber C, Zeiler K, Wessely P: Long-term outcome of patients with headache and drug abuse after inpatient withdrawal: Five year follow-up. Cephalalgia 1996;16:481–485.
50   De Marinis M, Janiri L, Agnoli A: Headache in the use and withdrawal of opiates and other associated substances of abuse. Headache 1991;31:159–163.
51   Isler H: Die Behandlung der Kopfschmerzen. Schweizerische Medizinische Wochenschrift 1984; 114:1174–1180.
52   Kudrow L: Paradoxical effects of frequent analgesic use; in Critchley M, Fridman AP, Gorini S, Sicuteri F (eds): Advances in Neurology, vol 33. New York, Raven Press, 1982, pp 335–341.
53   Russel MB, Rasmussen BK, Brennum J, Iversen HK, Jensen RA, Olesen J: Presentation of a new instrument: The diagnostic headache diary. Cephalalgia 1992;12:369–374.
54   Diener HC, Tfelt-Hansen P: Headache associated with chronic use of substances; in Olesen J, Tfelt-Hansen P, Welch KMA (eds): The Headaches. New York, Raven Press, 1993, pp–721–727.
55   Diener HC, Pfaffenrath V, Soyka D, Gerber W: Therapie des medikamenteninduzierten Kopf-schmerzes. Münch Med Wschr 1992;134:159–162.
56   Silberstein SD, Silberstein JR: Chronic daily headache: Long-term prognosis following inpatient treatment with repetitive i.v. DHE. Headache 1992;32:439–445.
57   Mathew NT, Ali S: Valproate in the treatment of persistent chronic daily headache. An open label study. Headache 1991;31:71–74.
58   Diener HC, Haab J, Peters C, Ried S, Dichgans J, Pilgrim A: Subcutaneous sumatriptan in the treatment of headache during withdrawal from drug-induced headache. Headache 1990;31:205–209.
59   Mathew NT: Amelioration of ergotamine withdrawal symptoms with naproxen. Headache 1987; 27:130–133.
60   Michultka DM, Blanchard EB, Appelbaum KA, Jaccard J, Dentinger MG: The refractory headache patient. II. High medication consumption (analgesic rebound) headache. Behav Res Ther 1989;27: 411–420.

Prof. Dr. H.C. Diener, Neurologische Universitäts-Klinik,
Hufelandstrasse 55, 45122 Essen (Germany)
Tel. +49 201 723 2460, Fax +49 201 723 5901, E-Mail h.diener@uni-essen.de

Diener HC (ed): Drug Treatment of Migraine and Other Headaches.
Monogr Clin Neurosci. Basel, Karger, 2000, vol 17, pp 357–362

....

Cervicogenic Headache

Nikolai Bogduk

Newcastle Bone and Joint Institute, University of Newcastle, Newcastle, Australia

Cervicogenic headache is a concept in search of endorsement. There is no doubt that pain from the upper cervical segments of the vertebral column can be referred to the head, where it is perceived as headache. Experiments in normal volunteers have repeatedly shown that this type of referral can occur from the upper cervical muscles [1, 2], the C2-3 zygapophysial joints [3], the lateral atlanto-axial and atlanto-occipital joints [4]. Clinical studies have shown that some patients can be relieved of their headaches by anaesthetizing one or other of the upper cervical joints [5–8]. However, the problems lie in recognizing this type of headache clinically.

Diagnosis

Aficionados of needle techniques to diagnose spinal pain have been content to diagnose cervicogenic headaches by using radiologically controlled diagnostic blocks of putative sources of pain in the upper cervical spine, usually the synovial joints at the occipito-cervical, C1-2, and C2-3 levels [4–8]. These techniques, however, are not without hazard, and require special expertise and facilities. Consequently, they have not been adopted by the headache community at large. Their availability is restricted to pain clinics and specialized spinal pain centers.

In contrast, headache specialists have sought to establish the diagnosis of cervicogenic headache by simpler and more expedient means such as history, physical examination or blocks of the greater occipital nerve or lesser occipital nerve which can be performed in an office setting. These techniques, however, have proved unable to discriminate patients with cervicogenic headache from those with other forms of headache. As a result the field is riddled with controversy and conflicting opinions [9, 10].

The leading proponents of history and clinical examination have listed several criteria for the diagnosis of cervicogenic headaches [11], but these do not distinguish between cervicogenic headache, migraine and other headaches [12]. There are no diagnostic radiologic features of cervicogenic headache [13, 14]. Blocks of the greater occipital nerve do not uniquely define cervicogenic headache [15, 16], for they also relieve pain in patients with migraine [17]. Moreover, the studies most often cited in this regard [15, 16], do not report complete relief of pain following diagnostic blocks; they report only some degree of relief. Incomplete relief from uncontrolled blocks cannot be respected as a diagnostic criterion.

The only study to have used double-blind, controlled diagnostic blocks addressed the C2-3 zygagophysial joint as a source of headache. This study followed earlier work in which uncontrolled blocks of the joint seemed to offer complete relief of headaches occurring anywhere in the region between the occiput and the fronto-orbital region [18–20]. However, response to controlled diagnostic blocks of the C2-3 zygapophysial joint has been documented only in patients with chronic headache following whiplash injury. In that context, referred pain from the C2-3 zygapophysial joint accounts for some 27% of patients with chronic pain after whiplash, and 53% of patients in whom headache is the dominant symptom [8]. Parallel studies, using controlled diagnostic blocks, have shown that in patients in whom headache is the dominant symptom, the joint responsible is most often C2-3 [21]; a minority of patients have headache stemming from C3-4 (fig. 1). In contrast, in patients in whom neck pain is the major complaint, and headache is only an incidental or lesser feature, the pain can arise from any cervical level, and the prevalence of pain from C2-3 is much less (fig. 1).

Patients with headache proven to arise from the zygapophysial joints do not exhibit any characteristic clinical features. The pain is most often felt in the occipital region but may radiate through the parietal or temporal region to the frontal and orbital regions. The pain may be unilateral or bilateral. In the latter case, diagnostic blocks on one side relieve the headache on that side but usually not on the other. The pain is dull and aching in quality. It is usually constant, or present for most of the waking hours. It is aggravated by neck movements but no particular pattern of movements aggravates it. Many patients are tender over the painful joint but this clinical sign has a positive likelihood ratio of only 2.1 [8]. Therefore, although it can be used to increase suspicion, it is not diagnostic of itself.

These clinical features serve to distinguish headache from the C2-3 joint from migraine, in that it is not throbbing in quality or periodic. Nor is C2-3

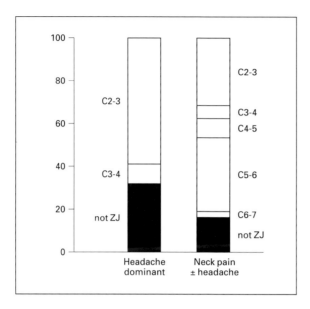

Fig. 1. The comparative prevalence of symptomatic zygapophysial joints (ZJ) in patients in whom headache was the dominant complaint after whiplash and in whom neck pain was the dominant complaint and headache only an incidental or lesser complaint. A diagnosis of zygapophysial joint pain was established if patients reported complete relief of their pain after double-blind controlled blocks of the joint at the segment indicated. Patients in whom diagnostic blocks did not relieve their pain are indicated as 'not ZJ'. Based on Lord and Bogduk [21].

joint pain associated with vomiting and photophobia. However, the features of C2-3 joint pain do not distinguish it from tension-type headache. The diagnosis is established only by controlled diagnostic blocks of the painful joint.

For this reason, the North American Cervicogenic Headache Society formulated diagnostic criteria for cervicogenic headache that do not rely on clinical features [22]. The criteria stipulate that the headache must be completely relieved by selective and controlled, diagnostic blocks of a structure in the cervical spine or of the nerves that innervate that structure. Although these criteria render the diagnosis unachievable by any except those equipped and able to perform radiologically controlled diagnostic blocks, they do provide for a rigorous definition of an entity that has defied clinical diagnosis. Proponents of other interpretations of cervicogenic headache, and other means of diagnosis, have yet to provide criteria that identify a unique form of headahce.

Treatment

Cervicogenic headache does not lend itself to pharmacotherapy. There are no data that support the use of anti-migraine drugs, analgesics, or even nonsteroidal anti-inflammatory agents. No studies have provided controlled data on the efficacy of drug therapy for suspected cervicogenic headache, let alone for proven cervicogenic headache. Those patients who have been the subject of studies typically have failed to respond to such measures of attempted pain control [8, 18–20].

Perhaps some patients with early or acute pain referred to the head from upper cervical joint might respond to manual therapy, but no studies have reported this. Not only are the data on physical therapy for neck pain at large meager [23, 24], no controlled studies of efficacy have been conducted explicitly in patients with proven cervicogenic headache. Manual and physical therapy have conspicuously been of no avail in those patients with chronic cervicogenic headache who have undergone controlled blocks to establish the diagnosis [8].

The intra-articular injection of corticosteroids has not been explicitly studied in the content of cervicogenic headache, but it has been studied for neck pain stemming from cervical zygapophysial joints. A randomized, double-blind, controlled trial showed that corticosteroids afforded no greater benefit than local anaesthetic alone [25]. Moreover, although some patients did have prolonged relief following administration of either agent, pain recurred within days in the vast majority of cases.

Surgical treatment is the only option that has been evaluated formally. In patients with headache due to osteoarthrosis of the lateral atlanto-axial joints, complete relief of headache has been reported following atlanto-axial arthrodesis [26, 28]. Although these studies had no control group, the relief was obtained in a large proportion of patients and has been sustained for several years. No similar studies have been published for the treatment by arthrodesis of pain stemming from other cervical joints.

A preliminary study of radiofrequency neurotomy of the treatment of C2-3 zygapophysial joint pain obtained mixed results [28]. Some patients obtained complete and lasting relief of their headaches, but they constituted only 30% of the patients in whom the procedure was attempted. The authors warned against adopting this form of treatment until results of greater efficacy were produced. Recent experience indicates that, following improvements in the technique used, radiofrequency neurotomy can achieve complete relief of headache in a greater proportion of patients [29], but this work has still to be submitted to peer review.

References

1 Feinstein B, Langton JBK, Jameson RM, Schiller F: Experiments on referred pain from deep somatic tissues. J Bone Joint Surg 1956;36A:981–997.
2 Campbell DG, Parsons CM: Referred head pain and its concomitants. J Nerve Ment Dis 1944;99: 544–551.
3 Dwyer A, Aprill C, Bogduk N: Cervical zygapophysial joint pain patterns. I: A study in normal volunteers. Spine 1990;15:453–457.
4 Drefuss P, Michaelsen M, Fletcher D: Atlanto-occipital and lateral atlanto-axial joint pain patterns. Spine 1994;19:1125–1131.
5 Ehni G, Benner B: Occipital neuralgia and the C1-2 arthrosis syndrome. J Neurosurg 1984;61: 961–965.
6 Busch E, Wilson PR: Atlanto-occipital and atlanto-axial injections in the treatment of headache and neck pain. Reg Anesth 1989;14(suppl 2):45.
7 McCormick CC: Arthrography of the atlanto-axial (C1-C2) joints: Technique and results. J Intervent Radiol 1987;2:9–13.
8 Lord S, Barnsley L, Wallis B, Bogduk N: Third occipital headache: A prevalence study. J Neurol Neurosurg Psychiat 1994;57:1187–1190.
9 Bogduk N: Headache and the neck; in Goadsby PJ, Silberstein SD (eds): Headache. Boston, Butterworth-Heinmann, 1997, pp 369–381.
10 Pöllman W, Keidel M, Pfaffenrath V: Headache and the cervical spine: A critical review. Cephalalgia 1997;17:801–816.
11 Sjaastad O, Fredriksen TA, Pfaffenrath V: Cervicogenic headache: Diagnostic criteria. Headache 1990;30:725–726.
12 Leone M, D'Amico D, Moschiano F, Farinotti M, Fillipini G, Bussone G: Possible identification of cervicogenic headache among patients with migraine: An analysis of 374 headaches. Headache 1995;35:461–464.
13 Fredriksen TA, Fougner R, Tangerund A, Sjaastad O: Cervicogenic headache. Radiological investigations concerning head/neck. Cephalalgia 1989;9:139–146.
14 Hinderaker J, Lord SM, Barnsley L, Bogduk N: Diagnostic value of C2-3 instantaneous axes of rotation in patients with headache of cervical origin. Cephalalgia 1995;15:391–395.
15 Bovim G, Berg R, Dale LG: Cervicogenic headache: Anaesthetic blockades of cervical nerves (C2-C5) and facet joint (C2/C3). Pain 1992;49:315–320.
16 Bovin G, Sand T: Cervicogenic headache, migraine without aura and tension-type headache. Diagnostic blockade of greater occipital and supra-orbital nerves. Pain 1992;51:43–48.
17 Caputi CA, Firetto V: Therapeutic blockade of greater occipital and supraorbital nerves in migraine patients. Headache 1997;37:174–179.
18 Bogduk N, Marsland A: Third occipital headache. Cephalalgia 1985;5(suppl 3):310–311.
19 Bogduk N, Marsland A: On the concept of third occipital headache. J Neurol Neurosurg Psychiat 1986;49:775–780.
20 Bogduk N, Marsland A: The cervical zygapophysial joint as a source of neck pain. Spine 1988;13: 610–617.
21 Lord SM, Bogduk N: The cervical synovial joints as sources of post-traumatic headache. J Musculoskel Pain 1996;4:81–94.
22 Rothbart P: Cervicogenic headache. Headache 1996;36:516.
23 Aker PD, Gross AR, Goldsmith CH, Peloso P: Conservative management of mechanical neck pain: Systematic overview and meta-analysis. Br Med J 1996;313:1291–1296.
24 Bogduk N: Treatment of whiplash injuries; in Malanga GA (ed.): Cervical Flexion-Extension/ Whiplash Injuries. Spine: State of the Art Reviews. Philadelphia, Hanley & Belfus, 1998, vol 12, pp 469–483.
25 Barnsley L, Lord SM, Wallis BJ, Bogduk N: Lack of effect of intraarticular corticosteroids for chronic pain in the cervical zygapophysial joints. N Engl J Med 1994;330:1047–1050.
26 Joseph B, Kumar B: Gallie's fusion for atlantoaxial arthrosis with occipital neuralgia. Spine 1994; 19:454–455.

27 Ghanayem AJ, Leventhal M, Bohlman HH: Osteoarthrosis of the atlanto-axial joints – Long-term follow-up after treatment with arthrodesis. J Bone Joint Surg 1996;78A:1300–1307.

28 Lord SM, Barnsley L, Bogduk N: Percutaneous radiofrequency neurotomy in the treatment of cervical zygapophysial joint pain: A caution. Neurosurgery 1995;36:732–739.

29 Macdonald G, Govind J, Lord S, Bogduk N: Percutaneous radiofrequency neurotomy for C2-3 zygapophysial joint pain. Proceedings of the Combined Meeting of the International Spinal Injection Society and the Australian Faculty of Musculoskeletal Medicine, Sydney, 26th–27th September, 1998, pp 14–15.

Professor Nikolai Bogduk, Newcastle Bone and Joint Institute, University of Newcastle, Royal Newcastle Hospital, Newcastle, NSW 2300 (Australia)
Tel. +61 2 49 236 172, Fax +61 2 49 236 103, E-Mail mgillam@mail.newcastle.edu.au

....
Author Index

Subject Index